Current Controversies in Neonatology

Editors

ROBERT M. KLIEGMAN
SUSAN S. COHEN

CLINICS IN PERINATOLOGY

www.perinatology.theclinics.com

Consulting Editor
LUCKY JAIN

March 2022 • Volume 49 • Number 1

ELSEVIER

1600 John F. Kennedy Boulevard • Suite 1800 • Philadelphia, Pennsylvania, 19103-2899

http://www.theclinics.com

CLINICS IN PERINATOLOGY Volume 49, Number 1
March 2022 ISSN 0095-5108, ISBN-13: 978-0-323-89698-6

Editor: Kerry Holland
Developmental Editor: Karen Solomon

Clinics in Perinatology (ISSN 0095-5108) is published quarterly by Elsevier Inc., 360 Park Avenue South, New York, NY 10010-1710. Months of issue are March, June, September, and December. Business and Editorial Offices: 1600 John F. Kennedy Blvd., Ste. 1800, Philadelphia, PA 19103-2899. Customer Service Office: 3251 Riverport Lane, Maryland Heights, MO 63043. Periodicals postage paid at New York, NY and additional mailing offices. Subscription prices are $331.00 per year (US individuals), $823.00 per year (US institutions), $376.00 per year (Canadian individuals), $860.00 per year (Canadian institutions), $448.00 per year (international individuals), $860.00 per year (international institutions), $100.00 per year (US and Canadian students), and $195.00 per year (International students). International air speed delivery is included in all Clinics subscription prices. All prices are subject to change without notice. **POSTMASTER:** Send address changes to *Clinics in Perinatology*, Elsevier Health Sciences Division, Subscription Customer Service, 3251 Riverport Lane, Maryland Heights, MO 63043. **Customer Service: Telephone: 1-800-654-2452** (U.S. and Canada); **1-314-447-8871** (outside U.S. and Canada). **Fax: 1-314-447-8029. E-mail: journalscustomerservice-usa@elsevier.com** (for print support); **journalsonlinesupport-usa@elsevier.com** (for online support).

Reprints. For copies of 100 or more, of articles in this publication, please contact the Commercial Reprints Department, Elsevier Inc., 360 Park Avenue South, New York, NY 10010-1710. Tel. 212-633-3874; Fax: 212-633-3820; E-mail: reprints@elsevier.com.

Clinics in Perinatology is also published in Spanish by McGraw-Hill Interamericana Editores S.A., P.O. Box 5-237, 06500 Mexico D.F., Mexico.

Clinics in Perinatology is covered in *MEDLINE/PubMed (Index Medicus) Current Contents, Excepta Medica, BIOSIS and ISI/BIOMED.*

Contributors

CONSULTING EDITOR

LUCKY JAIN, MD, MBA
George W. Brumley Jr Professor and Chairman, Emory University School of Medicine, Department of Pediatrics; Chief Academic Officer, Children's Healthcare of Atlanta; Executive Director, Emory + Children's Pediatric Institute, Atlanta, Georgia, USA

EDITORS

ROBERT M. KLIEGMAN, MD
Professor, Department of Pediatrics, Medical College of Wisconsin, Milwaukee, Wisconsin, USA

SUSAN S. COHEN, MD
Associate Professor, Department of Pediatrics, Division of Neonatology, Medical College of Wisconsin, Milwaukee, Wisconsin, USA

AUTHORS

SAMUEL J. ADAMS, MD
Neurology – Child Neurology, Medical College of Wisconsin, Children's Wisconsin, Milwaukee, Wisconsin, USA

NATALIE G. ALLEN, MD
Division of Endocrinology and Diabetes, Department of Pediatrics, Penn State Health Milton S. Hershey Medical Center, Hershey, Pennsylvania, USA

CARL H. BACKES, MD
Department of Pediatrics, The Ohio State University Wexner Medical Center, The Heart Center, Nationwide Children's Hospital, Center for Perinatal Research, The Abigail Wexner Research Institute at Nationwide Children's Hospital, Columbus, Ohio, USA

MEGAN BARCROFT, DO
Department of Pediatrics, The Ohio State University Wexner Medical Center, Columbus, Ohio, USA

JOHN D.E. BARKS, MD, FAAP
Professor, Department of Pediatrics, Division of Neonatal-Perinatal Medicine, Michigan Medicine–University of Michigan Medical School, C.S. Mott Children's Hospital, Ann Arbor, Michigan, USA

KATIE R. BAUGHMAN, MD
Professor, Department of Pediatrics, Children's Wisconsin, Medical College of Wisconsin, Milwaukee, Wisconsin, USA

DARREN P. BERMAN, MD
Department of Pediatrics, The Ohio State University Wexner Medical Center, The Heart Center, Nationwide Children's Hospital, Columbus, Ohio, USA

EMILY CALLAN, MD
Division of Neonatology, Department of Pediatrics, Medical College of Wisconsin, Children's Research Institute, Children's Wisconsin, Wauwatosa, Wisconsin, USA

HALA CHAABAN, MD
Associate Professor, Neonatal-Perinatal Medicine, The University of Oklahoma Health Sciences Center, Oklahoma City, Oklahoma, USA

LINA CHALAK, MD, MSCS
Professor of Pediatrics and Psychiatry, Department of Pediatrics, UT Southwestern Medical Center, Neonatal-Perinatal Medicine, University of Texas Southwestern Medical School, Dallas, Texas, USA

SCOTT COHEN, MD
Department of Internal Medicine, Division of Cardiovascular Medicine, Department of Pediatrics, Division of Pediatric Cardiology, Medical College of Wisconsin, Milwaukee, Wisconsin, USA

SUSAN S. COHEN, MD
Associate Professor, Department of Pediatrics, Division of Neonatology, Medical College of Wisconsin, Milwaukee, Wisconsin, USA

JAMES W. COLLINS Jr. MD, MPH
Medical Director, Neonatal Intensive Care Unit, Division of Neonatology, Associate Pediatric Program Director, Ann & Robert H. Lurie Children's Hospital of Chicago, Professor of Pediatrics, Northwestern University Feinberg School of Medicine, Chicago, Illinois, USA

RICHARD J. DAVID, MD
Division of Neonatology, Stroger Hospital of Cook County, University of Illinois at Chicago College of Medicine, Chicago, Illinois, USA

CHRISTA DEVETTE, MD, PhD
Department of Pediatrics, The University of Oklahoma Health Sciences Center, Oklahoma City, Oklahoma, USA

AFIF EL-KHUFFASH, MD
Department of Neonatology, The Rotunda Hospital, Department of Paediatrics, The Royal College of Surgeons in Ireland, Dublin, Ireland

JOHN FLIBOTTE, MD
Department of Pediatrics, Division of Neonatology, University of Pennsylvania Perelman School of Medicine, Philadelphia, Pennsylvania, USA

JOSEPH T. FLYNN, MD, MS
Department of Pediatrics, Division of Nephrology, Seattle Children's Hospital, Seattle, Washington

ANDREW B. FOY, MD
Associate Professor, Department of Pediatric Neurosurgery, Children's Wisconsin, Milwaukee, Wisconsin, USA

JENNIFER F. GERARDIN, MD
Department of Internal Medicine, Division of Cardiovascular Medicine, Department of Pediatrics, Division of Pediatric Cardiology, Medical College of Wisconsin, Milwaukee, Wisconsin, USA

REBECCA HJORTEN, MD
Department of Pediatrics, Division of Nephrology, Seattle Children's Hospital, Seattle, Washington

RUTH E. GRUNAU, PhD
Department of Pediatrics, University of British Columbia, BC Children's Hospital Research Institute, Vancouver, British Columbia, Canada

AARTHI GUNASEKARAN, MD
Assistant Professor, Neonatal-Perinatal Medicine, The University of Oklahoma Health Sciences Center, Oklahoma City, Oklahoma, USA

MARTIN KESZLER, MD, FAAP
Department of Pediatrics, Women & Infants Hospital of Rhode Island, Professor of Pediatrics, Warren Alpert Medical School of Brown University, Providence, Rhode Island, USA

G. GANESH KONDURI, MD
Division of Neonatology, Department of Pediatrics, Medical College of Wisconsin, Children's Research Institute, Children's Wisconsin, Wauwatosa, Wisconsin, USA

KANTHI BANGALORE KRISHNA, MD
Division of Endocrinology and Diabetes, Department of Pediatrics, Penn State Health Milton S. Hershey Medical Center, Hershey, Pennsylvania, USA

NAOMI T. LAVENTHAL, MD, MA, FAAP
Associate Professor, Department of Pediatrics, Division of Neonatal-Perinatal Medicine, Michigan Medicine–University of Michigan Medical School, C.S. Mott Children's Hospital, Ann Arbor, Michigan, USA

PETER A. LEE, MD, PhD
Division of Endocrinology and Diabetes, Department of Pediatrics, Penn State Health Milton S. Hershey Medical Center, Hershey, Pennsylvania, USA

STEVEN R. LEUTHNER, MD, MA
Professor, Department of Pediatrics, Children's Wisconsin, Medical College of Wisconsin, Wauwatosa, Wisconsin, USA

SAMUEL LEVIN, MD
Assistant Professor, Neonatal-Perinatal Medicine, The University of Oklahoma Health Sciences Center, Oklahoma City, Oklahoma, USA

JOHN P. MARQUART, MD
Pediatric Surgery Research Fellow, Children's Wisconsin, Milwaukee, Wisconsin, USA

CHRISTOPHER MCKEE, DO
Department of Pediatrics, The Ohio State University Wexner Medical Center, Department of Anesthesiology, The Heart Center, Nationwide Children's Hospital, Columbus, Ohio, USA

CHRISTOPHER MCPHERSON, PharmD
Department of Pharmacy, St. Louis Children's Hospital, Department of Pediatrics, Washington University School of Medicine, St Louis, Missouri, USA

MICHAEL MURIELLO, MD
Assistant Professor of Pediatrics, Division of Genetics, Medical College of Wisconsin, Milwaukee, Wisconsin, USA

JOSEF NEU, MD
Professor, Pediatrics, University of Florida, Gainesville, Florida, USA

JEFFREY M. PERLMAN, MB, ChB
Professor of Pediatrics, Division of Newborn, Weill Cornell Medicine, NewYork-Presbyterian Hospital, New York, New York, USA

ERIN L. RHOLL, MD, MA
Professor, Division of Hospital Medicine, PANDA Palliative Care Team, Children's National Medical Center, Washington, DC, USA

BRIAN K. RIVERA, MS
Center for Perinatal Research, The Abigail Wexner Research Institute at Nationwide Children's Hospital, Columbus, Ohio, USA

CHRISTINE SALVATORE, MD
Associate Professor of Clinical Pediatrics, Division of Pediatric Infectious Diseases, Weill Cornell Medicine, NewYork-Presbyterian Hospital, New York, New York, USA

MEGHA SHARMA, MD
Division of Neonatology, Department of Pediatrics, University of Arkansas for Medical Sciences, Little Rock, Arkansas, USA

JONATHAN L. SLAUGHTER, MD, MPH
Department of Pediatrics, The Ohio State University Wexner Medical Center, Center for Perinatal Research, The Abigail Wexner Research Institute at Nationwide Children's Hospital, Division of Epidemiology, College of Public Health, The Ohio State University, Columbus, Ohio, USA

ALICIA SPRECHER, MD
Pediatrics - Neonatology, Medical College of Wisconsin, Children's Wisconsin, Milwaukee, Wisconsin, USA

DIANA L. STANESCU, MD
Assistant Professor of Pediatrics, Division of Endocrinology, Department of Pediatrics, The Children's Hospital of Philadelphia, University of Pennsylvania Perelman School of Medicine, Philadelphia, Pennsylvania, USA

CHARLES A. STANLEY, MD
Professor of Pediatrics, Division of Endocrinology, Department of Pediatrics, The Children's Hospital of Philadelphia, University of Pennsylvania Perelman School of Medicine, Philadelphia, Pennsylvania, USA

RACHEL A. TAYLOR, MD
Department of Pediatrics, The Ohio State University Wexner Medical Center, The Heart Center, Nationwide Children's Hospital, Columbus, Ohio, USA

AMY J. WAGNER, MD
Professor of Surgery, Section Chief, Division of Pediatric Surgery, Children's Wisconsin, Milwaukee, Wisconsin, USA

Contents

Delirium in the Neonate　　　1

Samuel J. Adams and Alicia Sprecher

> Delirium is likely present in the neonatal intensive care unit and has been largely unrecognized. There are several risk factors for delirium including illness severity, neurosedative exposure, and environmental disruptions that put infants at risk for delirium. Regular use of scoring systems should be considered to improve delirium detection. When identified, initial steps in management should include resolving underlying causes and implementation of standard nonpharmacologic measures. Mounting pediatric evidence suggests that the atypical antipsychotics, as well as the α-2 agonists, may be additionally beneficial in treating delirium as well as improving the ability to wean off other neurosedative medications.

Treatment of Posthemorrhagic Hydrocephalus　　　15

Susan S. Cohen and John Flibotte

> The incidence of intraventricular hemorrhage (IVH) has overall declined to 15% to 20% of preterm infants with birth weight less than 1500 g. One of the major complications of severe IVH is posthemorrhagic ventricular dilation (PHVD). Nearly 10% of all infants with IVH and 20% of infants with severe IVH will develop progressive PHVD requiring surgical intervention to prevent parenchymal damage in the developing brain. This review focuses on the controversies regarding posthemorrhagic hydrocephalus interventions with a focus on how to interpret recent data from trials that some have seen as heralding a call toward more aggressive intervention.

Neonatal Hypertension　　　27

Rebecca Hjorten and Joseph T. Flynn

> Neonatal hypertension is uncommon but is becoming increasingly recognized. Normative blood pressure data are limited, as is research regarding the risks, treatment, and long-term outcomes. Therefore, there are no clinical practice guidelines and management is based on clinical judgment and expert opinion. Recognition of neonatal hypertension requires proper blood pressure measurement technique. When hypertension is present there should be a thorough clinical, laboratory, and imaging evaluation to promptly diagnose causes needing medical or surgical management. This review provides a practical overview for the practicing clinician

contemporary context of structural racism in the United States on the African–American women's birth outcome disadvantage. In the process, we propose a paradigm to address the racial health inequity in adverse birth outcome by considering the interplay of racism and social class.

Inhaled nitric oxide (iNO) therapy had a transformational impact on the management of infants with persistent pulmonary hypertension of the newborn (PPHN). iNO remains the only approved pulmonary vasodilator for PPHN; yet 30% to 40% of patients do not respond or have incomplete response to iNO. Lung recruitment strategies with early surfactant administration and high-frequency ventilation can optimize the response to iNO in the presence of parenchymal lung diseases. Alternate pulmonary vasodilators are used commonly as rescue, life-saving measures, though there is a lack of high-quality evidence supporting their efficacy and safety. This article reviews the available evidence and future directions for research in PPHN.

In cases whereby the continuation of life-sustaining medical therapies is not in the infant's best interest and does not align with the parents' goals, it is ethically and morally advisable to withhold/withdraw life-sustaining medical therapies. Withdrawing/withholding artificial nutrition hydration is not morally or ethically different from other medical treatments. Determination of what and when to withdraw should occur through shared decision-making considering the parents' values and the infant's physiology and comfort. The practice of physician recommendations followed by parental informed nondissent should be considered in these instances.

Mild therapeutic hypothermia has been extensively studied and validated as an effective and safe treatment for term and near-term infants with moderate and severe hypoxic encephalopathy meeting narrow inclusion criteria. Unanswered questions remain about whether cooling treatment can be optimized to improve outcomes even further, and whether it is reasonable to offer treatment to infants excluded from the foundational studies. Consideration of "off-protocol" cooling practices requires methical review of available evidence and analysis using both a clinical and a research ethical framework.

summarize currently used measures, and those showing future promise for prevention.

Differences of sex development (DSD) refer to rare conditions in which an individual's sex development is different from typical male or female development. The neonatologist is often the first health care provider to interact with parents of newborns with DSD and must be familiar with the approach to these conditions. In this article, we discuss the definition of DSD, initial workup of the patient with DSD, terminology, and controversies in care.

Extremely preterm infants who must suddenly support their own gas exchange with lungs that are incompletely developed and lacking adequate amount of surfactant and antioxidant defenses are susceptible to lung injury. The decades-long quest to prevent bronchopulmonary dysplasia has had limited success, in part because of increasing survival of more immature infants. The process must begin in the delivery room with gentle assistance in establishing and maintaining adequate lung aeration, followed by noninvasive support and less invasive surfactant administration. Various modalities of invasive and noninvasive support have been used with varying degree of effect and are reviewed in this article.

Chronic pain and agitation in neonatal life impact the developing brain. Oral sweet-tasting solutions should be used judiciously to mitigate behavioral responses to mild painful procedures, keeping in mind that the long-term impact is unknown. Rapidly acting opioids should be used as part of premedication cocktails for nonemergent endotracheal intubations. Continuous low-dose morphine or dexmedetomidine may be considered for preterm or term neonates exhibiting signs of stress during mechanical ventilation and therapeutic hypothermia, respectively. Further research is required regarding the pharmacokinetics, pharmacodynamics, safety, and efficacy of pharmacologic agents used to mitigate mild, moderate, and chronic pain and stress in neonates.

Fetal surgery is a constantly evolving field that showed noticeable progress with the treatment of myelomeningocele (MMC) using prenatal repair. Despite this success, there are ongoing questions regarding the optimal approach for fetal myelomeningocele repair, as well as which patients are eligible. Expansion of the inclusion and exclusion criteria is an important ongoing area of study for myelomeningocele including the recent

PROGRAM OBJECTIVE
The goal of *Clinics in Perinatology* is to keep practicing perinatologists, neonatologists, obstetricians, practicing physicians and residents up to date with current clinical practice in perinatology by providing timely articles reviewing the state of the art in patient care.

TARGET AUDIENCE
Perinatologists, neonatologists, obstetricians, practicing physicians, residents and healthcare professionals who provide patient care utilizing findings from *Clinics in Perinatology.*

LEARNING OBJECTIVES
Upon completion of this activity, participants will be able to:
1. Recognize the identification of disorders that contribute to neonatal complications in the NICU setting using the appropriate assessment, screening, and diagnostic tools to assist in developing care management based on best practices and ethical considerations.
2. Discuss current controversies in perinatology and its impact on neonates, families, health care providers, and culture.
3. Review the efficacy, risks, and benefits of treatment and prevention strategies, including the use of assistive technology, surgical intervention, genomic testing, and pharmacotherapy.

ACCREDITATION
The Elsevier Office of Continuing Medical Education (EOCME) is accredited by the Accreditation Council for Continuing Medical Education (ACCME) to provide continuing medical education for physicians.

The EOCME designates this journal-based CME activity for a maximum of 19 *AMA PRA Category 1 Credit*(s)™. Physicians should claim only the credit commensurate with the extent of their participation in the activity.

All other health care professionals requesting continuing education credit for this enduring material will be issued a certificate of participation.

DISCLOSURE OF CONFLICTS OF INTEREST
The EOCME assesses conflict of interest with its instructors, faculty, planners, and other individuals who are in a position to control the content of CME activities. All relevant conflicts of interest that are identified are thoroughly vetted by EOCME for fair balance, scientific objectivity, and patient care recommendations. EOCME is committed to providing its learners with CME activities that promote improvements or quality in healthcare and not a specific proprietary business or a commercial interest.

The planning committee, staff, authors, and editors listed below have identified no financial relationships or relationships to products or devices they or their spouse/life partner have with commercial interest related to the content of this CME activity:
Samuel J. Adams, MD; Natalie G. Allen, MD; Carl H. Backes, MD; Megan Barcroft, DO; John D. E. Barks, MD, FAAP; Katie R. Baughman, MD; Darren P. Berman, MD; Emily Callan, MD; Hala Chaaban, MD; Lina Chalak, MD; Susan S. Cohen, MD; Scott Cohen, MD; James W. Collins Jr, MD, MPH; Richard J. David, MD; Crista Devette, MD, PhD; Afif El-Khuffash, MD; John Flibotte, MD; Joseph T. Flynn, MD, MS; Andrew B. Foy, MD; Jennifer F. Gerardin, MD; Ruth E. Grunau, PhD; Aarthi Gunasekaran, MD; Rebecca Hjorten, MD; Robert M. Kliegman, MD; G. Ganesh Konduri, MD; Kanthi Bangalore Krishna, MD; Naomi T. Laventhal, MD, MA, FAAP; Peter A. Lee, MD, PhD; Steven R. Leuthner, MD, MA; Samuel Levin, MD; John Marquart, MD; Christopher McKee, DO; Christopher McPherson, PharmD; Michael Muriello, MD; Josef Neu, MD; Jeffrey M. Perlman, MB ChB; Erin L. Rholl, MD, MA; Brian K. Rivera, MS; Christine Salvatore, MD; Megha Sharma, MD; Jonathan L. Slaughter, MD, MPH; Alicia Sprecher, MD; Diana L. Stanescu, MD; Charles A. Stanley, MD; Jeyanthi Surendrakumar; Rachel A. Taylor, MD; Doreen Thomas-Payne, MSN, BSN, RN, PMHNP-BC; Amy J. Wagner, MD

The planning committee, staff, authors, and editors listed below have identified financial relationships or relationships to products or devices they or their spouse/life partner have with commercial interest related to the content of this CME activity:
Martin Keszler, MD, FAAP: *Researcher*: Draeger Medical, Inc.

UNAPPROVED/OFF-LABEL USE DISCLOSURE
The EOCME requires CME faculty to disclose to the participants:
1. When products or procedures being discussed are off-label, unlabelled, experimental, and/or investigational (not US Food and Drug Administration [FDA] approved); and

2. Any limitations on the information presented, such as data that are preliminary or that represent ongoing research, interim analyses, and/or unsupported opinions. Faculty may discuss information about pharmaceutical agents that is outside of FDA-approved labelling. This information is intended solely for CME and is not intended to promote off-label use of these medications. If you have any questions, contact the medical affairs department of the manufacturer for the most recent prescribing information.

TO ENROLL

To enroll in the *Clinics in Perinatology* Continuing Medical Education program, call customer service at 1-800-654-2452 or sign up online at http://www.theclinics.com/home/cme. The CME program is available to subscribers for an additional annual fee of USD 265.00.

METHOD OF PARTICIPATION

In order to claim credit, participants must complete the following:
1. Complete enrolment as indicated above.
2. Read the activity.
3. Complete the CME Test and Evaluation. Participants must achieve a score of 70% on the test. All CME Tests and Evaluations must be completed online.

CME INQUIRIES/SPECIAL NEEDS

For all CME inquiries or special needs, please contact elsevierCME@elsevier.com.

CLINICS IN PERINATOLOGY

SERIES OF RELATED INTEREST

Obstetrics and Gynecology Clinics of North America
https://www.obgyn.theclinics.com

THE CLINICS ARE AVAILABLE ONLINE!
Access your subscription at:
www.theclinics.com

CLINICS IN PERINATOLOGY

FORTHCOMING ISSUES

June 2022
Neonatal and Perinatal Nutrition
Akhil Maheshwari and Jonathan R.
Swanson, Editors

September 2022
Advances in Imaging of the Fetus and
Newborn
Sangam Kanekar and Sarah Sarvis Milla,
Editors

December 2022
Advances and Updates in Fetal and Neonatal
Surgery
KuoJen Tsao and Hanmin Lee, Editors

RECENT ISSUES

December 2021
Advances in Respiratory Management
Manuel Sanchez-Luna, Editor

September 2021
Care for the Term Newborn
Anup Katheria and Lisa Stellwagen,
Editors

June 2021
Perinatal and Neonatal Infections
Joseph B. Cantey and Andi L. Shane,
Editors

SERIES OF RELATED INTEREST

Obstetrics and Gynecology Clinics of North America
http://www.obgyn.theclinics.com

THE CLINICS ARE AVAILABLE ONLINE!
Access your subscription at:
www.theclinics.com

Foreword

Controversies Will Always Be There: They Need to Be Managed

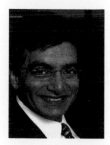

Lucky Jain, MD, MBA
Consulting Editor

More than twenty years after the publication of the landmark report *To Err Is Human*,[1] much progress has been made in making health care safe. Institutions across the country have focused on improving quality and patient safety through standardization of practices. In a follow-up publication in 2005, Drs Leape and Berwick[2] commented on the progress made after the original report and future expectations. They predicted that the pace of change would accelerate with implementation of electronic medical records, coupled with more widespread adoption of best practices to improve patient safety and outcomes. They also surmised that access to more reliable data will allow us to weed out unwarranted variability in care and reduce waste.

The jury is still out on how well the health care system has kept these promises twenty years later. Indeed, it is far from clear if pesky old controversies that impact day-to-day management are being resolved expeditiously and new ones contained to a manageable pace. In a recent article on quality of care and disparities in obstetrics, experts paint a worrisome picture.[3] They contend that even though the United States spends more on maternity care than any other country in the world, the extra spending has not translated into improved outcomes, and our maternal and infant mortalities continue to be among the highest in the industrialized world. Not just that, according to them, data suggest that quality of obstetric care continues to vary widely across the country. Unresolved controversies and variability of care persist in some of the most used interventions, such as use of oxytocin, timing of delivery, episiotomy, and general anesthesia.[3] It is not surprising that these uncertainties translate into wide variation in care provided to patients and result in equally unpredictable outcomes.

Such is the case in neonatal care as well. From use of oxygen, feeding practices, to adequate level of analgesia, challenges persist in nearly every area of the discipline. Clinicians struggle when there are no evidence-based recommendations. However, randomized controlled trials are hard to conduct, and meaningful data trickle in at

Clin Perinatol 49 (2022) xvii–xix
https://doi.org/10.1016/j.clp.2021.12.002
0095-5108/22/© 2021 Published by Elsevier Inc.

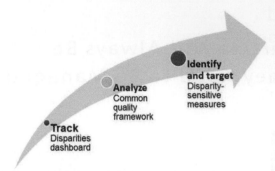

Fig. 1. Three strategies to reduce disparities by focusing on quality of care. (*From* Howell EA, Zeitlin J. Quality of care and disparities in obstetrics. Obstet Gynecol Clin North Am 2017;44(1):13-25.)

an even slower pace to impact change. There is also the culture of medicine we are all so familiar with, which relies on high standards of autonomous individual performance but struggles with the complexity of medicine and propensity for errors.[2]

Let us also not forget the racial and ethnic disparities in care and outcomes. Variability in care is magnified in care delivered to underserved and ethnically diverse populations and correlates well with poorer outcomes. This is important since half of all US births are to minority women. A study from a few years ago showed that women who delivered in hospitals with a high number of black patients had higher rates of severe morbidity compared with women who delivered in hospitals with a low number of black patients.[3] The authors propose a three-pronged approach to reducing disparities by focusing on quality of care and closely tracking outcomes (**Fig. 1**).[3]

In this issue of the *Clinics in Perinatology*, Drs Cohen and Kliegman have collated an important set of articles on current controversies in neonatal-perinatal medicine. Despite the challenges posed by the pandemic, this has been an outstanding year for the *Clinics in Perinatology*, and I am grateful to you for making us your trusted source of state-of-the-art information. I am also thankful to the publishing staff at Elsevier, including Kerry Holland and Karen Justine Solomon, for their support in bringing this wonderful publication to you.

Lucky Jain, MD, MBA
Department of Pediatrics
Emory University School of Medicine, and
Children's Healthcare of Atlanta
1760 Haygood Drive, W409
Atlanta, GA 30322, USA

E-mail address:
LJAIN@EMORY.EDU

REFERENCES

1. Kohn KT, Corrigan JM, Donaldson MS. To err is human: building a safer health system. Washington, DC: National Academy Press; 1999.
2. Leape LL, Berwick DM. Five years after to err is human. What have we learned? JAMA 2005;293:2384–90.
3. Howell EA, Zeitlin J. Quality of care and disparities in obstetrics. Obstet Gynecol Clin North Am 2017;44:13–25.

Preface

Current Controversies in Perinatology

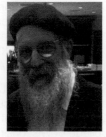 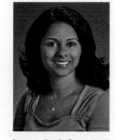

Robert M. Kliegman, MD   Susan S. Cohen, MD
Editors

In the modern era of perinatology, controversy exists in the daily clinical management of the most vulnerable infants in the neonatal intensive care unit (NICU). Infants who may not have survived beyond the perinatal period in the past now survive, and their comorbidities create clinical conundrums in both the short term and the long term. Therefore, we are always in search of new and better ways to care for these infants. We have become increasingly aware though that innovation requires continued critical evaluation and review. Such evaluations have always been important because of the potential dangers of introducing untested therapies to the high-risk infant. More so now than ever, we are charged with the responsibility to inform families of the risks and benefits of the treatments we offer so that they can make the best decisions for their child.

The NICU has not been spared from the controversies that our culture has faced: implicit bias as it affects the care of babies of color, newborn sex designation as it pertains to disorders of sex development, and withholding care in infants facing end of life, to name a few. We are faced with therapeutic drift of treatments that were tested in one population, but its use has been extended to others without validation of safety or efficacy. We are left to speculate perinatal outcomes of infants born during a global pandemic, when disinformation is abundant and the clinical stakes are high. These are just a few topics that will be addressed in this issue of *Clinics in Perinatology*. We have selected contributors to this issue who have been working actively on the problems they discuss. We are thankful to them for the time they have spent critically analyzing these important topics. Our hope is that the topics and issues raised in this issue will stimulate further discussions and inquiry, challenge current practice and dogma, and provide fodder for future research.

This is the seventh issue of "Controversies in Perinatology" for Dr Kliegman and the first for Dr Cohen. We appreciate that no great advance in any field has been made

Clin Perinatol 49 (2022) xxi–xxii
https://doi.org/10.1016/j.clp.2021.12.001
0095-5108/22/© 2021 Published by Elsevier Inc.

perinatology.theclinics.com

without controversy. We embrace the opportunity to continue a tradition of examining, questioning, and validating new and innovative practices in the NICU together. We would like to express our appreciation to Carolyn Redman for her outstanding editorial assistance and dedication to this issue.

Robert M. Kliegman, MD
Department of Pediatrics
Children's Wisconsin
Medical College of Wisconsin
Children's Corporate Center
999 North 92nd Street
Suite 410
Milwaukee, WI 53226, USA

Susan S. Cohen, MD
Department of Pediatrics
Children's Wisconsin
Medical College of Wisconsin
Children's Corporate Center
999 North 92nd Street
Suite 410
Milwaukee, WI 53226, USA

E-mail addresses:
rkliegma@mcw.edu (R.M. Kliegman)
scohen@mcw.edu (S.S. Cohen)

Delirium in the Neonate

Samuel J. Adams, MD[a],*, Alicia Sprecher, MD[b]

KEYWORDS

- Delirium • Neonatal • Quetiapine • Risperidone • Dexmedetomidine

KEY POINTS

- Delirium is a well-recognized phenomenon in adult and pediatric intensive care and is very likely to be present and underrecognized in neonatal intensive care.
- Delirium comes in 3 forms, the most easily recognized and most rare form being hyperactive and the more subtle hypoactive and mixed forms.
- Scoring systems, including the Cornell Assessment for Pediatric Delirium, can be applied to infants and improve detection of delirium in this population.
- When delirium is detected, initial steps in management should include resolving underlying causes and implementation of standard nonpharmacologic measures.
- There are no set guidelines for pharmacologic management, as randomized controlled trials are lacking, but there is mounting evidence that the atypical antipsychotics and the α-2 agonists are both safe and effective in the neonatal population.

INTRODUCTION

Delirium is an increasingly recognized complication of hospitalization, particularly in intensive care units (ICU). Although delirium is well described in the adult population and an area of ongoing research within the pediatric population, its recognition within the neonatal ICU (NICU) is limited. Many of the risk factors for delirium in older populations are present within the NICU, and it stands to reason that infants cared for in the NICU would have the potential to develop this complication. This article explores the features of delirium, particularly as they relate to the neonate, the possible pathways to delirium, the incidence in the ICU environment, methods for detection, an approach to treatment, and the consequences of delirium.

DEFINITION

Delirium is a disorder of neurocognition characterized by alterations in attention and awareness. The *Diagnostic and Statistical Manual of Mental Disorders*, 5th ed.

a Neurology – Child Neurology, Medical College of Wisconsin, Children's Wisconsin, 8915 W. Connell Ct Milwaukee, WI 53226, USA; b Pediatrics - Neonatology, Medical College of Wisconsin, Children's Wisconsin, 8915 W. Connell Ct, Milwaukee, WI 53226, USA
* Corresponding author.
E-mail address: sjadams@mcw.edu

Clin Perinatol 49 (2022) 1–14
https://doi.org/10.1016/j.clp.2021.11.001
perinatology.theclinics.com

describes it as a disturbance that presents over a subacute timeline that represents an alteration from the patient's baseline and may fluctuate throughout the day.[1] These alterations cannot be explained by a preexisting condition or evolving primary neurologic disorder. The diagnosis of delirium can be further divided into 3 subtypes: hyperactive, hypoactive, and mixed.[2]

PRESENTATION

The onset of delirium typically occurs over the course of hours or days. The individual presentation depends on the patient baseline and the subtype of delirium present: hyperactive, hypoactive, or mixed.

The symptoms of delirium are related to changes in patient consciousness and cognition. In the adult or pediatric population, this may result in altered sleeping patterns or decreased interaction. Thought processes may be deranged, and confusion may be obvious. These alterations may be more difficult to detect in the neonate. It is normal for an infant to spend much of their day sleeping, but failure to respond to painful stimuli or lack of any period of calm wakefulness could be an indication of delirium.[3] Abrupt changes in sleeping or feeding patterns may be present.[3,4] As the infant matures, day-night differentiation becomes more apparent, and failure in this differentiation can be a sign of delirium.[3] In addition, limitations in eye contact and an inability to soothe indicate altered consciousness in the newborn.[4] Further, poorly coordinated, excessive, or slow movements may indicate altered cognition. Even newborn infants show a preference for parents or frequent caregivers, and failure to differentiate between individuals may also reflect issues with cognition.[3,4] As the infant develops, new metrics can be used to assess cognition including the ability to follow past midline at 8 weeks or the emergence of more purposeful reaching.[3]

Much of the current literature regarding delirium in the NICU comes from case reports describing difficult to sedate, chronically ventilated infants. Groves and colleagues describe 3 cases of delirium in NICU infants. The infants in this case series ranged from 4 to 17 weeks corrected gestational age. All required surgical interventions for congenital anomalies and were receiving pharmacologic sedation.[5] In all 3 cases, infants were noted to have increasing agitation that was nonresponsive to pharmacologic intervention. A diagnosis of delirium was made in collaboration with child psychology, and symptoms improved with initiation of quetiapine (an atypical antipsychotic), which facilitated weaning of other neurosedative agents. Additional case reports from Brahmbhatt and Whitgob, Edwards and colleagues, and Madden and colleagues, all describe cases of infants at 6 to 7 months of age being managed on multiple neurosedatives either postoperatively or due to chronic ventilation who demonstrated an increase in agitation from baseline. Agitation in these cases persisted despite environmental measures, medication adjustments, and diagnostic evaluations. After a diagnosis of delirium rendered by child psychiatry, each of these patients were initiated on atypical antipsychotics with improvement in symptoms.[6–8]

Despite the frequency of hyperactive delirium in case reports, hypoactive delirium is the most common subtype in prevalence studies. Hypoactive delirium may be difficult to recognize, as infants and children with decreased consciousness may represent "easy" patients, where an investigation into the potential for delirium is less likely to occur.[9] Hyperactive delirium is the least common subtype but the most obvious to the observer.[4]

INCIDENCE

Currently, the incidence of delirium in the NICU is difficult to ascertain. In adult ICUs, the incidence ranges between 40% and 80%.[9] Several recent studies have explored the incidence of delirium within the pediatric ICU (PICU). In one study, the incidence of delirium was 17.3% as diagnosed by the Cornell Assessment of Pediatric Delirium (CAPD) score, with 46.4% being hypoactive delirium, 8.4% hyperactive, and 45.2% mixed.[10] Another study reported CAPD scores positive for delirium among 44% of PICU admissions and 69% of admissions with a length of stay greater than 48 hours.[11] In an international point prevalence study, 25% of PICU patients were positive for delirium via CAPD scores, which increased to 54% for patients hospitalized for more than 6 days.[12] Factors that seem to increase the risk of delirium in these studies include patient age less than 2 years, baseline cognitive dysfunction, need for invasive ventilation, severe illness, use of restraints, inadequate pain or agitation management, and exposure to neurosedatives, particularly benzodiazepines.[10–12] Many of these risk factors are present in NICU patients, suggesting the potential for a high incidence of delirium.

PATHOPHYSIOLOGY

The pathophysiology of delirium is poorly understood; indeed, there are likely several pathways, all terminating in dysregulation of neuronal activity. Several of the proposed mechanisms overlap and include derangement related to neuroinflammation, neuroendocrine abnormalities, diurnal dysregulation, oxidative stress, and neurotransmitter imbalance.[13]

Systemic inflammation increases the expression of cytokines within the brain and can compromise the blood-brain barrier, leading to neuronal and synaptic dysfunction. The stress of illness and systemic inflammation elevates glucocorticoids that increase brain vulnerability, particularly within the hippocampus. Inflammation also disrupts the production of melatonin, leading to diurnal dysregulation. Melatonin has several important functions including free radical scavenging and anti-apoptotic and anti-inflammatory effects.[13] In the study by Traube and colleagues, delirium rates were highest among children admitted with infectious or inflammatory causes.[12] In addition, exposure to exogenous corticosteroids increases the risk of delirium.[4]

In the course of acute illness, the central nervous system may be subject to periods of hypoperfusion either due to hypotension or due to local capillary injury. Hypoperfusion results in an energy deficit and the development of free radicals that may cause further injury. Central nervous system energy failure can impair the clearance of toxic metabolites, affect neurotransmitter synthesis and metabolism, and lead to spreading depolarization due to an inability to maintain ion gradients,[13] and this may explain some of the correlation between illness severity and delirium risk.[4,12]

Neurotransmitter imbalances have been documented in delirium and include decreased levels of acetylcholine and increased dopamine and glutamine, among others. Acetylcholine synthesis is particularly sensitive to energy deficits. In addition, increased anticholinergic activity has been documented in delirious patients in the absence of exposure to exogenous anticholinergic agents. Finally, inflammation can decrease the activity of acetylcholine. Dopamine reuptake and metabolism are impaired in the energy-deficient nervous system. Elevated levels of glutamine are thought to result from spreading depolarization when the central nervous system cannot maintain ion gradients and results in calcium ion–mediated neuronal injury.[13] Many of the medications associated with delirium affect neurotransmitters including anticholinergics and benzodiazepines (which enhance the effect of gamma-aminobutyric acid [GABA]).[4,6,9]

Although the exact pathogenesis of delirium is not understood, studies have identified many risk factors regarding environment, medications, and patient characteristics. Patient characteristics that tend to increase the risk of delirium include severity of illness, infectious causes, metabolic derangements, direct central nervous system injury, need for mechanical ventilation, and baseline cognitive deficits.[2,4,6,9] Medications commonly associated with delirium include benzodiazepines, anticholinergics, and corticosteroids as described earlier, as well as opiates, particularly short-acting agents, and vasopressors.[4,6,9] Environmental factors include lights and sound, use of restraints, lack of family, lack of a schedule, and multiple caregivers.[9] A useful system for remembering these factors is the BRAIN MAPS mnemonic as shown in **Table 1**.[9]

DIAGNOSIS

In case reports, the diagnosis of delirium within the NICU has been made with the assistance of child psychiatry. Unfortunately, this method is likely to underrecognize infants suffering from delirium. Hyperactive delirium is the least common form but the easiest to recognize.[9] Infants with hypoactive delirium are more likely to go undiagnosed. Regular use of a delirium scoring systems increases the chance delirium will be recognized and is recommended in adult and pediatric ICUs.[2]

Many of the current tools for delirium assessment require verbal communication with the patient. Few scoring systems are well validated for the pediatric population, and fewer are validated for the neonatal population. The CAPD score is one of the only scores validated in the newborn period. It is designed to detect hyperactive, hypoactive, and mixed delirium. The score is derived from asking 8 questions regarding the child's attention, awareness, actions, and general state as described in **Fig. 1**. It is designed to be assigned by a nurse at the end of each shift to reflect several hours of observations. Scores of 9 or higher suggest delirium, but care should be taken to compare with the patient's baseline. In validation studies in the pediatric population, the score demonstrated 94.1% sensitivity and 79.2% specificity.[14]

Delirium scores must be interpreted in the context of potential behavioral regression during illness, baseline developmental delay, and age-appropriate behavioral expectations. The CAPD score has a set of anchor points that allow the scorer to apply the questions of the scoring system in a developmentally appropriate manner, which are summarized **Fig. 2**.[3] For example, when assessing eye contact, the newborn is expected only to fixate on the face, whereas the 8-week-old infant should follow a point of interest past midline. Movements and actions are increasingly expected to be purposeful and smooth as the infant ages. These anchor points were used for the validation of the CAPD score.[3] Accordingly, the CAPD score is among the most widely used scoring systems for the assessment of delirium in the child and infant population.

TREATMENT

The first steps in management of any delirious patient lies in attempting to discover and resolve the inciting cause. As evidenced earlier, the cause of delirium is often multifactorial, but working to eliminate potential sources as they are determined often will lead to rapid improvement. In the NICU, this includes evaluation and rectification of new or worsening medical diagnoses, including infections, pain, respiratory instability, and withdrawal.[15] In addition, the possibility of an epileptic encephalopathies or non-convulsive status epilepticus, as a mimic of delirium, should prompt consideration of consultation with neurology for possible electroencephalographic monitoring. The ICU environment poses its own risks for development of delirium, but NICU protocols to limit noise, cluster cares to promote ideal sleep cycles, and surrounding the patient with familiar objects, scents, and caregivers, all promote recovery from delirium

Table 1		
BRAIN MAPS mnemonic of contributors to delirium		
B	Bring oxygen	Treat hypoxia, improve oxygen delivery by augmenting cardiac output or correcting anemia
R	Remove/Reduce deliriogenic medications	Medications of interest include benzodiazepines, anticholinergics, corticosteroids, and short-acting narcotics
A	Atmosphere	Control light and noise, use restraints sparingly, keep family involved, limit the number of caregivers, make a daily schedule
I	Infection, Immobilization, and Inflammation	Evaluate and treat for infection and inflammation. Encourage early mobility
N	New organ dysfunction	Investigate for evolving organ dysfunction
M	Metabolic disturbance	Evaluate and correct metabolic disturbances including abnormalities in serum sodium, potassium, glucose, calcium, acidosis, and alkalosis
A	Awake	Establish a normal sleep-wake cycle. Use appropriate light cycling and encourage clustering of care
P	Pain	Evaluate for uncontrolled pain. For patients on pain medications, ensure dosing reflects pain scores and medications are titrated to effect
S	Sedation	Ensure sedation medications are minimized by titrating to effect. Use sedation scores to assess sedation

Adapted from Smith HAB, Brink E, Fuchs DC, Ely EW, Pandharipande PP. Pediatric Delirium: Monitoring and management in the pediatric intensive care unit. Pediatr Clin North Am. 2013 Jun;60(3):741-60; with permission.

providing reorientation. These measures are also helpful when implemented early to prevent the development of symptoms. Careful assessment to the current medication regimen should also be conducted, and steps to decrease or cease use of known deleriogenic medications, including benzodiazepines, opioids, corticosteroids, and anticholinergics, should be considered.

When the attempts discussed earlier do not lead to improvement in symptoms, pharmacologic management is often deliberated. Data on safety and efficacy in the pediatric population are expectedly lacking, and there are no FDA-approved medications for use in the pediatric population. Owing to the difficulties of underrecognition of delirium in the NICU, specific recommendations regarding pharmacologic treatment are based on relatively small retrospective case studies or series, and use is off-label. A summary of the medications outlined later is compiled in **Table 2**.

A recent pharmacologic synopsis by Liviskie and McPherson discussed the current state of interventions available in the NICU population.[4] The most commonly used medications for delirium in the adult population have been the antipsychotics. The broad division into first-generation (typical) and second-generation (atypical) still

RASS Score _____ (if -4 or -5 do not proceed)						
Please answer the following questions based on your interactions with the patient over the course of your shift:						
	Never	Rarely	Sometimes	Often	Always	Score
	4	3	2	1	0	
1. Does the child make eye contact with the caregiver?						
2. Are the child's actions purposeful?						
3. Is the child aware of his/her surroundings?						
4. Does the child communicate needs and wants?						
	Never	Rarely	Sometimes	Often	Always	
	0	1	2	3	4	
5. Is the child restless?						
6. Is the child inconsolable?						
7. Is the child underactive—very little movement while awake?						
8. Does it take the child a long time to respond to interactions?						
					TOTAL	

Fig. 1. Cornell Assessment of Pediatric Delirium score. (*From* Silver G, Kearney J, Traube C, Hertzig M. Delirium screening anchored in child development: The Cornell Assessment for Pediatric Delirium. Palliat Support Care. 2015 Aug;13(4):1005-1011; with permission.)

applies, as does the general principle of increased risk of side effects in the former due to the stronger affinity at the Dopamine D_2 receptors. As such, use in the pediatric population has predominately focused on the atypical antipsychotic class. Should any medication in the antipsychotic class be used to treat neonatal delirium, baseline and repeat electrocardiogram (EKG) assessments should be performed while on therapy, and treatment duration should be limited to as short a course as possible.

The greatest benefit of the first-generation antipsychotics class, specifically haloperidol, remains its intravenous formulation availability. However, with up to a nearly 40% rate of adverse effects, including hypotension, decreased consciousness, extrapyramidal symptoms (EPS), or neuroleptic malignant syndrome (NMS),[16] use should be reserved to those with confirmed extreme symptoms or the inability to tolerate enteral medication administration, and steps to limit duration of use are recommended. There are no documented reports of use in the NICU; however, several reports document use in patients younger than 1 year, in former premature infants, and with the youngest age 3 months in a child with multiple congenital malformations presenting with an emerging delirium.[17] Dosing recommendations do have some variability, ranging from 0.003 to 0.278 mg/kg/dose (0.005–0.15 mg/kg/d) with dosing divided every 6 to 12 hours.[18]

In the second-generation atypical antipsychotic class, olanzapine has been one of the most studied overall in the pediatric population (>125 cases); however, none

	NB	4 wk	6 wk	8 wk	28 wk	1 y	2 y
1. Does the child make eye contact with the caregiver?	Fixates on face	Holds gaze briefly. Follows 90 degrees	Holds gaze	Follows moving object/caregiver past midline, regards examiner's hand holding object, focused attention	Holds gaze. Prefers primary parent. Looks at speaker.	Holds gaze. Prefers primary parent. Looks at speaker.	Holds gaze. Prefers primary parent. Looks at speaker
2. Are the child's actions purposeful?	Moves head to side, dominated by primitive reflexes	Reaches (with some discoordination)	Reaches	Symmetric movements, will passively grasp handed object	Reaches with coordinated smooth movement	Reaches and manipulates objects, tries to change position, if mobile may try to get up.	Reaches and manipulates objects, tries to change position, if mobile may try to get up and walk
3. Is the child aware of his/her surroundings?	Calm awake time	Awake alert time. Turns to primary caretaker's voice. May turn to smell of primary care taker	Increasing awake alert time. Turns to primary caretaker's voice. May turn to smell of primary care taker	Facial brightening or smile in response to nodding head, frown to bell, coos	Strongly prefers mother, then other familiars. Differentiates between novel and familiar objects	Prefers primary parent, then other familiars, upset when separated from preferred care takers. Comforted by familiar objects especially favorite blanket or stuffed animal	Prefers primary parent, then other familiars, upset when separated from preferred care takers. Comforted by familiar objects, especially favorite blanket or stuffed animal
4. Does the child communicate needs and wants?	Cries when hungry or uncomfortable	Cries when hungry or uncomfortable	Cries when hungry or uncomfortable	Cries when hungry or uncomfortable	Vocalizes /indicates about needs, e.g., hunger, discomfort, curiosity in objects, or surroundings	Uses single words or signs	3 to 4 word sentences, or signs. May indicate toilet needs, calls self or me
5. Is the child restless?	No sustained awake alert state	No sustained calm state	No sustained calm state	No sustained awake alert state	No sustained calm state	No sustained calm state	No sustained calm state
6. Is the child inconsolable?	Not soothed by parental rocking, singing, feeding, comforting actions	Not soothed by parental rocking, singing, feeding, comforting actions	Not soothed by parental rocking, singing, feeding, comforting actions	Not soothed by parental rocking, singing, comforting actions	Not soothed by usual methods, e.g., singing, holding, talking	Not soothed by usual methods, e.g., singing, holding, talking, reading	Not soothed by usual methods, e.g. singing, holding, talking, reading (may tantrum, but can organize)
7. Is the child underactive—very little movement while awake?	Little if any flexed and then relaxed state with primitive reflexes (Child should be sleeping comfortably most of the time)	Little if any reaching, kicking, grasping (still may be somewhat discoordinated)	Little if any reaching, kicking, grasping (may begin to be more coordinated)	Little if any purposive grasping, control of head and arm movements, such as pushing things that are noxious away	Little if any reaching, grasping, moving around in bed, pushing things away	Little if any play, efforts to sit up, pull up, and if mobile crawl or walk around	Little if any more elaborate play, efforts to sit up and move around, and if able to stand, walk, or jump
8. Does it take the child a long time to respond to interactions?	Not making sounds or reflexes active as expected (grasp, suck, moro)	Not making sounds or reflexes active as expected (grasp, suck, moro)	Not kicking or crying with noxious stimuli	Not cooing, smiling, or focusing gaze in response to interactions	Not babbling or smiling/laughing in social interactions (or even actively rejecting an interaction)	Not following simple directions. If verbal, not engaging in simple dialogue with words or jargon	Not following 1–2 step simple commands. If verbal, not engaging in more complex dialogue

Fig. 2. Newborn to 2-year-old anchor points for the Cornell Assessment of Pediatric Delirium score. (*From* Silver G, Kearney J, Traube C, Hertzig M. Delirium screening anchored in child development: The Cornell Assessment for Pediatric Delirium. Palliat Support Care. 2015 Aug;13(4):1005-1011; with permission.)

specifically in the NICU population.[18] Reported improvement were related to the ability to wean off other neurosedative medications and improved scores on the Delirium Ratings Scale—R-98 (DRS-R-98). It seems to have a very favorable side effect profile in the pediatric population, with dystonia being one of the only reported effects. Although the class as a whole carries additional risks, specifically for QTc prolongation, prior studies were limited in how well this was monitored or tracked. Weight-based dosing recommendations for the younger population was limited, instead studies used standard dosing for age ranges, including a 0.625 mg daily to BID dose for infants, leaving it difficult to extrapolate in an NICU population.

Quetiapine is currently the next most studied atypical antipsychotic, with at least 82 published pediatric use cases,[18] and has the most studies in the NICU population, with Groves and colleagues reporting on a 3-child case series,[5] and multiple other studies including patients younger than 1 year. One of the largest studies was a retrospective review of 50 patients treated with quetiapine in the PICU, ranging in age from 2 months to 20 years, with a median patient age of 4.5 years.[19] Diagnosis was made via CAPD scoring, treated first with nonpharmacologic measures before dosing with quetiapine according to a predetermined protocol, with a total of greater than 2400 doses given, of which greater than 950 were in children younger than 2 years. Side-effect profile in this study was very favorable, with no incidences of torsades de pointes, EPS, or NMS. All patients were monitored on telemetry with no instances of ventricular dysrhythmias, and only 3 patients with a prolonged QTc, none of which were found to be clinically significant, one resolving on own on repeat testing, another resolving with a modest 20% decrease in quetiapine. Dosing recommendations were derived from adult studies for delirium combined with recommendations for nondelirium indications. Initial dosing was set at 0.5 mg/kg every 8 hours, with an option for an as

Table 2
Summary of medications with potential use for neonatal and pediatric delirium

Medication	Receptor Targets	Initial Dosing	Maximum Daily Dosing	Short-Term Use Side Effects	Special Notes
Haloperidol	D_2 ++++ α_1 ++ $5HT_{2a}$ +	0.005 mg/kg/d divided q6-q12 h	0.15 mg/kg/d	EPS, NMS, hypotension, anticholinergics, somnolence	More evidence for hyperactive delirium subtype than other medications. High risk of side effects (>30%–40%)
Olanzapine	H_1 ++++ $5HT_{2a}$ +++ D_2, $M_{1\&2}$ ++ α_1 +	0.625 mg daily	0.625 mg BID	QTc prolongation, EPS, somnolence	Limited reports of weight-based dosing
Quetiapine	H_1 +++ α_1, $5HT_{2a}$ ++ D_2, $M_{1\&2}$ +	1.5 mg/kg/d divided q8 hours	6 mg/kg/d	QTc prolongation, EPS, somnolence	Most available reports for atypical antipsychotic use specifically in the neonatal population
Risperidone	$5HT_{2a}$ ++++ α_1, D_2, H_1 +++	0.01–0.04 mg/kg	0.1 mg/kg max 0.5 mg daily divided BID	QTc prolongation, EPS, somnolence	Oral liquid forms readily available
Dexmedetomidine	α_1 ++++	Loading dose 0.05–0.2 µg/kg	Reports from 0.6-1.2 µg/kg/h	Hypotension, bradycardia, tachyphylaxis,	Dosing recommendations based on studies for sedation/analgesia, and not specific to delirium
Gabapentin	$\alpha_2\delta$ VDCCs antagonist	15 mg/kg/d divided TID	35 mg/kg/d divided TID	Dizziness, sleepiness, ataxia, nystagmus, myoclonus	No reports for neonatal delirium but has been studied in pain management in the NICU

| Melatonin | MT$_{1\&2}$ | 0.05 mg/kg | NR^a | Rare | Limited evidence for direct effects on delirium, may largely help as an adjunctive to regulate sleep decreasing development of delirium |

+ + + + = higher affinity. + = lower affinity.

Abbreviations: 5HT$_{2a}$, Serotonergic receptors; D$_2$, Dopaminergic receptors; EPS, extrapyramidal symptoms (akathisia, dystonia, rigidity, parkinsonisms); H$_1$, histaminergic receptors; M$_{1\&2}$ muscarinic receptors; MT$_{1\&2}$ melatonin receptors; NMS, neuroleptic malignant syndrome (fever, confusion, rigidity variable BP, sweating, tachycardia); NR, not reported; α$_{1 \text{ or } 2}$ adrenergic alpha receptors; α2δ VDCCs, voltage-dependent calcium channels.

^{a} Max dosing in neonates not established. Dosing up to 10 mg have been used as young as 1 year of age.

needed 0.5 mg/kg dose, with escalation based on clinical reassessments, and a maximum dosing of 6 mg/kg/d.

The last in the group of atypical antipsychotics with reported pediatric use for delirium, Risperidone also has been used in the PICU setting in at least 51 children, and one report of use in the neonatal ICU setting, although in a former 32 week gestational age infant who was corrected to approximately 4 months.[4] Again, early studies documented improvement based on clinical evaluations by child psychiatrists or in weaning off sedative drips; however, later studies did use the DRS-R-98 or CAPD scores, improving reliability.[18] Risk for side effects increases with prolonged use, and in these short-duration studies treating delirium, the side-effect profile was very favorable, with only 2 children having a clinically nonsignificant QTc prolongation that did not hinder continued use, although it is important to note that this was with less than 50% receiving formal EKG readings but all patients on continuous telemetry.[20] No extrapyramidal symptoms or dystonic events were reported. Dosing was variable, with early studies relying on flat daily dosing and later development of weight-based dosing. Capino and colleagues summarized the 4 recent studies involving risperidone for delirium in the PICU with dosing reported at 0.1 to 0.2 mg daily.[18] Around the same time Campbell and colleagues published their report on risperidone dosing for pediatric delirium in 17 children younger than 2 years, with initial daily dosing at 0.01 to 0.04 mg/kg, with a mean of 0.02 mg/kg. They also noted more than 80% of patients required a dose increase during their therapy, with maximum dosing listed at 0.1 mg/kg with a median of 0.039 mg/kg.[20]

Dexmedetomidine is commonly used in the NICU for sedation and opioid-sparing analgesia, and in fact, many of the aforementioned studies were conducted in patients already receiving dexmedetomidine as part of the ICU sedation protocols. The ability to avoid or decrease use of opioids likely contributes to prevention of delirium. As an acute pharmacologic intervention to treat delirium, there is limited evidence. It has been studied head to head and as a rescue medication for delirium in cases of failed use of haloperidol.[21,22] A placebo-controlled, randomized trial is currently underway in the adult population[23]; however, no such trials are currently underway in the pediatric or neonatal populations. With its established use already in the neonates for sedation, the side-effect profile is relatively benign, with risks for hypotension and bradycardia that are ameliorated with dosing titration as needed. Loading doses have been used at a range from 0.05 to 0.2 µg/kg, with maximum rates of at least 1.2 µg/kg/h reported.[24,25]

Other medications that could potentially prove beneficial in the management of delirium include gabapentin and melatonin. Gabapentin has seen increasing use in the neonatal population for postoperative pain management, agitation related to chronic lung disease and prolonged intubation, and other visceral hyperalgesia states.[26,27] Gabapentin is a structural GABA analogue, but despite its naming and structure, it does not bind to GABA receptors, convert into GABA, or interfere with GABA transmission or metabolism.[28] Although not extensively studied for ICU delirium in the pediatric population, it has been used as a preoperative medication to prevent postoperative emergence delirium.[29,30] Side effects seem well tolerated with only transient sleepiness during dosing initiation and provoked nystagmus at elevated doses (toward the upper end of the typical ranges of 10–35 mg/kg/d). A handful of patients seemed to develop findings concerning for dysautonomia after abrupt discontinuation of gabapentin, which resolved with resumption of lower dosing and a more prolonged wean.[26] Calandriello and colleagues's review of sleep and delirium in the pediatric ICU highlighted that clear evidence for a causal relationship between sleep disturbance and delirium is lacking, even in the adult literature; however, as both have similar risks for development as well as similar proposed management, addressing concerns for both is prudent. Melatonin was reviewed by Laudone and colleagues regarding its role in therapy delirium as a prophylaxis as well as treatment.[31] Primary outcome measures to decrease the cumulative days of antipsychotic exposure were not met; however, after melatonin initiation, there was a decrease in cumulative sedation medication exposure, with lighter sedation via RASS scores and improvement in pain FLACC scores, but formal delirium scoring was not performed. The most common dose in their study was 3 mg nightly; however, as the Food and Drug Administration classifies melatonin as a dietary supplement, specific dosing ranges are limited. It has been shown that smaller doses of 0.1 to 0.5 mg can be useful for both sleep onset and sleep cycle phase shifting, with higher dosing of up to 10 mg nightly likely contributing to more hypnotic as opposed to chronobiotic effects.[32] Neonatal weight–based dosing is not available, but older pediatric patient dosing has been reported from 0.05 to 0.15 mg/kg, and even as high as 0.4 mg/kg in preprocedural sedation or emergence delirium studies.[31,33,34]

Again, noting the variability in studies discussed earlier, drastic improvements in the safety and efficacy profiles of essentially all of the medications listed earlier would be achieved with regimented blinded clinical trials. Two pediatric randomized controlled trials looking at the efficacy of quetiapine for delirium were unfortunately closed due to enrollment difficulties.[35,36] Thus, it is likely that a multicenter collaboration will be required to answer these important questions in the sensitive NICU population.

OUTCOMES

As studies to diagnose and treat delirium in the NICU are lacking as outlined earlier, studies on outcomes are also in short supply, and therefore, extrapolation from the older PICU population serves as proxy. There have been many reports supporting concerns that delirium in the PICU leads to prolonged mechanical ventilation, increased length of PICU admission and hospital stay in general, higher rates of morbidity and mortality, and increased medical care cost.[37] For instance, Traube and colleagues outlined the effects of delirium on PICU in-hospital outcomes and mortality in a cohort of 267 patients.[10] After controlling for confounders such as mechanical ventilation and probability of mortality, children with delirium stayed in the PICU 2.3 times longer than those without delirium. In-hospital mortality in their study was 5.24% versus 0.94% even after adjusting for probability of mortality on admission. They made special note that the in-hospital mortality was only a witnessed association without causality implied, although in their study it was a stronger predictor of mortality than the validated Pediatric Index of Mortality 3 score. This would be congruent with findings in adult ICUs, where delirium is now part of prognostic scoring.[38,39] However, long-term outcomes do leave room for hope, with Schieveld and colleagues noting when delirium is identified, it resolved in all 38 study patients treated with antipsychotic medications.[17] After discharge, Meyburg and colleagues found no association between PICU delirium and long-term (18 month) cognition or behavioral assessments, although the study was limited by a smaller sample size of 41 patients, and the effects of some recall bias on questionnaires. With these discrepancies, it will be prudent to include long-term outcomes that control for exposure to any medications used for treatment of delirium in the design of future clinical trials.

SUMMARY

Delirium is likely present in the NICU and has been largely underrecognized. There are several risk factors for delirium including illness severity, neurosedative exposure, and environmental disruptions that put infants at risk for delirium. Regular use of scoring systems should be considered to improve delirium detection. When identified, initial steps in management should include resolving underlying causes and implementation of standard nonpharmacologic measures. Mounting pediatric evidence suggests that the atypical antipsychotics as well as the α-2 agonists may be additionally beneficial in treating delirium as well as improving the ability to wean off other neurosedative medications.

Best Practices Box

What is the current practice?
Currently, there is limited attention to the prevalence, treatment, and prevention of delirium in the neonate.

Best practice/guideline/care path objectives
Consideration should be given to routine screening of infants in the NICU for delirium using validated screening tools, particularly term corrected infants. When delirium is detected, initial steps in management should include resolving underlying causes and implementation of standard nonpharmacologic measures. There are no set guidelines for pharmacologic management, as randomized controlled trials are lacking, but there is mounting evidence that the atypical antipsychotics and the α-2 agonists are both safe and effective in the neonatal population.

DISCLOSURE

The authors have nothing to disclose.

REFERENCES

1. American Psychiatric Association., American Psychiatric Association. DSM-5 Task Force. Diagnostic and statistical manual of mental disorders : DSM-5. 5th edition. Washington, DC: American Psychiatric Association; 2013.
2. Harris J, Ramelet AS, van Dijk M, et al. Clinical recommendations for pain, sedation, withdrawal and delirium assessment in critically ill infants and children: an ESPNIC position statement for healthcare professionals. Intensive Care Med 2016;42(6):972–86.
3. Silver G, Kearney J, Traube C, et al. Delirium screening anchored in child development: the Cornell assessment for pediatric delirium. Palliat Support Care 2015; 13(4):1005–11.
4. Liviskie C, McPherson C. Delirium in the NICU: risk or reality? Neonatal Netw 2021;40(2):103–12.
5. Groves A, Traube C, Silver G. Detection and management of delirium in the neonatal unit: a case series. Pediatrics 2016;137(3):e20153369.
6. Brahmbhatt K, Whitgob E. Diagnosis and management of delirium in critically ill infants: case report and review. Pediatrics 2016;137(3):e20151940.
7. Edwards LE, Hutchison LB, Hornik CD, et al. A case of infant delirium in the neonatal intensive care unit. J Neonatal Perinatal Med 2017;10(1):119–23.
8. Madden K, Turkel S, Jacobson J, et al. Recurrent delirium after surgery for congenital heart disease in an infant. Pediatr Crit Care Med 2011;12(6):e413–5.
9. Smith HA, Brink E, Fuchs DC, et al. Pediatric delirium: monitoring and management in the pediatric intensive care unit. Pediatr Clin North Am 2013;60(3): 741–60.

10. Traube C, Silver G, Gerber LM, et al. Delirium and mortality in critically ill children: epidemiology and outcomes of pediatric delirium. Crit Care Med 2017;45(5): 891–8.
11. Dervan LA, Di Gennaro JL, Farris RWD, et al. Delirium in a Tertiary PICU: risk factors and outcomes. Pediatr Crit Care Med 2020;21(1):21–32.
12. Traube C, Silver G, Reeder RW, et al. Delirium in critically ill children: an international point prevalence study. Crit Care Med 2017;45(4):584–90.
13. Maldonado JR. Neuropathogenesis of delirium: review of current etiologic theories and common pathways. Am J Geriatr Psychiatry 2013;21(12):1190–222.
14. Traube C, Silver G, Kearney J, et al. Cornell Assessment of Pediatric Delirium: a valid, rapid, observational tool for screening delirium in the PICU. Crit Care Med 2014;42(3):656–63.
15. Patel AK, Bell MJ, Traube C. Delirium in pediatric critical care. Pediatr Clin North Am 2017;64(5):1117–32.
16. Slooff VD, van den Dungen DK, van Beusekom BS, et al. Monitoring haloperidol plasma concentration and associated adverse events in critically ill children with delirium: first results of a clinical protocol aimed to monitor efficacy and safety. Pediatr Crit Care Med 2018;19(2):e112–9.
17. Schieveld JN, Leroy PL, van Os J, et al. Pediatric delirium in critical illness: phenomenology, clinical correlates and treatment response in 40 cases in the pediatric intensive care unit. Intensive Care Med 2007;33(6):1033–40.
18. Capino AC, Thomas AN, Baylor S, et al. Antipsychotic use in the prevention and treatment of intensive care unit delirium in pediatric patients. J Pediatr Pharmacol Ther 2020;25(2):81–95.
19. Joyce C, Witcher R, Herrup E, et al. Evaluation of the safety of quetiapine in treating delirium in critically ill children: a retrospective review. J Child Adolesc Psychopharmacol 2015;25(9):666–70.
20. Campbell CT, Grey E, Munoz-Pareja J, et al. An evaluation of risperidone dosing for pediatric delirium in children less than or equal to 2 years of age. Ann Pharmacother 2020;54(5):464–9.
21. Carrasco G, Baeza N, Cabre L, et al. Dexmedetomidine for the treatment of hyperactive delirium refractory to haloperidol in nonintubated ICU patients: a nonrandomized controlled trial. Crit Care Med 2016;44(7):1295–306.
22. Reade MC, O'Sullivan K, Bates S, et al. Dexmedetomidine vs. haloperidol in delirious, agitated, intubated patients: a randomised open-label trial. Crit Care 2009; 13(3):R75.
23. (U.S.). NLoM. Effects of Dexmedetomidine on Delirium Duration of Non-intubated ICU Patients (4D Trial). In: Available at: https://ClinicalTrials.gov/show/NCT03317067. Accessed June 22, 2021.
24. Louis C, Godet T, Chanques G, et al. Effects of dexmedetomidine on delirium duration of non-intubated ICU patients (4D trial): study protocol for a randomized trial. Trials 2018;19(1):307.
25. O'Mara K, Gal P, Wimmer J, et al. Dexmedetomidine versus standard therapy with fentanyl for sedation in mechanically ventilated premature neonates. J Pediatr Pharmacol Ther 2012;17(3):252–62.
26. Abdi HH, Maitre NL, Benninger KL, et al. Gabapentin use for hospitalized neonates. Pediatr Neurol 2019;97:64–70.
27. Edwards L, DeMeo S, Hornik CD, et al. Gabapentin use in the neonatal intensive care unit. J Pediatr 2016;169:310–2.
28. Sills GJ. The mechanisms of action of gabapentin and pregabalin. Curr Opin Pharmacol 2006;6(1):108–13.

29. Pinto Filho WA, Silveira LHJ, Vale ML, et al. Gabapentin in improvement of procedural sedation and analgesia in oncologic pediatric patients: a clinical trial. Anesth Pain Med 2019;9(5):e91197.
30. Badawy AA, Kasem SA, Rashwan D, et al. The role of Gabapentin oral solution in decreasing desflurane associated emergence agitation and delirium in children after stabismus surgery, a prospective randomized double-blind study. BMC Anesthesiol 2018;18(1):73.
31. Laudone TW, Beck SD, Lahr HJ. Evaluation of melatonin practices for delirium in pediatric critically ill patients. J Pediatr Pharmacol Ther 2021;26(4):361–5.
32. Parvataneni T, Srinivas S, Shah K, et al. Perspective on melatonin use for sleep problems in autism and attention-deficit hyperactivity disorder: a systematic review of randomized clinical trials. Cureus 2020;12(5):e8335.
33. Calandriello A, Tylka JC, Patwari PP. Sleep and delirium in pediatric critical illness: what is the relationship? Med Sci (Basel) 2018;6(4).
34. Mason KP. Paediatric emergence delirium: a comprehensive review and interpretation of the literature. Br J Anaesth 2017;118(3):335–43.
35. (U.S.). NLoM. Efficacy of quetiapine for pediatric delirium. 2015-2016. Available at: https://ClinicalTrials.gov/show/NCT02056171. Accessed June 23, 2021.
36. (U.S.). NLoM. Quetiapine treatment for pediatric delirium. 2019-2020. Available at: https://clinicaltrials.gov/ct2/show/NCT03572257. Accessed June 23, 2021.
37. Egbuta C, Mason KP. Current state of analgesia and sedation in the pediatric intensive care unit. J Clin Med 2021;10(9):1847.
38. Scarpi E, Maltoni M, Miceli R, et al. Survival prediction for terminally ill cancer patients: revision of the palliative prognostic score with incorporation of delirium. Oncologist 2011;16(12):1793–9.
39. Shehabi Y, Riker RR, Bokesch PM, et al. Delirium duration and mortality in lightly sedated, mechanically ventilated intensive care patients. Crit Care Med 2010; 38(12):2311–8.

Treatment of Posthemorrhagic Hydrocephalus

Susan Cohen, MD[a],*, John Flibotte, MD[b]

KEYWORDS

- Intraventricular hemorrhage (IVH) • Posthemorrhagic ventricular dilation (PHVD)
- Posthemorrhagic hydrocephalus (PHH)

KEY POINTS

- Severe intraventricular hemorrhage continues to be a significant comorbidity of prematurity.
- Occurrence of hemorrhage and subsequent posthemorrhagic ventricular dilation is associated with poor neurodevelopmental outcomes.
- Controversy exists regarding impact and timing of neurosurgical interventions to drain or divert cerebrospinal fluid, but recent clinical trials suggest that there may be benefit to earlier intervention.

CONTROVERSIES WITH POSTHEMORRHAGIC HYDROCEPHALUS TREATMENT OPTIONS

Management of posthemorrhagic hydrocephalus in the premature infant remains a clinical conundrum.[1,2] When, how, and with what strategy has been debated for decades. As improved neuroimaging modalities have emerged, the ability to delineate injury and follow the progression has led to medical and surgical practice variation. For this article, clear definitions of intraventricular hemorrhage (IVH), posthemorrhagic ventricular dilation (PHVD), and posthemorrhagic hydrocephalus (PHH) are necessary to fully explain the controversies that exist and provide context for next steps to resolve them.

INTRAVENTRICULAR HEMORRHAGE

The periventricular region is selectively vulnerable to hemorrhage in premature infants predominantly in the first 48 hours of life. IVH most commonly occurs in the germinal

a Department of Pediatrics, Division of Neonatology, Medical College of Wisconsin, 999 North 92nd Street, CCC 410, Milwaukee, WI 53226, USA; b Department of Pediatrics, Division of Neonatology, Children's Hospital of Phildealphia & the Perelman School of Medicine at the University of Pennsylvania, 34th & Civic Center Boulevard, Philadelphia, PA 19104, USA
* Corresponding author.
E-mail address: scohen@mcw.edu

Clin Perinatol 49 (2022) 15–25
https://doi.org/10.1016/j.clp.2021.11.002
0095-5108/22/© 2021 Elsevier Inc. All rights reserved.

matrix, the site where neuroblast and glioblast mitotic activity occurs before cells migrate to other parts of the brain.[3] The germinal matrix is located on the head of the caudate nucleus and underneath the ventricular ependyma and has a transient blood supply that typically involutes by 26 to 32 weeks. Many factors contribute to the fragility of the germinal matrix, including the circular morphology of the vasculature, insufficiency of key secreted products within the neurovascular unit, immaturity of the vascular basal lamina, and a paucity of stabilizing pericytes for the microvasculature.[4] When this intrinsic vulnerability to bleeding is coupled with disturbances in cerebral autoregulation due to prematurity, it is the perfect clinical scenario for a germinal matrix hemorrhage. When this hemorrhage is substantial, the ependyma breaks and the cerebral ventricle fills up with blood leading to IVH. IVH is often progressive and is graded using a neuroimaging grading system developed by Papile and colleagues[5] and modified by Volpe.[6,7] The diagnosis of IVH is made on screening ultrasonography, which is performed in very preterm infants (born at ≤30 weeks of gestation) in neonatal intensive care units (NICUs) during the first weeks of life.[8] The clinical presentation of IVH is variable and typically silent. In rare cases infants can present with a catastrophic syndrome of neurologic disturbance consisting of abrupt pupillary and behavior changes and cardiovascular instability and acidosis. Alternatively, some may have a saltatory presentation with subtle behavior changes and the potential development of seizures. The risk of severe IVH is inversely related to gestational age, with infants born at less than 24 weeks' gestation at highest risk. The incidence of IVH was 4.7% before the 1960s and increased to 50% from 1975 to 1980 following the introduction of novel positive pressure mechanical ventilation, later declining by three-quarters to 12.5% in 2005 probably as a result of improvements in NICU clinical practices such as surfactant and antenatal corticosteroids.[9] The global incidence of IVH among preterm infants ranges from 14.7% to 44.7% with considerable variation across gestational age groups, NICUs, and countries.[9]

POSTHEMORRHAGIC VENTRICULAR DILATION

One of the major complications resulting from IVH is the development of PHVD. Following a large IVH, multiple small clots throughout the ventricular system may obstruct cerebrospinal fluid (CSF) flow and resorption, all in the face of ongoing production of CSF in the choroid plexus in the lateral ventricles and the roof of the third ventricle.[10] Days after a large IVH, there may be a period of reduced CSF production, but when CSF production returns, the lateral ventricles enlarge. The progressive accumulation of CSF changes the shape of the lateral ventricles from a slit to a balloon. The expanding ventricles distort the developing brain and pressure eventually starts to increase. Normal CSF pressure does not exceed 6 mmHg.[11] As the preterm skull is compliant, the ventricles can expand without pressure increasing initially but eventually can result in increased intracranial pressure (ICP). PHVD develops in 30% to 50% of infants with severe IVH and is mostly asymptomatic in presentation. Therefore, sequential cranial ultrasonography facilitates early detection. PHVD can progress either slowly or rapidly; in most cases slowly progressing ventricular dilation is followed by spontaneous arrest and even reduction.[12] In the remaining 30% to 35% of infants with PHVD, ventricular size increases rapidly over several days to weeks.[13] The term ventriculomegaly is occasionally used for both infants with ventricular enlargement following IVH and those without hemorrhage. In infants without IVH, ventricular enlargement is more likely due to white matter loss rather than an accumulation of CSF. Therefore, it is preferable to use the term PHVD when ventricular enlargement follows IVH.

POSTHEMORRHAGIC HYDROCEPHALUS

PHH of prematurity is a common form of pediatric hydrocephalus, accounting for 20% of the shunted hydrocephalus in the United States.[14] Hydrocephalus represents an alteration in fluid balance within the brain and cranial cavity leading to increased ICP. Under normal conditions, CSF is primarily secreted into the cerebral ventricles by the choroid plexus and moves via bulk flow through the ventricular system and subarachnoid space before being absorbed at the arachnoid villi/granulations, which are fully developed after 35 weeks.[15] An increase in CSF production or reduction in CSF absorption may result in ventricular enlargement if the system cannot compensate for the changes. Secondary white matter injury resulting from ventricular dilation is likely exacerbated by compression and ischemia from increased ICP of symptomatic PHH.[16] The clinical presentation of symptomatic PHH in preterm infant is generally like that of symptomatic hydrocephalus in term neonates, with allowances for the preterm infant's relative immaturity. Orbitofrontal head circumference, fontanel fullness, and the splaying of sutures all show limited reliability when studied as measures among numerous practitioners of varied skill levels, but these clinical signs can be reliable when used by experienced practitioners to assess progression of disease in the same infant. Progressive splaying of the sagittal suture width is the most reliable sign of increased pressure.[16] A subset of infants with increased ICP will also present with nonspecific signs such as apnea, bradycardia, lethargy, and decreased activity. Some preterm infants with PHH develop only transient symptomatic hydrocephalus and require CSF diversion for only a few weeks. Others require longer and more permanent treatments. Herein lies the controversy for selection of neuroimaging surveillance, timing for intervention, and choice of surgical intervention.

LONG-TERM OUTCOMES OF POSTHEMORRHAGIC HYDROCEPHALUS

The risk of a poor neurodevelopmental outcome is significantly higher when severe IVH is complicated with PHVD (40%–60%) and more so for infants who eventually require a shunt (75%–88%).[12,17] Significant cognitive and motor impairments were found among infants with PHVD at 18 to 24 months corrected age in many retrospective studies and in a limited number of randomized controlled trials.[18–21] In the presurfactant era, up to 82% of infants with PHH who survived developed significant neurologic impairments with cerebral palsy being the most common clinical sequela (74%).[19] A population-based study of children with hydrocephalus in the 1990s demonstrated that learning disabilities were present in 47% of children with infantile hydrocephalus compared with 16% of those with myelomeningocele, cerebral palsy in 27% versus 0%, and epilepsy in 43% versus 11%. Hydrocephalus present at birth, low gestational age, a perinatal origin, enlarged ventricles at follow-up, and several shunt revisions all indicated risk factors for poor outcome.[20] The Drainage, Irrigation and Fibrinolytic Therapy (DRIFT) trial, conducted between 2003 and 2006, performed neurocognitive assessments at both 2 and 10 years after birth and demonstrated improved cognitive ability when considering birth weight, IVH grade, and sex.[21] The investigators reported that infants who received DRIFT were almost twice as likely to survive without severe cognitive disability than those who received standard treatment. The Early versus Late Ventricular Intervention Study (ELVIS) trial was a randomized controlled study performed from 2006 to 2016 that compared the effectiveness of intervention at low versus high threshold of ventricular dilation in preterm infants with PHVD on death and severe neurodevelopmental disability.[18] In this study, 35% of the low threshold group had an adverse composite outcome defined as death, cerebral palsy, or a Bayley Scale of Infant and Toddler Development (BSID) examination composite cognitive or motor score of less than 2 SD compared with 51% in the high-threshold group. The posthoc analysis of this study demonstrated that infants in the low-threshold group with a ventriculoperitoneal shunt had cognitive and motor scores similar to those without ($P = .3$ for both), whereas in the high-threshold group those with a ventriculoperitoneal shunt had significantly lower scores than those without a ventriculoperitoneal shunt ($P = .01$ and $P = .004$, respectively).[18] Using a standardized mean composite score of 100 (SD 15) on the BSID examination,[22] both groups scored in the low 90s in cognitive testing and the high 80s for motor testing, suggesting that even though overall survival has improved in children with PHVD in this modern cohort, there is still room for improvement for developmental outcomes.

APPROACHES TO TREATMENT OF POSTHEMORRHAGIC HYDROCEPHALUS

Because of the significant impact that PHH has on later neurodevelopmental outcomes, identifying therapies that improve these outcomes has been a high priority. The mainstay of treatment is to reduce the evolution of increased ICP; this has been attempted through both medical and surgical approaches.

Although oral medications are effective in temporization of hydrocephalus in older children and adults, a randomized controlled trial from the 1990s demonstrated that the addition of acetazolamide and furosemide with the intent of diminishing CSF production did not decrease the need for permanent shunt insertion and unfortunately increased the likelihood of death and neurologic morbidity at 1 year.[23,24] Hence, no medications are currently recommended to treat symptomatic PHH. Direct removal or diversion of CSF therefore remains the basis of current approaches to therapy.

Serial lumbar punctures (LPs) represent one potential option for removal of CSF from below. However, this is only possible when the lumbar subarachnoid space communicates with the ventricular system, and they are often viewed as time-limited options to bridge to a point of surgical intervention. Daily LPs can be used if it is necessary to stabilize the head circumference, and usually up to 10 mL CSF is removed per LP.[16] The most recent Cochrane review concluded that serial LPs do not contribute to avoidance of shunt.[25] However, a retrospective study showed that early intervention with serial LPs (with "early" defined as before the ventricular index crossed Levene's 97th percentile + 4-mm line) reduced the need for surgical intervention.[26] Interestingly, hydrocephalus stabilized without any surgical intervention in about 25% of the infants studied.

Surgical intervention largely includes placement of a catheter into the ventricular space to facilitate CSF removal or diversion. Several approaches are possible that have been explored in prior studies. For small infants, not yet at a size that would facilitate placement of a ventricular peritoneal shunt, CSF can be drained through an implanted subcutaneous ventricular access device (VAD, reservoir) in the lateral ventricle. Treating providers then proceed with intermittent drainage of CSF until such time a more permanent diversion may be undertaken. Some centers pursue early ventricular subgaleal shunts (VSGS) to avoid the need for intermittent tapping and CSF removal. Prior work has shown both these approaches to be equivalent with respect to rates of infection and complication.[27] Both the VAD and the VSGS are temporary interventions, though, that require conversion to more permanent CSF diversion via a ventricular shunt into either the peritoneum (most common) or to a vascular site (such as the jugular or atria) or pleural space in some infants when a peritoneal site is not possible; this may be the case for infants with complex surgical history and high intra-abdominal pressures from necrotizing enterocolitis or other comorbidity of prematurity.

Shunting and CSF diversion are ways to manage increased pressure that is established after IVH. However, they do not represent permanent cures and carry with them expected complications that include infection and mechanical dysfunction that led to future interventions for these children. Therefore, there is immense interest in potential early therapies that may fundamentally alter the pathophysiology and allow avoidance of shunt altogether. One potentially promising approach is represented in the DRIFT trial.[28] This approach involved placement of an anterior and posterior ventricular catheter in infants shortly after development of IVH. Artificial CSF was then infused through the ventricles and also contained tissue plasminogen activator until such time as the draining fluid was no longer cola colored. The benefits of this approach were purported to be multifactorial: it decreased physical obstruction from the intraventricular clot due to both the flushing and the anticoagulant, and it removed cytokines that contributed to tissue remodeling and additional obstruction. The phase II version of the study demonstrated increased occurrence of repeat bleeds in patients randomized to DRIFT without meaningful difference in avoidance of shunt.[29] As described earlier, ongoing follow-up of the trial subjects demonstrated in later childhood improved outcomes among those infants randomized to DRIFT intervention.[21] These encouraging later results prompt the question of whether further study is warranted for this invasive and technically demanding intervention.

TREATMENT TIMING OF POSTHEMORRHAGIC HYDROCEPHALUS

Although prior work has focused on what to do for these infants with PHH, another central and controversial question in their management is when to intervene. Prior work has explored the potential value of physiologic measurements that might reflect increasing ICP for guiding management, including the use of near-infrared spectroscopy in some clinical settings,[30] as well as auditory brainstem response changes[31] and amplitude-integrated electroencephalogram and visual evoked responses in some small studies.[32] However, none of these tools has been definitive. Most neonatal practitioners make judgments about timing of intervention based on neuroimaging and clinical markers of increasing ICP including head circumference, quality of the suture examination, and qualitative impression of fontanel.[33] Some schools of thought argue that waiting for such clinical signs to evolve is too late.[34]

Cranial ultrasonography is a mainstay of clinical management for infants with ventricular hemorrhage and potential for PHVD. There are no direct measures of ICP to currently guide management that are reasonably used for this population. Therefore, several standard measures of ventricular size have been defined to serve as surrogate markers of ICP and guide management decisions. Many of these have been described across a range of gestational ages to provide normative measures. However, there are inconsistencies between studies for some, largely reflecting the small number of infants included. This adds to the challenge of interpretation for specific patients and also defining uniform care guidelines based on them. Finally, data are just now emerging that associate intervention at specific cutoffs with later outcomes.

The most common measures of ventricular size are summarized in **Table 1**. There are others in addition to these; however, they are not commonly used to guide management for a variety of reasons, principally related to feasibility. The interested reader is referred to a systematic review by Brouwer and colleagues[35] for thorough review of ultrasound measurements and normative values. For visual reference, **Fig. 1** provides the measurements described in this article.

Perhaps the longest standing and most used measure of ventricular size is the ventricular index (VI) defined by Levene and Starte.[36] This measure changes over the

Table 1
Table summarizing commonly used measures of ventricular size on ultrasound, how they are calculated and normative/ actionable values

Ultrasound Measure	How Calculated	Normative/Actionable Value	Key References
VI	• Coronal view at the level of the foramen of Monro • Greatest distance from falx to the lateral wall of the lateral ventricle	• Cohort-derived "growth curve" norms defined by percentile • Interventions based on measures at or above 97th percentile (study specific)	• Levene MI. Measurement of the growth of the lateral ventricles in preterm infants with real-time ultrasound. Arch Dis Child. 1981 Dec;56(12):900-4. doi: 10.1136/adc.56.12.900. PMID: 7332336; PMCID: PMC1627506. • [36]
AHW	• Coronal view at the level of the foramen of Monro • Greatest width between the medial wall and floor of the lateral ventricle	• Cohort-derived norms • Controversy regarding gestational age dependency of norms	• Davies MW, Swaminathan M, Chuang SL, Betheras FR. Reference ranges for the linear dimensions of the intracranial ventricles in preterm neonates. Arch Dis Child Fetal Neonatal Ed. 2000 May;82(3):F218-23. doi: 10.1136/fn.82.3.f218. PMID: 10794790; PMCID: PMC1721078.
TOD	• Oblique parasagittal view with entire lateral ventricle and the anterior horn of the atrium and the temporal and occipital horns in view • Outermost point of the thalamus to outermost part of the occipital horn posteriorly	• Cohort-derived norms • Controversy regarding gestational age dependency of norms	• ADD REFERENCE ABOVE

(continued on next page)

Table 1 (continued)			
Ultrasound Measure	How Calculated	Normative/Actionable Value	Key References
FOHR	• Axial cUS, at level of foramen of Monroe • Average of the frontal and occipital horn width divided by interparietal diameter	• Normal = 0.4 • Mild HC = 0.55 • Moderate HC = 0.60 • Severe HC = 0.7	• O'Hayon BB, Drake JM, Ossip MG, Tuli S, Clarke M. Frontal and occipital horn ratio: A linear estimate of ventricular size for multiple imaging modalities in pediatric hydrocephalus. Pediatr Neurosurg. 1998 Nov;29(5):245-9. doi: 10.1159/000028730. PMID: 9917541. • [43] • [42]
FTHR	• Coronal cUS, at level of foramen of Monroe • Average of the frontal and temporal horn width divided by interparietal diameter	• Normal = 0.4 • Mild HC = 0.55 • Moderate HC = 0.60 • Severe HC = 0.7	• [43]

Abbreviations: VI, ventricular index; AHW, anterior horn width; TOD, thalamo-occipital distance; FOHR, fronto-occipital horn ratio; FTHR, fronto-temporal horn ratio.

course of development, and normative values based on postmenstrual age are available.[37] Anterior horn width (AHW) and thalamo-occipital distance (TOD) are 2 additional measures often evaluated in conjunction with VI. The VI and AHW are of particular importance because of their use in several published retrospective and randomized controlled trials of intervention for PHVD.[18,26,38,39] Although it is generally accepted that norms for VI change with postmenstrual age, there is some controversy

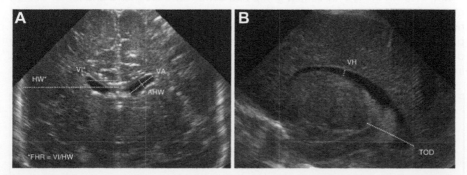

Fig. 1. Ventricular parameters measured in the (A) coronal and (B) sagittal planes by cranial ultrasonography. HW, hemispheric width; VA, ventricular axis; VH, ventricular height. (From Brouwer MJ, de Vries LS, Pistorius L, et al. Ultrasound measurements of the lateral ventricles in neonates: why, how and when? A systematic review. Acta Paediatr. 2010;99(9):1298–306.)

regarding the norms for AHW and TOD. Some case series have demonstrated changing values with postmenstrual age,[40] whereas others have shown relatively unchanging values over time.[37]

Additional measures of ventricular size have been developed largely by the neurosurgical community and include the frontal and occipital horn ratio (FOHR) and the frontal and temporal horn ratio (FTHR). The FOHR was initially developed for measurement of ventricular size in patients with established hydrocephalus[41] and was correlated with ventricular volumetric calculations on axial slice imaging. This initial study also included ultrasound scan evaluations. Follow-up work showed that FOHR has a high degree of interrater reliability and established cutoffs that approximated severity of hydrocephalus.[42] To facilitate assessment of ventricular size based on coronal ultrasonography, the FTHR was developed later and closely approximates FOHR[43] and correlates with calculations of ventricular volume.[44] The FOHR and FTHR have been used less to define intervention trials for neonates with hydrocephalus. However, the FOHR was used to guide management within a prospective cohort study in the Hydrocephalus Clinical Research Network (HCRN)[27] as well as in some clinical settings.[45] Although the association between intervention for PHVD at specific FOHR/FTHR thresholds and later outcomes have not been established, the recently published ELVIS trial (see later) did demonstrate larger FOHR in infants with adverse outcomes.[18] The ease and reproducibility of the FOHR/FTHR make these potentially attractive measures around which to define timing of therapeutic intervention.

Until recently, there was little to no evidence base to inform timing of interventions based on specific measurement thresholds, creating significant practice variation across clinical environments.[33] However, a Dutch working group has been exploring defining specific thresholds for intervention based on the VI. Initial retrospective work comparing early versus late LP, with early LP being before the VI exceeding the 97th percentile compared with late, when the VI exceeds 4 mm beyond the 97th percentile, reported decreased need for VP shunt with early intervention.[26] This work was followed by a large, randomized trial comparing early versus late intervention, again based on the VI and AHW. Early intervention was defined as when the VI crossed the 97th percentile and the AHW was greater than 6 mm. Late intervention was defined as waiting until the VI was 97th percentile + 4 mm and AHW greater than 10 mm. Intervention consisted of early LPs followed by insertion of a ventricular reservoir and subsequent intermittent removal of CSF.[39] The initial results of this trial showed no difference in the primary outcome of VP shunt placement or death.[39] However, later outcomes were recently reported, and among infants who required a VP shunt, those in the low-threshold group had better BSID Cognitive and Motor Scores at 24 months corrected age. These outcomes were equivalent to those who did not need VP shunt in both the low- and high-threshold groups.[18] Although this was an unplanned secondary analysis of the original trial, it has, nonetheless, reignited the debate around the potential value of earlier intervention to preserve later outcomes in this population of infants.[34]

Best Practice Box

- PHVD is associated with impaired later outcomes. Despite this, consensus around best approach to treatment is lacking.
- Monitoring for the evolution of PHVD in infants with severe IVH is necessary and largely based on intermittent cranial ultrasonographies.
- Formal measurements of ventricular size provide some objectivity to degree of enlargement that is superior to qualitative radiologist impressions.

- CSF removal or diversion is the mainstay of treatment to avoid impact from increased ICP. However, debate continues around when to intervene.
- Recent trial data suggest that more aggressive intervention may offer improved 2-year outcomes and have been the basis for a proposed approach to therapy based on VI and AHW enlargement.

DISCLOSURE

The authors have nothing to disclose.

REFERENCES

1. Christian EA, Jin DL, Attenello F, et al. Trends in hospitalization of preterm infants with intraventricular hemorrhage and hydrocephalus in the United States, 2000-2010. J Neurosurg Pediatr 2016;17(3):260–9.
2. Alan N, Manjila S, Minich N, et al. Reduced ventricular shunt rate in very preterm infants with severe intraventricular hemorrhage: an institutional experience. J Neurosurg Pediatr 2012;10(5):357–64.
3. Del Bigio MR. Cell proliferation in human ganglionic eminence and suppression after prematurity-associated haemorrhage. Brain 2011;134(Pt 5):1344–61.
4. Ballabh P. Intraventricular hemorrhage in premature infants: mechanism of disease. Pediatr Res 2010;67(1):1–8.
5. Papile LA, Burstein J, Burstein R, et al. Incidence and evolution of subependymal and intraventricular hemorrhage: a study of infants with birth weights less than 1,500 gm. J Pediatr 1978;92(4):529–34.
6. Volpe JJ. Intraventricular hemorrhage in the premature infant–current concepts. Part II. Ann Neurol 1989;25(2):109–16.
7. Volpe JJ. Intraventricular hemorrhage in the premature infant–current concepts. Part I. Ann Neurol 1989;25(1):3–11.
8. Hand IL, Shellhaas RA, Milla SS, et al. Routine neuroimaging of the preterm brain. Pediatrics 2020;146(5). e2020029082.
9. Egesa WI, Odoch S, Odong RJ, et al. Germinal matrix-intraventricular hemorrhage: a tale of preterm infants. Int J Pediatr 2021;2021:6622598.
10. Whitelaw A, Aquilina K. Management of posthaemorrhagic ventricular dilatation. Arch Dis Child Fetal Neonatal Ed 2012;97(3). F229-3.
11. Kaiser AM, Whitelaw AG. Cerebrospinal fluid pressure during post haemorrhagic ventricular dilatation in newborn infants. Arch Dis Child 1985;60(10):920–4.
12. Leijser LM, de Vries LS. Preterm brain injury: germinal matrix-intraventricular hemorrhage and post-hemorrhagic ventricular dilatation. Handb Clin Neurol 2019;162:173–99.
13. Murphy BP, Inder TE, Rooks V, et al. Posthaemorrhagic ventricular dilatation in the premature infant: natural history and predictors of outcome. Arch Dis Child Fetal Neonatal Ed 2002;87(1):F37–41.
14. Riva-Cambrin J, Kestle JR, Holubkov R, et al. Risk factors for shunt malfunction in pediatric hydrocephalus: a multicenter prospective cohort study. J Neurosurg Pediatr 2016;17(4):382–90.
15. Gómez DG, DiBenedetto AT, Pavese AM, et al. Development of arachnoid villi and granulations in man. Acta Anat (Basel) 1982;111(3):247–58.
16. Robinson S. Neonatal posthemorrhagic hydrocephalus from prematurity: pathophysiology and current treatment concepts. J Neurosurg Pediatr 2012;9(3):242–58.

17. Shankaran S, Bajaj M, Natarajan G, et al. Outcomes following post-hemorrhagic ventricular dilatation among infants of extremely low gestational age. J Pediatr 2020;226:36–44.e3.
18. Cizmeci MN, Groenendaal F, Liem KD, et al. Randomized controlled early versus late ventricular intervention study in posthemorrhagic ventricular dilatation: outcome at 2 years. J Pediatr 2020;226:28–35.e3.
19. Fernell E, Hagberg G, Hagberg B. Infantile hydrocephalus in preterm, low-birth-weight infants—a nationwide Swedish cohort study 1979–1988. Acta Paediatr 1993;82(1):45–8.
20. Persson EK, Hagberg G, Uvebrant P. Disabilities in children with hydrocephalus–a population-based study of children aged between four and twelve years. Neuropediatrics 2006;37(6):330–6.
21. Luyt K, Jary SL, Lea CL, et al. Drainage, irrigation and fibrinolytic therapy (DRIFT) for posthaemorrhagic ventricular dilatation: 10-year follow-up of a randomised controlled trial. Arch Dis Child Fetal Neonatal Ed 2020;105(5):466–73.
22. Vohr BR, Stephens BE, Higgins RD, et al. Are outcomes of extremely preterm infants improving? Impact of Bayley assessment on outcomes. J Pediatr 2012; 161(2):222–8.e3.
23. Kennedy CR, Ayers S, Campbell MJ, et al. Randomized, controlled trial of acetazolamide and furosemide in posthemorrhagic ventricular dilation in infancy: follow-up at 1 year. Pediatrics 2001;108(3):597–607.
24. Whitelaw A, Kennedy CR, Brion LP. Diuretic therapy for newborn infants with post-hemorrhagic ventricular dilatation. Cochrane Database Syst Rev 2001;(2):Cd002270.
25. Whitelaw A, Lee-Kelland R. Repeated lumbar or ventricular punctures in newborns with intraventricular haemorrhage. Cochrane Database Syst Rev 2017;(4):CD000216.
26. de Vries LS, Liem KD, van Dijk K, et al. Early versus late treatment of posthaemorrhagic ventricular dilatation: results of a retrospective study from five neonatal intensive care units in The Netherlands. Acta Paediatr 2002;91(2):212–7.
27. Wellons JC 3rd, Shannon CN, Holubkov R, et al. Shunting outcomes in posthemorrhagic hydrocephalus: results of a Hydrocephalus Clinical Research Network prospective cohort study. J Neurosurg Pediatr 2017;20(1):19–29.
28. Whitelaw A, Pople I, Cherian S, et al. Phase 1 trial of prevention of hydrocephalus after intraventricular hemorrhage in newborn infants by drainage, irrigation, and fibrinolytic therapy. Pediatrics 2003;111(4):759–65.
29. Whitelaw A, Evans D, Carter M, et al. Randomized clinical trial of prevention of hydrocephalus after intraventricular hemorrhage in preterm infants: brain-washing versus tapping fluid. Pediatrics 2007;119(5):e1071–8.
30. Whittemore BA, Swift DM, Thomas JM, et al. A neonatal neuroNICU collaborative approach to neuromonitoring of posthemorrhagic ventricular dilation in preterm infants. Pediatr Res 2021. https://doi.org/10.1038/s41390-021-01406-9.
31. Lary S, De Vries LS, Kaiser A, et al. Auditory brain stem responses in infants with posthaemorrhagic ventricular dilatation. Arch Dis Child 1989;64(1 Spec No):17–23.
32. Klebermass-Schrehof K, Rona Z, Waldhör T, et al. Can neurophysiological assessment improve timing of intervention in posthaemorrhagic ventricular dilatation? Arch Dis Child Fetal Neonatal Ed 2013;98(4):F291–7.
33. Cohen S, Mietzsch U, Coghill C, et al. Survey of quaternary neonatal management of posthemorrhagic hydrocephalus. Am J Perinatol 2021. https://doi.org/10.1055/s-0041-1732417x.

34. El-Dib M, Limbrick DD Jr, Inder T, et al. Management of post-hemorrhagic ventricular dilatation in the infant born preterm. J Pediatr 2020;226:16–27.e3.
35. Brouwer MJ, de Vries LS, Pistorius L, et al. Ultrasound measurements of the lateral ventricles in neonates: why, how and when? A systematic review. Acta Paediatr 2010;99(9):1298–306.
36. Levene MI, Starte DR. A longitudinal study of post-haemorrhagic ventricular dilatation in the newborn. Arch Dis Child 1981;56(12):905–10.
37. Brouwer AJ, Brouwer MJ, Groenendaal F, et al. European perspective on the diagnosis and treatment of posthaemorrhagic ventricular dilatation. Arch Dis Child Fetal Neonatal Ed 2012;97(1):F50–5.
38. Leijser LM, Miller SP, van Wezel-Meijler G, et al. Posthemorrhagic ventricular dilatation in preterm infants: when best to intervene? Neurology 2018;90(8): e698–706.
39. de Vries LS, Groenendaal F, Liem KD, et al. Treatment thresholds for intervention in posthaemorrhagic ventricular dilation: a randomised controlled trial. Arch Dis Child Fetal Neonatal Ed 2019;104(1):F70–5.
40. Sondhi V, Gupta G, Gupta PK, et al. Establishment of nomograms and reference ranges for intra-cranial ventricular dimensions and ventriculo-hemispheric ratio in newborns by ultrasonography. Acta Paediatr 2008;97(6):738–44.
41. O'Hayon BB, Drake JM, Ossip MG, et al. Frontal and occipital horn ratio: a linear estimate of ventricular size for multiple imaging modalities in pediatric hydrocephalus. Pediatr Neurosurg 1998;29(5):245–9.
42. Kulkarni AV, Drake JM, Armstrong DC, et al. Measurement of ventricular size: reliability of the frontal and occipital horn ratio compared to subjective assessment. Pediatr Neurosurg 1999;31(2):65–70.
43. Antes S, Kiefer M, Schmitt M, et al. Frontal and temporal horn ratio: a valid and reliable index to determine ventricular size in paediatric hydrocephalus patients? Acta Neurochir Suppl 2012;114:227–30.
44. Antes S, Welsch M, Kiefer M, et al. The frontal and temporal horn ratio to assess dimension of paediatric hydrocephalus: a comparative volumetric study. Acta Neurochir Suppl 2013;118:211–4.
45. Flanders TM, Kimmel AC, Lang S-S, et al. Standardizing treatment of preterm infants with post-hemorrhagic hydrocephalus at a single institution with a multidisciplinary team. Childs Nervous Syst 2020;36(8):1737–44.

Neonatal Hypertension

Rebecca Hjorten, MD, Clinical Assistant Professor, Department of
Pediatrics, University of Washington School of Medicine,
Joseph T. Flynn, MD, MS, Professor, Department of Pediatrics, University of
Washington School of Medicine*

KEYWORDS

• Hypertension • Blood pressure • Antihypertensives • Neonates

KEY POINTS

- There are limited normative data and research on risk factors, treatment, and long-term outcomes of neonatal hypertension; therefore, management is based on clinical experience and expert opinion.
- Identification of neonatal hypertension is difficult given that it is often asymptomatic and requires attention to vital sign data, careful blood pressure measurement, and comparison with normative values for postmenstrual age.
- When hypertension is identified it should prompt thorough evaluation to diagnose neonates requiring additional surgical or medical management.
- Most cases resolve in the first few years of life but for some there is risk for hypertension into adulthood requiring long-term follow-up.

INTRODUCTION

Advances in neonatology have led to increased recognition of neonatal hypertension. Additionally, neonatal hypertension may become more prevalent with increasing survival rates of infants at risk for developing hypertension, such as those with prematurity, bronchopulmonary dysplasia (BPD), or congenital heart disease. There may also be more infants experiencing iatrogenic causes of hypertension, such as those with acute kidney injury or those needing extracorporeal membrane oxygenation (ECMO).

However, the diagnosis, management, and treatment of neonatal hypertension has been fraught with difficulty given that measurement of blood pressure in the neonatal period is challenging and information on normal blood pressure values in premature and term infants remains limited. Similarly, given the low prevalence of hypertension in neonates and their exclusion from clinical trials, information is limited on optimal treatment and long-term outcomes.

Department of Pediatrics, Division of Nephrology, Seattle Children's Hospital, 4800 Sand Point Way NE, OC.9.820 – Nephrology, Seattle, WA 98105, USA
* Corresponding author.
E-mail address: joseph.flynn@seattlechildrens.org

Clin Perinatol 49 (2022) 27–42
https://doi.org/10.1016/j.clp.2021.11.003
0095-5108/22/© 2021 Elsevier Inc. All rights reserved.
perinatology.theclinics.com

This review provides a practical overview for the practicing physician regarding the identification, evaluation, and management of neonatal hypertension.

INCIDENCE

Generally, the incidence of hypertension in the neonatal period has focused primarily on those in the neonatal intensive care unit (NICU) within small single-center populations using different thresholds for defining hypertension. Such studies have reported incidences of 0.8% to 2%.[1-5] The largest study used the Pediatric Health Information System to look for diagnosis of hypertension within 123,847 NICU encounters finding an incidence of 1%.[2]

Recently there was a large, multicenter study of neonatal hypertension using patients from the Assessment of Worldwide Acute Kidney Injury Epidemiology in Neonates (AWAKEN) cohort study. The study looked at the incidence of hypertension and its associated risk factors in 2162 neonates recruited from 24, level 2 to 4, NICUs around the world. It showed a similar incidence of hypertension diagnosis, with an incidence of 1.8% within the entire cohort. The study also looked at undiagnosed hypertension, which they defined as having more than 50% of the blood pressure readings throughout the admission greater than the 95th percentile for postmenstrual age. The incidence of undiagnosed hypertension was 3.7%, with either diagnosed or undiagnosed hypertension being present in more than 5% of infants.[6] One caveat regarding these figures is that the AWAKEN investigators derived their own blood pressure percentiles from a literature review, as opposed to using the blood pressure data published by Dionne and colleagues that were endorsed in the 2017 American Academy of Pediatrics pediatric hypertension guideline.[7,8]

The AWAKEN study also looked at the incidence of diagnosed and undiagnosed hypertension by gestational age. The highest incidence of hypertension was in those that were the most premature or those closer to term. The rate of undiagnosed hypertension increased with gestation age. The population was divided into the following gestational ages: (1) less than 29 weeks, (2) 30 to 35 weeks, and (3) greater than 36 weeks. The incidence of diagnosed hypertension was 4%, 0.6%, and 1.8%, respectively; whereas the incidence of undiagnosed hypertension was 1.4%, 3.2%, and 5%, respectively.[6] It is notable that a large number of patients were excluded from this cohort including those with severe congenital abnormalities of the kidney and urinary tract (CAKUT), those with congenital heart disease requiring surgery at less than 7 days of life, and those who did not require intravenous fluids.[6]

DIFFERENTIAL DIAGNOSIS AND RISK FACTORS

The first studies focusing on neonatal hypertension were written in the 1970s and focused on severe, renin-mediated hypertension most often caused by renal artery thromboembolism associated with prolonged use of umbilical artery catheterization.[9-11] With increased interest in the area of neonatal hypertension many different maternal and perinatal factors potentially playing a role in neonatal hypertension have been described. Evidence suggests that there is increased risk for neonatal hypertension with increased maternal blood pressure and use of antenatal steroids. Many other potential risk factors have been identified, such as preeclampsia, maternal obesity, smoking, socioeconomic status, and prenatal drug and air pollution exposure. However, many studies are small and at times the data are contradictory.[4,12-14]

In terms of the underlying cause of neonatal hypertension, there is a large list of potential causes (Table 1). Among the published small cohorts of neonates with hypertension, no specific diagnosis was found in about 9% to 60% of patients.[1,3,15,16] In the

Table 1	
Causes of neonatal hypertension	
Renovascular	Medications/intoxications
Thromboembolism	Infant
Renal artery stenosis	Dexamethasone
Midaortic syndrome	Adrenergic agents
Renal venous/arterial thrombosis	Vitamin D intoxication
Renal artery compression	Theophylline
Idiopathic arterial calcification	Caffeine
Congenital rubella syndrome	Pancuronium
Renal parenchymal disease	Phenylephrine
Congenital	Maternal
Polycystic kidney (ARPKD, ADPKD)	Cocaine
Multicystic dysplastic kidney disease	Heroin
Severe renal dysplasia	Antenatal steroids
Ureteropelvic junction obstruction	Neoplasia
Unilateral renal hypoplasia	Wilms tumor
Congenital nephrotic syndrome ACE inhibitor fetopathy	Mesoblastic nephroma
Acquired	Neuroblastoma
Acute kidney injury	Pheochromocytoma
Cortical necrosis	Chorioangioma
Interstitial nephritis	Neuropathic
Hemolytic-uremic syndrome	Pain
Obstruction (stones, tumors)	Intracranial hypertension
Pulmonary	Seizures
Bronchopulmonary dysplasia	Familial dysautonomia
Pneumothorax	Subdural hematoma
Cardiac	Other causes
Aortic dissection	Volume overload
Endocrine	Abdominal wall defect closure
Congenital adrenal hyperplasia	Adrenal hemorrhage
Hyperaldosteronism	Hypercalcemia
Hyperthyroidism	Traction
Pseudohypoaldosteronism type II	Birth asphyxia ECMO
Glucocorticoid-remediable aldosteronism	

Abbreviations: ACE, angiotensin-converting enzyme; ADPKD, autosomal dominant polycystic kidney disease; ARPKD, autosomal recessive polycystic kidney disease.

largest two studies, the most commonly identified causes were respiratory (53%–65%), cardiovascular (0%–4%), neurologic (1%–13%), endocrine (0%–6%), and renal (11%–25%), with renovascular hypertension making up only less than 2% of the total cases of hypertension. Approximately 25% to 60% were believed to be either idiopathic or iatrogenic from such causes as medications or ECMO.[3,15]

Renal parenchymal causes of hypertension include CAKUT, autosomal-recessive polycystic kidney disease, and acute kidney injury or cortical necrosis.[17] In obstructive uropathies, hypertension can persist after surgical correction.[18] Although uncommon, hypertension is seen with unilateral multicystic dysplastic kidney caused by excessive renin production.[19] The most common cause of renovascular hypertension in neonates is that associated with umbilical artery catheterization. Reduced prominence of arterial thromboembolism as an underlying cause of neonatal hypertension is likely caused by reduced use and duration of umbilical artery catheterization.[20,21] Thrombus formation occurs in about 26% of neonates with umbilical artery catheters; however, hypertension is present in neonates even without demonstrated thrombus, and therefore it is believed that disruption of the vascular endothelium might lead to small clots that embolize to the kidney resulting in hypertension.[21] There is increased risk of thrombus formation with the length of use but not with the catheter position.[20,22] Other causes of renovascular hypertension are renal vein thrombosis, fibromuscular dysplasia, arterial calcification, and external compression of the renal artery.[23–26] Compression by a mass or abdominal wall closure can result in release of catechol-amines driving hypertension, and some tumors may directly secrete vasoactive substances.[27,28]

One of the largest causes of neonatal hypertension is chronic lung disease, ac-counting for about 50% of neonatal hypertension. About 43% of those with BPD have hypertension with more than half not being diagnosed until after discharge.[15,29] Hypertension is related to the severity of lung disease and thought to be related to hypoxemia possibly driving changes in aortic wall thickness and vasomotor func-tion.[30,31] However, it is also possible that exposure to phthalates, a common additive to plastic intravenous and ventilator tubing, may also be playing a role. Given that it is not integrated into the plastic scaffold, it can leach out of plastic and levels of phtha-late metabolites are found in neonatal urine. They have been shown to inhibit 11-βHSD2, which usually converts cortisol to a less potent cortisol; inhibition of this enzyme in other situations (eg, excessive consumption of black licorice) can cause hy-pertension. The impact of phthalate exposure may be greater on neonates given their likely slower metabolism and smaller size.[32–36] In one small study of 18 patients in whom phthalate levels were measured, nine patients developed hypertension and systolic blood pressure was associated with phthalate exposure. In another study of 129 neonates at two different centers, they evaluated the most likely underlying cause of hypertension, the time course of their hypertension, and their estimated phthalate exposure. Those with medication-related or lung disease–associated hypertension had significant phthalate exposure. The center with phthalate-containing products had a significantly higher rate neonatal hypertension. In the center that eliminated phthalate from their products during the study period the rate of lung disease associ-ated hypertension dropped significantly.[15,29,37] All of these reports come from the same group of investigators and require further validation on other cohorts.

In terms of iatrogenic causes of neonatal hypertension, ECMO and medications are common causes. Hypertension is present in many of the patients receiving ECMO, although the prevalence varies widely depending on the study. In one study of 500 consecutive infants treated with ECMO there was hypertension in 38%.[2,38–40] Commonly used medications resulting in hypertension are dexamethasone, theophyl-line, phenylephrine eye drops, and pancuronium.[41,42] Elevation in blood pressure may also occur during withdrawal from sedative or analgesic medications or in neonatal abstinence syndrome.[2,43,44] Neonates receiving vitamin supplementation or paren-teral nutrition may become hypertensive because of salt or volume overload. They may also get hypertension because of hypercalcemia from excessive vitamin A or vitamin D intake.[45]

Blood Pressure Measurement

Measurement of accurate blood pressures in neonates and infants is difficult. In an ideal world, diagnosis of hypertension would be made based on measurements by de-vices that produce accurate and precise values approximating the intra-arterial blood pressure. Unfortunately, blood pressure measurement devices are inaccurate and imprecise, and these issues are exacerbated in neonates given that measurement dif-ferences between techniques may be more significant than in older children and adults.

Although intra-arterial blood pressure measurement is the gold standard, oscillometric blood pressure measurement is the most common given that it is noninvasive and easy to use. Intra-arterial measurement, although accurate, carries risk of thrombosis, ischemia, and infection. Oscillometric devices measure the blood pressure by inflating past the systolic pressure, gradually deflating and then determining the pressure with the maximum arterial pulsation amplitude. This is the mean arterial pressure. Using device-specific algorithms, the systolic and diastolic blood pressures are calculated from the mean arterial pressure. For devices to be validated they may vary up to 5 mm Hg with a standard deviation of up to 8 mm Hg. Given that mean arterial blood pressures are generally 30 to 50 mm Hg in neonates, this degree of variability is clinically significant. A recent systematic review of the literature looked at optimal measurement and variability of blood pressure using oscillometric devices in the neonatal population. Data continue to be limited, with only 34 studies meeting criteria for inclusion. The reliability of blood pressure measurement was improved with the optimal cuff width to arm ratio of 0.5 (0.44–0.55) with greater likelihood of error when this ratio was less than 0.45 or greater than 0.7 with a consistent risk for overestimating blood pressure when the ratio was too small. Additionally, blood pressures differed in accuracy and variability by location of blood pressure measurement. Arm blood pressures most consistently correlated with invasive blood pressure measurement. Those taken in the thigh were not similar to those in the arms and calves and are not recommended. Calf blood pressures may be similar to those in the arm within the first few days of life but after that are more variable, initially giving lower measurements but becoming higher than arm blood pressures by 6 to 9 months.

In addition to variability coming from the device and the technique of measurement, there is variability depending on patient activity level and position. Blood pressures are higher when infants are awake, feeding, sucking, crying, or if their head is elevated. Additionally, they may be affected by medical interventions, such as suctioning. Screening may be performed using individual blood pressures with the appropriate cuff and position, when the child is asleep or quietly awake. However, if the blood pressure does not correlate with what is expected, further measurements should be taken. A standard blood pressure method has been shown to provide lower and less variable blood pressures than routine nurse measurements.[46] Measurements are more reliable when the cuff is placed and then the infant is allowed to settle. When the infant is asleep or quietly awake, three successive blood pressure measurements should be taken around 2 minutes apart and the resulting values averaged for analysis. The first measurement may be higher and should be discarded if discrepant from the second two measurements.[47]

DEFINITION OF NEONATAL HYPERTENSION

There is a lack of robust normative data for term and preterm infants. Currently the definition of hypertension is similar to that in older children. Hypertension in neonates is generally defined as persistent blood pressure elevation greater than the 95th percentile for postmenstrual age. Those with blood pressure values greater than the 95th percentile should be closely monitored. Those with blood pressure greater than the 99th percentile should have further evaluation with treatment depending on the clinical situation.[8] Those with evidence of end-organ dysfunction have acute severe hypertension and intravenous antihypertensives should be used.[48]

In neonates providing these normative values has proved challenging given that studies of neonatal blood pressure are in small heterogenous populations with varying blood pressure measurement techniques. In addition, there are many factors that affect blood pressure amplitude and the pattern of rise. Blood pressure in newborns at 1 day after birth increases linearly with gestational age and birthweight.[49,50] After birth blood pressure rises, most rapidly in the first few days of life and then continues to rise in the first 2 months of life, with systolic blood pressure becoming more constant for the remaining year of life, whereas diastolic blood pressure continues to rise steadily. The rate of rise in the first week of life is greatest in the most premature and lowest birth weight infants with blood pressure values eventually reaching those of term infants by around 1 month of age.[50–52] Data from individual small studies of neonatal blood pressure have been combined to create a reference table of normative mean arterial blood pressure values by postmenstrual age after 2 weeks of life, which is the best current reference[7]; its use was endorsed by the American Academy of Pediatrics pediatric hypertension guideline.[8] If blood pressures are noted to be outside of what is expected, care should be taken to optimize the technique with which the blood pressure measurements are taken to ensure that the diagnosis of hypertension is an accurate one.

PRESENTATION OF NEONATAL HYPERTENSION

Generally, hypertension is discovered when blood pressures are found to be persistently elevated on routine vital sign monitoring. However, hypertension may show subtle or even more severe nonspecific signs, which are often difficult to recognize as symptoms of hypertension. Therefore, when there is a clinical change, it is important to review the blood pressure data for evidence of hypertension. Subtle signs of hypertension can include irritability, poor feeding, and vomiting. Although more severe signs can include symptoms of congestive heart failure and cardiogenic shock including respiratory distress, tachypnea, and hypoxemia, they can also include neurologic changes, such as lethargy, tremors, seizure, or apnea. Older infants may demonstrate poor weight gain.[53–55]

EVALUATION

Given the expansive list of conditions that can cause hypertension, a careful history and physical examination must be done to appropriately guide laboratory and imaging work-up. A thorough history often reveals risk factors contributing to the development of hypertension and should include a maternal and perinatal history; comorbidities; medication exposures; events that may cause acute kidney injury; and procedures, such as umbilical artery catheter placement.

Once elevated blood pressures are confirmed by proper measurement, it is important that four limb blood pressures are performed to screen for coarctation or aortic thrombus. If there is a concern for coarctation, it can only be excluded or confirmed with echocardiogram because there is a great deal of variability in neonatal blood pressure between limbs.[56] Careful physical examination should be performed. One should look for evidence of a genetic syndrome, which may be associated with hypertension; presence of murmur on cardiac examination; or abdominal bruit, edema concerning for volume overload, or evidence of abdominal mass that could indicate the presence of urinary tract obstruction, tumor, or polycystic kidney disease. There may also be evidence of sequelae of hypertension, such as symptoms of heart failure or neurologic dysfunction.

Initial evaluation in all infants should include chest radiograph to look at heart size; complete blood count with platelet count looking for evidence of thrombosis or thrombophilia; and evaluation for underlying kidney disease with urinalysis, basic metabolic panel including calcium, and a renal ultrasound with Doppler. Renal ultrasound with

Doppler can help evaluate for CAKUT, cystic kidney disease, and arterial or venous thrombus.

Unfortunately, many children with renal artery stenosis may only have involvement in smaller intrarenal branch vessels that are too small to be seen on Doppler ultrasound.[57] Computed tomography angiography and magnetic resonance angiography are difficult to perform in neonates and there are little data regarding their use in infants. Radionucleotide imaging has also been used to assess for perfusion abnormalities caused by thrombus, but its use is limited by immature kidney function in the neonatal population. Although angiography is the gold standard for detection of thrombus or renal artery stenosis, given the risk for vascular injury, radiation exposure, and the need for general anesthesia its use is limited in neonates. Also, one of the benefits of angiography is the opportunity for intervention with angioplasty or another endovascular repair. However, angioplasty, although reported in neonates, is not commonly performed and many centers may lack the expertise or experts to perform it.[58] Therefore, in those neonates with extreme blood pressure elevation in whom diagnosis of renovascular hypertension should be considered, medical management is necessary until they are old enough to get definitive imaging diagnosis and treatment with endovascular intervention.[59]

Additional laboratory or imaging should be driven by findings on history, physical, or laboratory examination. In particular, given the variability of plasma renin activity in neonates, it should be sent only if there is laboratory evidence, such as hypokalemia and metabolic alkalosis, indicating a possible monogenic form of hypertension.[29,60,61]

TREATMENT
When to Treat

In general, asymptomatic hypertensive neonates with blood pressure measurements persistently greater than the 95th percentile but not greater than the 99th percentile should be monitored. Those who have developed symptoms or sequelae of hypertension or who have blood pressure measurements persistently greater than the 99th percentile should have further evaluation and treatment should be considered. If possible, before treatment, correctable causes of hypertension should be addressed, such as volume overload, hypercalcemia or modifiable medications. In those with severe acute hypertension, defined as showing evidence of end-organ dysfunction, intravenous agents should be used.[48] To avoid cerebral ischemia or hemorrhage, care should be taken to avoid rapid reduction of blood pressure, particularly in those with severe acute hypertension and in premature infants who are at higher risk because of immaturity of the periventricular circulation.[62]

As with other medications in the neonatal population pharmacokinetic data and information on drug efficacy and side effect profiles within the neonatal population are generally lacking. This is in addition to the lack of robust data regarding normative blood pressure values in infancy and regarding long-term adverse effects of hypertension in infancy. Therefore, there are no evidence-based guidelines for the treatment of neonatal hypertension. Given lack of guidelines, clinical expertise must be used when determining when to initiate treatment.

Antihypertensives Used Today

More robust data regarding pharmacokinetics in neonates would be helpful because they have a lower kidney perfusion pressure, increased renal vascular resistance, lower glomerular filtration rate, and immature tubular function at birth. In addition, neonates are at high risk of hypovolemia. Therefore, when using antihypertensives that are cleared by the kidney, younger neonates may be at greater risk for adverse side effects. Glomerular filtration increases over the first 2 weeks postbirth and therefore this risk may be the highest within the first 2 weeks of life; however, infants do not reach adult levels of glomerular filtration rate until around 12 months of age.[63]

One of the larger studies looking at what antihypertensives are currently used to treat neonatal hypertension was performed using the Pediatric Health Information System database. Within 764 encounters where patients were diagnosed with hypertension, the antihypertensives used spanned all pharmacologic categories. The most common agents used were vasodilators and angiotensin-converting enzyme (ACE) inhibitors followed by calcium channel blockers, used in 64%, 51%, and 24% of patients, respectively. α-Blockers or β-blockers were used in 18%, whereas clonidine was used in 5% of patients. They found that the median duration of exposure was 10 days, and 45% of neonates were treated with two or more agents.[2]

General Approach

When determining which agent to use, it is good to determine the acuity of the patient and the speed at which blood pressure control is desired. In those with acute severe hypertension displaying evidence of end-organ damage, intravenous agents should be used. In the absence of severe hypertension, oral agents are considered. Some agents, such as amlodipine, may have a slower onset with a longer duration of action, making them more appropriate for stable patients in whom the blood pressure can be slowly lowered as the medication takes effect.

Overall, it is reasonable to follow a similar treatment approach as is taken in the treatment of pediatric hypertension aside from concerns specific to the neonatal infant population. For those in whom oral therapy is considered safe, calcium channel blockers, such as amlodipine and isradipine, are a reasonable first choice, as are the vasodilators hydralazine and minoxidil. Amlodipine is commercially available as a suspension, and isradipine is easily compounded into a 1 mg/mL solution, making administration easy.[64–66] Diuretics, although not useful as first-line antihypertensive, may be useful as second-line agents in the setting of BPD.[29,67] β-Adrenergic blockers, however, can cause bronchospasm and bradycardia and should be avoided if there is concurrent chronic lung disease.[29,37]

ACE inhibitors are one of the most common agents used in older children, but there are few data available regarding their use in neonates.[68] In fact, neonates may be at higher risk for side effects from ACE inhibitors, with one case series describing prolonged, excessive hypotension with risk for acute kidney injury with oliguria unresponsive to fluid resuscitation in premature infants treated with captopril.[69–71] Given their known effects on renal development in utero, there is also concern that there could be effects on ongoing postnatal renal development. Currently animal data suggest that use of ACE inhibitors could impair ongoing nephrogenesis, reducing glomerular number and increasing risk for hypertension later in life.[72,73] The safety data regarding use of ACE inhibitors within the neonatal population are primarily from those with congenital cardiac disease. In one study looking at the use of enalapril within 662 neonates without congenital heart disease from 348 different NICUs, they found that 21% experienced an adverse event, such as hyperkalemia, elevated creatinine, or death. Other adverse effects were cough, swelling, hypotension, and renal failure. Those who were less than 30 days of age were more likely to experience elevated creatinine, hyperkalemia, and hypotension. Those with longer exposure were at greater risk for hyperkalemia and death.[74] Given risk for side effects in general it is helpful to avoid using ACE inhibitors until after infants have reached a corrected postmenstrual age of 44 weeks.[2,74,75]

In neonates with acute severe hypertension, continuous intravenous infusions, such as nicardipine, sodium nitroprusside, esmolol, and labetalol, have the important benefit of being easily titratable to keep the blood pressure within the desired range.[39,75–82] When used, blood pressure should be monitored continuously using an indwelling intra-arterial catheter or if necessary, an automated oscillometric device taking regular repeat blood pressure measurements. When choosing which continuous antihypertensive infusion to use, note that although sodium nitroprusside has been used safely in neonates it may rarely result in cyanide toxicity in those with renal dysfunction, when given at higher doses or when given for a prolonged duration.[79,80] Given that neonates have reduced kidney function, particularly in the first 2 weeks of life it may be beneficial to start with other agents. Nicardipine is well tolerated given that it is safe, has a rapid onset of action, and short half-life allowing it to easily be titrated.[75,78] The largest study in the neonatal population included 20 term and preterm neonates, showing good efficacy with no side effects.[77] Given the high rate of hypertension in neonates receiving ECMO one group looked at the safety and efficacy of nicardipine in a retrospective cohort of eight neonates, for a mean duration of 51 hours. Dosing started at a mean of 0.5 µg/kg/min up to a max of 1.1 µg/kg/min with significant decreases in blood pressure and no adverse side effects.[39] A larger study looking at nicardipine use in a pediatric cohort of 29 patients, ranging from 2 days old to 18 years old, showed similar efficacy without side effects other than a clinically insignificant increase in heart rate.[78]

Surgical Management

For some infants, such as those with coarctation of the aorta or urinary obstruction,[83] surgery is necessary to relieve the underlying cause of hypertension. For those with severe elevation of blood pressure caused by renal artery stenosis, medical management is preferred until the patient is old enough to undergo arteriography and endovascular repair.[84] However, if the blood pressure is unable to be medically managed nephrectomy may be performed and has also been reported in cases of severe hypertension caused by a multicystic dysplastic kidney.[83,85,86] If hypertension is caused by malignancy, such as Wilms tumor or neuroblastoma, tumor debulking may be needed.

Outcomes

Most studies examining the long-term outcome of neonatal hypertension are small, with limited duration of follow-up, often less than 1 year. In most studies, most neonatal hypertension resolved by 6 months of age.[4,16,87–89] The largest study with the longest follow-up included 122 neonates from 13 different children's hospitals in the United States showing that 79% of infants were able to discontinue their antihypertensive medications by 2 years of age. In those that remained on antihypertensives, calcium channel blockers were the most used agents.[89] In general, those with hypertension secondary to medications, chronic lung disease, or deemed idiopathic, may be more likely to resolve. Persistent hypertension is seen in those with genetic forms of hypertension; unresolved renal artery stenosis; or other underlying kidney disease, such as CAKUT or polycystic kidney disease.

Ideally all patients on antihypertensive medications should be sent home with an oscillometric blood pressure measurement device for safety to monitor blood pressure and titrate medications between visits. Although medications may need to be adjusted for growth in the immediate neonatal period, in those with hypertension that is likely to resolve, it is reasonable to follow blood pressures while either weaning their antihypertensives or no longer adjusting their dose for growth.

Less data are available regarding longer term outcomes. For those with either renal vein thrombosis or coarctation of the aorta, there is evidence of effects into late childhood requiring long-term follow-up. For those with renal vein thrombosis there is a risk of persistent hypertension and development of chronic kidney disease.[90,91] One study of long-term outcomes in the setting of renal vein thrombosis including 85 neonates with renal vein thrombosis followed for a mean of 15 years, found that 39% had persistent hypertension and 46% had chronic kidney disease.[91] In the case of coarctation of the aorta it seems there is longer term risk for hypertension even if it resolves in the neonatal period. A follow-up study of 119 children with repaired coarctation of the aorta with a mean follow-up of 12 years showed that 30% had elevated mean blood pressure on 24-hour ambulatory blood pressure monitoring. Nineteen percent of those with no residual obstruction still had elevated mean blood pressure.[92] Additionally, even in the absence of neonatal hypertension, neonates with such conditions as BPD, kidney disease, congenital heart disease, premature birth, or intrauterine growth restriction are at risk for developing hypertension later in childhood or in adulthood.[29,93–95] Therefore, long-term monitoring for development of hypertension is important given that there is evidence that those with hypertension as children are more likely to have hypertension as adults.[96]

DISCUSSION

Neonatal hypertension is uncommon but is becoming increasingly recognized. Accurate blood pressure measurement is challenging and requires careful attention to technique and comparison with normative data, which varies by postmenstrual age. Therefore, neonatal hypertension may go unrecognized.

Neonatal hypertension has a diverse range of underlying risk factors and causes, varying by several factors including maternal health, postnatal exposures, birth history, and underlying medical illnesses. Monitoring blood pressure for possible hypertension detects neonates in need of additional evaluation with more timely diagnosis and management of secondary hypertension from such causes as renal artery thrombosis, cardiovascular disease, or renal disease. In those cases, hypertension may require surgical intervention, long-term treatment, and monitoring. Most neonatal hypertension is secondary to medications, lung disease, or is idiopathic. In most of those neonates the hypertension resolves within the first 6 months to 2 years of life. Some patients with BPD, kidney disease, congenital cardiac disease, premature birth, or intrauterine growth restriction may not have hypertension in the neonatal period but are at risk for hypertension later in life.

Similar to the lack of normative data regarding neonatal blood pressure, there are few studies evaluating the long-term outcomes of neonatal hypertension or on the safety and efficacy of antihypertensive medications in the neonatal population. There is a clear need for additional research on short- and long-term outcomes, and optimal treatment approaches.

SUMMARY

Identification of neonatal hypertension is difficult given that it requires accurate blood pressure measurement. When present it should prompt thorough evaluation to diagnose causes that require additional surgical or medical management. Most neonatal hypertension resolves in the first few years of life but for some there is risk for hypertension into adulthood. More study is needed to better define neonatal hypertension, and understand its optimal treatment and its long-term outcomes.

CLINICS CARE POINTS

- Neonates with hypertension may demonstrate nonspecific signs ranging from subtle to severe and so care must be taken to monitor vital sign data for evidence of hypertension.
- Identification of neonatal hypertension requires accurate blood pressure measurement, optimally taken in an upper extremity with an oscillometric device, using an appropriately sized cuff when the child is sleeping or restfully awake.
- The mean arterial pressure should be compared with normative data for neonates of a similar postmenstrual age.
- Neonatal hypertension should prompt thorough examination including four limb blood pressures, careful clinical history and physical examination, laboratory testing, and imaging.
- Most neonatal hypertension resolves within the first 6 to 24 months of life.
- Long-term follow-up is recommended, particularly in those with conditions that place the infant at risk for hypertension later in life.

Best Practices

■ **What is the current practice for managing neonatal hypertension?**

1. Detection of neonatal hypertension Monitor for blood pressure elevation above the 95th percentile for postmenstrual age. If elevated on routine measurement, retake them assuring optimized techniqueo in the upper extremity with an oscillometric device, using an appropriately sized cuff in terms of both length and width for the patiento Place the cuff and then allow the infant to settle. When the infant is asleep or quietly awake, three successive blood pressure measurements should be taken around two minutes apart. The first measurement may be higher and should be discarded if discrepant from the second two. If elevated blood pressures are confirmed perform four limb blood pressures are performed to screen for coarctation or aortic thrombus. If there is a concern for coarctation, it can only be excluded or confirmed with echocardiogram.

2. Monitoring versus evaluation and treatment Monitoringo Asymptomatic hypertensive neonates with blood pressure measurements above the 95th percentile but not greater than the 99th percentile. Further evaluation and treatment in those with:o Symptoms or sequelae of hypertension o Blood pressure measurements persistently over the 99th percentile.

3. Initial evaluation: Detailed history and physical exam including four limb blood pressures Chest x-ray, complete blood count, urinalysis, basic metabolic panel including calcium and a renal ultrasound with Doppler.

4. Treatment In those with acute severe hypertension displaying evidence of end organ damage, intravenous agents should be used. In the absence of severe hypertension, oral agents can be considered. Agents with a slower onset and longer duration of action are more appropriate for relatively stable patients in whom the blood pressure can be slowly lowered as the medication takes effect.

5. Long-term monitoringEven if elevated blood pressures resolve those at risk for developing hypertension later in childhood should continue to be monitored for development of hypertension such as those with BPD, kidney disease, congenital heart disease, premature birth or IUGR.

DISCLOSURE

The authors have nothing to disclose.

REFERENCES

1. Singh HP, Hurley RM, Myers TF. Neonatal hypertension: incidence and risk factors. Am J Hypertens 1992;5(2):51–5.
2. Blowey DL, Duda PJ, Stokes P, et al. Incidence and treatment of hypertension in the neonatal intensive care unit. J Am Soc Hypertens 2011;5(6):478–83.
3. Sahu R, Pannu H, Yu R, et al. Systemic hypertension requiring treatment in the neonatal intensive care Unit. J Pediatr 2013;163(1):84–8.
4. Seliem WA, Falk MC, Shadbolt B, et al. Antenatal and postnatal risk factors for neonatal hypertension and infant follow-up. Pediatr Nephrol 2007;22(12):2081.
5. Ravisankar S, Kuehn D, Clark RH, et al. Antihypertensive drug exposure in premature infants from 1997 to 2013. Cardiol Young 2017;27(5):905–11.
6. Kraut EJ, Boohaker LJ, Askenazi DJ, et al. Incidence of neonatal hypertension from a large multicenter study (Assessment of Worldwide acute kidney injury Epidemiology in neonates—AWAKEN). Pediatr Res 2018;84(2):279–89.
7. Dionne JM, Abitbol CL, Flynn JT. Hypertension in infancy: diagnosis, management and outcome. Pediatr Nephrol 2011;27(1):17–32.
8. Flynn JT, Kaelber DC, Baker-Smith CM, et al. Clinical practice guideline for screening and management of high blood pressure in children and adolescents. Pediatrics 2017;140(3):e20171904.
9. Adelman RD. Neonatal hypertension. Pediatr Clin North Am 1978;25(1):99–110.
10. Neal WA, Reynolds JW, Jarvis CW, et al. Umbilical artery catheterization: demonstration of arterial thrombosis by aortography. Pediatrics 1972;50(1):6–13.
11. Vailas GN, Brouillette RT, Scott JP, et al. Neonatal aortic thrombosis: recent experience. J Pediatr 1986;109(1):101–8.
12. Dionne JM. Determinants of blood pressure in neonates and infants: predictable variability. Hypertension 2021;77(3):781–7.
13. Kent AL, Chaudhari T. Determinants of neonatal blood pressure. Curr Hypertens Rep 2013;15(5):426–32.
14. Sadoh WE, Ibhanesehbor SE, Monguno AM, et al. Predictors of newborn systolic blood pressure. West Afr J Med 2010;29(2):86–90.
15. Farnbach K, Iragorri S, Al-Uzri A, et al. The changing spectrum of hypertension in premature infants. J Perinatol 2019;39(11):1528–34.
16. Fridman AL, Hustead VA. Hypertension in babies following discharge from a neonatal intensive care unit. Pediatr Nephrol 1987;1(1):30–4.
17. Selewski DT, Charlton JR, Jetton JG, et al. Neonatal acute kidney injury. Pediatrics 2015;136(2):e463–73.
18. Gilboa N, Urizar RE. Severe hypertension in newborn after pyeloplasty of hydronephrotic kidney. Urology 1983;22(2):179–82.
19. Moralıoğlu S, Celayir AC, Bosnalı O, et al. Single center experience in patients with unilateral multicystic dysplastic kidney. J Pediatr Urol 2014;10(4):763–8.
20. Boo N, Wong N, Zulkifli SS, et al. Risk factors associated with umbilical vascular catheter-associated thrombosis in newborn infants. J Paediatr Child Health 1999; 35(5):460–5.
21. Seibert J, Taylor B, Williamson S, et al. Sonographic detection of neonatal umbilical-artery thrombosis: clinical correlation. Am J Roentgenol 1987;148(5): 965–8.
22. Barrington KJ. Umbilical artery catheters in the newborn: effects of position of the catheter tip. Cochrane Db Syst Rev 1999;1:CD000505.

23. Marks SD, Massicotte MP, Steele BT, et al. Neonatal renal venous thrombosis: clinical outcomes and prevalence of prothrombotic disorders. J Pediatr 2005; 146(6):811–6.
24. Lau KK, Stoffman JM, Williams S, et al. Neonatal renal vein thrombosis: review of the English-language literature between 1992 and 2006. Pediatrics 2007;120(5): e1278–84.
25. Tullus K, Brennan E, Hamilton G, et al. Renovascular hypertension in children. Lancet 2008;371(9622):1453–63.
26. Izraelit A, Kim M, Ratner V, et al. Mid-aortic syndrome in two preterm infants. J Perinatol 2012;32(5):390–2.
27. Peranteau WH, Tharakan SJ, Partridge E, et al. Systemic hypertension in giant omphalocele: an underappreciated association. J Pediatr Surg 2015;50(9): 1477–80.
28. Fujishiro J, Sugiyama M, Ishimaru T, et al. Cyclic fluctuation of blood pressure in neonatal neuroblastoma. Pediatr Int 2014;56(6):934–7.
29. Jenkins RD, Aziz JK, Gievers LL, et al. Characteristics of hypertension in premature infants with and without chronic lung disease: a long-term multi-center study. Pediatr Nephrol 2017;32(11):2115–24.
30. Abman SH. Monitoring cardiovascular function in infants with chronic lung disease of prematurity. Arch Dis Child - Fetal Neonatal Ed 2002;87(1):F15.
31. Sehgal A, Malikiwi A, Paul E, et al. Systemic arterial stiffness in infants with bronchopulmonary dysplasia: potential cause of systemic hypertension. J Perinatol 2016;36(7):564–9.
32. Stroustrup A, Bragg JB, Busgang SA, et al. Sources of clinically significant neonatal intensive care unit phthalate exposure. J Expo Sci Environ Epidemiol 2020;30(1):137–48.
33. Téllez-Rojo MM, Cantoral A, Cantonwine DE, et al. Prenatal urinary phthalate metabolites levels and neurodevelopment in children at two and three years of age. Sci Total Environ 2013;461:386–90.
34. Kim Y, Ha E, Kim E, et al. Prenatal exposure to phthalates and infant development at 6 months: prospective Mothers and children's Environmental health (MOCEH) study. Environ Health Persp 2011;119(10):1495–500.
35. Cho S-C, Bhang S-Y, Hong Y-C, et al. Relationship between environmental phthalate exposure and the intelligence of school-age children. Environ Health Persp 2010;118(7):1027–32.
36. Fischer CJ, Graz MB, Muehlethaler V, et al. Phthalates in the NICU: is it safe? J Paediatr Child H 2013;49(9):E413–9.
37. Jenkins R, Tackitt S, Gievers L, et al. Phthalate-associated hypertension in premature infants: a prospective mechanistic cohort study. Pediatr Nephrol 2019;34(8): 1413–24.
38. Becker JA, Short BL, Martin GR. Cardiovascular complications adversely affect survival during extracorporeal membrane oxygenation. Crit Care Med 1998; 26(9):1582–6.
39. Liviskie CJ, DeAvilla KM, Zeller BN, et al. Nicardipine for the treatment of neonatal hypertension during extracorporeal membrane oxygenation. Pediatr Cardiol 2019;40(5):1041–5.
40. Boedy RF, Goldberg AK, Howell CG, et al. Incidence of hypertension in infants on extracorporeal membrane oxygenation. J Pediatr Surg 1990;25(2):258–61.
41. Merritt JC, Kraybill EN. Effect of mydriatics on blood pressure in premature infants. J Pediatr Ophthalmol Strabismus 1981;18(5):42–6.

42. Marinelli KA, Burke GS, Herson VC. Effects of dexamethasone on blood pressure in premature infants with bronchopulmonary dysplasia. J Pediatr 1997;130(4): 594–602.
43. Bailey NA, Diaz-Barbosa M. Effect of maternal substance abuse on the fetus, neonate, and child. Pediatr Rev 2018;39(11):550–9.
44. Horn PT. Persistent hypertension after prenatal cocaine exposure. J Pediatr 1992; 121(2):288–91.
45. Rodd C, Goodyer P. Hypercalcemia of the newborn: etiology, evaluation, and management. Pediatr Nephrol 1999;13(6):542.
46. Nwankwo MU, Lorenz JM, Gardiner JC. A standard protocol for blood pressure measurement in the newborn. Pediatrics 1997;99(6):e10.
47. Dionne JM, Bremner SA, Baygani SK, et al. Method of blood pressure measurement in neonates and infants: a systematic review and analysis. J Pediatr 2020; 221:23–31.e5.
48. Dionne JM, Flynn JT. Management of severe hypertension in the newborn. Arch Dis Child 2017;102(12):1176.
49. Zubrow AB, Hulman S, Kushner H, et al. Determinants of blood pressure in infants admitted to neonatal intensive care units: a prospective multicenter study. Philadelphia Neonatal Blood Pressure Study Group. J Perinatol 1995;15(6):470–9.
50. Pejovic B, Peco-Antic A, Marinkovic-Eric J. Blood pressure in non-critically ill preterm and full-term neonates. Pediatr Nephrol 2006;22(2):249–57.
51. Report of the second Task Force on blood pressure control in children–1987. Task Force on blood pressure control in children. National Heart, Lung, and Blood Institute, Bethesda, Maryland. Pediatrics 1987;79(1):1–25.
52. Lurbe E, Garcia-Vicent C, Torro I, et al. First-year blood pressure increase steepest in low birthweight newborns. J Hypertens 2007;25(1):81–6.
53. Skalina M, Kliegman R, Fanaroff A. Epidemiology and management of severe symptomatic neonatal hypertension. Am J Perinatol 1986;3(03):235–9.
54. Louw J, Brown S, Eyskens B, et al. Neonatal circulatory failure due to acute hypertensive crisis: clinical and echocardiographic clues. Cardiovasc J Afr 2013; 24(3):73–7.
55. Xiao N, Tandon A, Goldstein S, et al. Cardiogenic shock as the initial presentation of neonatal systemic hypertension. J Neonatal-perinatal Med 2013;6(3):267–72.
56. Crossland DS, Furness JC, Abu-Harb M, et al. Variability of four limb blood pressure in normal neonates. Arch Dis Child - Fetal Neonatal Ed 2004;89(4):F325.
57. Vo NJ, Hammelman BD, Racadio JM, et al. Anatomic distribution of renal artery stenosis in children: implications for imaging. Pediatr Radiol 2006;36(10):1032–6.
58. Daehnert I, Hennig B, Scheinert D. Percutaneous transluminal angioplasty for renovascular hypertension in a neonate. Acta Paediatr 2005;94(8):1149–52.
59. Roth CG, Spottswood SE, Chan JCM, et al. Evaluation of the hypertensive infant a rational approach to diagnosis. Radiol Clin North Am 2003;41(5):931–44.
60. Sulyok E, Németh M, Tényi I, et al. Postnatal development of renin-angiotensin-aldosterone system, RAAS, in relation to electrolyte balance in premature infants. Pediatr Res 1979;13(7):817–20.
61. Ingelfinger JR. Monogenic and polygenic contributions to hypertension. In: Flynn JT, Ingelfinger JR, Redwine KR, editors. Pediatric hypertension. 2018. p. 113–34.
62. Perlman JM. The relationship between systemic hemodynamic perturbations and periventricular-intraventricular hemorrhage: a historical perspective. Semin Pediatr Neurol 2009;16(4):191–9.

63. Rodieux F, Wilbaux M, van den Anker JN, et al. Effect of kidney function on drug kinetics and dosing in neonates, infants, and children. Clin Pharm 2015;54(12): 1183–204.
64. Flynn JT, Warnick SJ. Isradipine treatment of hypertension in children: a single-center experience. Pediatr Nephrol 2002;17(9):748–53.
65. Miyashita Y, Peterson D, Rees JM, et al. Isradipine for treatment of acute hypertension in hospitalized children and adolescents. J Clin Hypertens 2010;12(11): 850–5.
66. Flynn JT, Pasko DA. Calcium channel blockers: pharmacology and place in therapy of pediatric hypertension. Pediatr Nephrol 2000;15(3–4):302–16.
67. Kao LC, Durand DJ, McCrea RC, et al. Randomized trial of long-term diuretic therapy for infants with oxygen-dependent bronchopulmonary dysplasia. J Pediatr 1994;124(5):772–81.
68. Snauwaert E, Walle JV, Bruyne PD. Therapeutic efficacy and safety of ACE inhibitors in the hypertensive paediatric population: a review. Arch Dis Child 2017; 102(1):63.
69. Tack ED, Perlman JM. Renal failure in sick hypertensive premature infants receiving captopril therapy. J Pediatr 1988;112(5):805–10.
70. Pandey R, Koshy RG, Dako J. Angiotensin converting enzyme inhibitors induced acute kidney injury in newborn. J Maternal-fetal Neonatal Med 2016;30(6):1–3.
71. O'Dea RF, Mirkin BL, Alward CT, et al. Treatment of neonatal hypertension with captopril. J Pediatr 1988;113(2):403–6.
72. Tufro-McReddie A, Romano LM, Harris JM, et al. Angiotensin II regulates nephrogenesis and renal vascular development. Am J Phy 1995;269(1):F110–5.
73. Frölich S, Slattery P, Thomas D, et al. Angiotensin II-AT1–receptor signaling is necessary for cyclooxygenase-2–dependent postnatal nephron generation. Kidney Int 2017;91(4):818–29.
74. Ku LC, Zimmerman K, Benjamin DK, et al. Safety of enalapril in infants admitted to the neonatal intensive care unit. Pediatr Cardiol 2017;38(1):155–61.
75. Gouyon JB, Geneste B, Semama DS, et al. Intravenous nicardipine in hypertensive preterm infants. Arch Dis Child - Fetal Neonatal Ed 1997;76(2):F126.
76. Treluyer JM, Hubert P, Jouvet P, et al. Intravenous nicardipine in hypertensive children. Eur J Pediatr 1993;152(9):712–4.
77. Milou C, Debuche-Benouachkou V, Semama DS, et al. Intravenous nicardipine as a first-line antihypertensive drug in neonates. Intensive Care Med 2000;26(7): 956–8.
78. Flynn JT, Mottes TA, Brophy PD, et al. Intravenous nicardipine for treatment of severe hypertension in children. J Pediatr 2001;139(1):38–43.
79. Thomas C, Svehla L, Moffett BS. Sodium nitroprusside induced cyanide toxicity in pediatric patients. Expert Opin Drug Saf 2009;8(5):599–602.
80. Benitz WE, Malachowski N, Cohen RS, et al. Use of sodium nitroprusside in neonates: efficacy and safety. J Pediatr 1985;106(1):102–10.
81. Tabbutt S, Nicolson SC, Adamson PC, et al. The safety, efficacy, and pharmacokinetics of esmolol for blood pressure control immediately after repair of coarctation of the aorta in infants and children: a multicenter, double-blind, randomized trial. J Thorac Cardiovasc Surg 2008;136(2):321–8.
82. Thomas CA, Moffett BS, Wagner JL, et al. Safety and efficacy of intravenous labetalol for hypertensive crisis in infants and small children. Pediatr Crit Care Me 2011;12(1):28–32.
83. Rajpoot DK, Duel B, Thayer K, et al. Medically resistant neonatal hypertension: revisiting the surgical causes. J Perinatol 1999;19(8):582–3.

84. Bendel-Stenzel M, Najarian JS, Sinaiko AR. Renal artery stenosis in infants: long-term medical treatment before surgery. Pediatr Nephrol 1996;10(2):147–51.
85. Kiessling SG, Wadhwa N, Kriss VM, et al. An unusual case of severe therapy-resistant hypertension in a newborn. Pediatrics 2007;119(1):e301–4.
86. Abdulhannan P, Stahlschmidt J, Subramaniam R. Multicystic dysplastic kidney disease and hypertension: clinical and pathological correlation. J Pediatr Urol 2011;7(5):566–8.
87. Sheftel DN, Hustead V, Friedman A. Hypertension screening in the follow-up of premature infants. Pediatrics 1983;71(5):763–6.
88. Buchi KF, Siegler RL. Hypertension in the first month of life. J Hypertens 1986; 4(5):525–8.
89. Xiao N, Hamdani G, Michelle S, et al. SAT-318 blood pressure outcomes in neonatal intensive care unit graduates with idiopathic hypertension. Kidney Int Rep 2019;4(7):S141.
90. Mocan H, Beattie TJ, Murphy AV. Renal venous thrombosis in infancy: long-term follow-up. Pediatr Nephrol 1991;5(1):45–9.
91. Ouellette AC, Darling EK, Sivapathasundaram B, et al. Incidence, risk factors, and outcomes of neonatal renal vein thrombosis in Ontario: population-based cohort study. Kidney360 2020;1(7):640–7.
92. O'Sullivan JJ, Derrick G, Darnell R. Prevalence of hypertension in children after early repair of coarctation of the aorta: a cohort study using casual and 24 hour blood pressure measurement. Heart 2002;88(2):163.
93. Sutherland MR, Bertagnolli M, Lukaszewski M-A, et al. Preterm birth and hypertension risk. Hypertension 2014;63(1):12–8.
94. Sutherland M, Ryan D, Black MJ, et al. Long-term renal consequences of preterm birth. Clin Perinatol 2014;41(3):561–73.
95. Greenberg JH, McArthur E, Thiessen-Philbrook H, et al. Long-term risk of hypertension after surgical repair of congenital heart disease in children. JAMA Netw Open 2021;4(4):e215237.
96. Bao W, Threefoot SA, Srinivasan SR, et al. Essential hypertension predicted by tracking of elevated blood pressure from childhood to adulthood: the Bogalusa heart study. Am J Hypertens 1995;8(7):657–65.

Counseling for Perinatal Outcomes in Women with Congenital Heart Disease

Jennifer F. Gerardin, MD[a,b], Scott Cohen, MD[a,b],*

KEYWORDS

- Adult congenital heart disease • Pregnancy • Cardiac complications

KEY POINTS

- Women with congenital heart disease may be at an increased risk of cardiovascular morbidity and mortality, as well as, neonatal complications.
- Preconceptual risk stratification of women with underlying congenital heart is vital to decreasing the risk of pregnancy related cardiovascular morbidity.
- Women with congenital heart disease should be cared for by a multidisciplinary team during pregnancy.

ADULT CONGENITAL HEART DISEASE POPULATION

As the adult congenital heart disease (ACHD) population continues to grow, most women born with congenital heart disease (CHD) now reach childbearing age. In 2010, it was estimated that there were 1.4 million adults with CHD living in the United States with almost a half million women of childbearing age.[1] The type of CHD and comorbidities that these women have determines their risk during pregnancy. Women with simple CHD may have the same risk as other women their age without CHD, whereas women with complex CHD may be at risk of significant morbidity, preterm delivery. They also may have a higher risk of mortality during pregnancy. Regular preconceptual ACHD care, contraception counseling, and multidisciplinary care during a pregnancy can help minimize the risk during pregnancy for both mother and baby[2] (Fig. 1).

The authors do not have any financial disclosures.
^a Department of Internal Medicine, Division of Cardiovascular Medicine, Medical College of Wisconsin, 8915 W. Connell Ct, PO Box 1997, Milwaukee, WI 53226, USA; ^b Department of Pediatrics, Division of Pediatric Cardiology, Medical College of Wisconsin, 8915 W. Connell Ct, PO Box 1997, Milwaukee, WI 53226, USA
* Corresponding author. Department of Internal Medicine, Division of Cardiovascular Medicine, Medical College of Wisconsin, 8915 W. Connell Ct, PO Box 1997, Milwaukee, WI 53226.
E-mail address: Scohen@chw.org

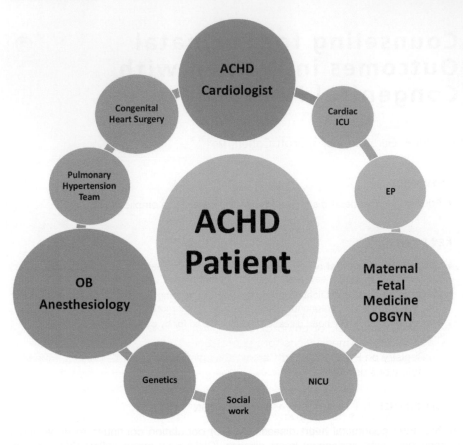

Fig. 1. A multidisciplinary team is needed to care for a patient with ACHD during pregnancy.

NORMAL CARDIOVASCULAR CHANGES DURING PREGNANCY

In order to understand how pregnancy affects patients with CHD, it is essential to understand the normal hemodynamic changes pregnancy can have on a normal heart. During pregnancy, the maternal blood volume increases by 40%[2] and the cardiac output by 30% to 50%.[3] The systemic vascular resistance and blood pressure decrease early in pregnancy. In cardiac patients, a bimodal distribution of heart failure symptoms peaks at late second and early third trimester and shortly after delivery. The maternal blood volume and cardiac output demands peak in late second trimester and early third trimester. Then systemic vascular resistance increases quickly after delivery. This sudden change in afterload in addition to an increase in preload related to relief of caval compression by the uterus may exacerbate heart failure in the postpartum period. The heart rate typically increases by 10 to 20 beats per minute, and the lower threshold for developing arrhythmias during pregnancy decreases.[2] Women with structural heart disease have been shown to develop more atrial arrhythmias during the second trimester,[4] and ventricular tachycardia most commonly occurs in the third trimester in women with heart failure.[5]

PREPREGNANCY COUNSELING

Ideally, patients with ACHD should be up to date on their recommended screening and seen regularly at an ACHD comprehensive care center.[6] (**Fig. 2**). During routine ACHD

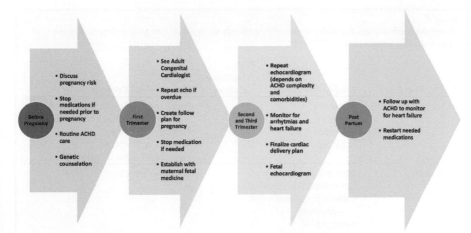

Fig. 2. Recommended cardiac management for pregnant patients with ACHD.

care, contraception and family planning should be discussed, including explaining the individual patient's risk of complications during pregnancy.[2] Patients should be warned if they are on medications not compatible with pregnancy (**Table 1**). According to the Registry on Pregnancy and Cardiac Disease (ROPAC), the most common cardiac medications used during pregnancy are β-blockers, antiplatelet agents, diuretics angiotensin-converting enzyme (ACE) inhibitors, and statins.[7] Some of the medications patients with ACHD use may be beneficial in pregnancy. Low-dose aspirin after the first trimester has been shown to decrease preeclampsia and should be restarted at 12 weeks gestation.[8] Other medications are contraindicated in pregnancy. The highest fetal complications were associated with ACE inhibitors (8%).[7] ACE inhibitors and angiotensin receptor blockers are not recommended in pregnancy because they increase the risk of congenital anomalies and oligohydramnios and decrease renal function.[9] β-blockers may cause fetal growth restriction; the only one that is contraindicated in pregnancy is atenolol.[2,9] Anticoagulation for a mechanical valve has to be well planned during pregnancy, and each medication regiment's risk benefits should be discussed with the patient.[10] A weaning plan should be established if the patient becomes pregnant or would like to try to conceive while on a contraindicated medication. In general, if the mother's cardiac function is improved with heart failure medications or antiarrhythmics, it may help the fetus get adequate blood flow and nutrition for growth.

Besides reviewing medications, a prepregnancy evaluation may include echocardiogram, cardiac MRI, cardiopulmonary exercise stress testing, and an electrocardiogram. The 2018 American Heart Association/American College of Cardiology ACHD guidelines give disease-specific recommendations on screenings.[6] Echocardiogram alone may miss extracardiac complications[11] that are important in pregnancy. For example, patients with coarctation of the aorta are recommended to have advanced imaging every 3 to 5 years because echocardiography alone may miss late complications such as discreet aortic aneurysm or recoarctation at the site of a prior repair as the patient ages (**Fig. 3**). Modifiable risk factors such as severe ascending aorta dilation or recoarctation may need intervention before pregnancy to reduce complications during pregnancy. Preconception cardiopulmonary exercise testing can help predict a women's ability to tolerate the cardiovascular demands of pregnancy.[2]

Table 1
Common medications typically used with patients with adult congenital heart disease and safety during pregnancy[2,7–10,23]

Medication Class	Medication Name	FDA Pregnancy Category	Known Fetal Complications
ACE inhibitors/ARB	Captopril	D	Fetal demise Congenital anomalies Renal impairment
	Enalapril	D	
	Lisinopril	D	Oligohydramnios
	Losartan	D	Growth restriction Need fetal echo if exposed
β-blockers	Atenolol	D	Growth restriction
	Carvedilol	C	
	Labetalol (β- and α-blocker)	C	
	Metoprolol	C	
	Propranolol	C	
Diuretics	Furosemide	C	—
	Spironolactone	C	Not recommended in pregnancy
Antiplatelet	Aspirin full dose	D (third trimester)	Premature ductus arteriosus closure
	Aspirin (<100 mg/d)	—	May decrease preeclampsia risk
Anticoagulation	Enoxaparin	C	Need to follow levels in pregnancy Does not cross the placenta
	Heparin	C	Does not cross the placenta
	Warfarin	X	Fetal warfarin syndrome Low-dose warfarin increases risk of miscarriage Crosses the placenta
Antiarrhythmics	Amiodarone	D	Thyroid complications
	Digoxin	C	—
	Flecainide	C	—
	Procainamide	C	—
	Sotalol	B	—
Endothelin receptor antagonists	Bosentan	X	—
	Ambrisentan	X	—
	Macitentan	X	—
Vasodilators	Epoprostenol	B	—
	Hydralazine	C	—
	Sildenafil	B	—

Abbreviation: ACE, angiotensin-converting enzyme.

Finally, preconception genetic screening and counseling may be offered to the family before pregnancy.[12] Depending on type of CHD the mother has, the risk of their offspring having CHD can be between 2% and 21%, which is higher than the general population.[12] In general, if a mother is affected with CHD, there is a slightly higher risk of passing on CHD to the infant than if the father is affected. For example, a mother with tetralogy of Fallot has a 2% to 2.5% chance of passing CHD to her infant compared with a father with tetralogy of Fallot with a reported risk of 1.5%. Left-sided obstructive disease has a high rate of penetrance. A woman with coarctation of the aorta, aortic stenosis, and hypoplastic left heart syndrome has a 4% to 6.5%, 8% to 18%, and 21% chance of passing on CHD to her infant, respectively. Women with atrioventricular septal defects can have up to 11.5% to 14% risk of passing on

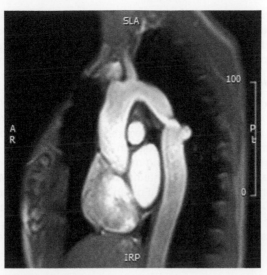

Fig. 3. Cardiac MRI of a 36-year-old woman at 20 weeks gestation. Arrow points to a pseudoaneurysm at prior coarctation site not found in routine echocardiography.

CHD to infant. CHD associated with autosomal dominate genetic syndromes such as Alagille, Holt-Oram and 22q11 deletion can have up to 50% penetrance to the infant. A fetal echocardiogram is recommended at 18 to 22 weeks gestation to evaluate for CHD in the fetus because infants of women with CHD are at high risk of developing CHD.[2,12] Fetal echocardiograms have a 69% sensitivity at identifying CHD before birth and have greater than 99% specificity.[13] The fetal echocardiogram gives parents, pediatric cardiologists, and the neonatal team to prepare the best delivery plan for the infant, including if they need to deliver at a tertiary care center. If prenatal screening does not catch CHD in the infant, pulse oximetry screening for critical CHD and physical examination are the final screening tests that can be done before the infant goes home.[14]

MATERNAL RISK STRATIFICATION

There are 3 major stratification systems to assess risk of complications during pregnancy in patients with ACHD.

CARPREG and CARPREG II

CARPREG was the original attempt to risk stratify cardiac risk during pregnancy.[15] It developed in 2001 and described maternal and neonatal risk of almost 600 women. In this original group 13% of women had cardiac complications, including arrhythmias, pulmonary edema, stroke, or death. It just looked at several predictors of poor outcomes. Risk factors included arrhythmias, poor functional status, left-sided obstructive disease, and poor left ventricular systolic function. Twenty percent of infants had complications including prematurity and small for gestational age.

In 2018, the CARPREG II study updated the original risk stratification score.[16] During this study almost 2000 pregnant women with heart disease were followed-up for cardiac complications during pregnancy. About 16% of the cohort developed cardiac complications, most commonly arrhythmias (9.3%) and heart failure (6.4%). Mortality during this study was still low (0.3%). In this iteration of CARPREG, prior cardiac events, arrhythmias, functional status and cyanosis, and mechanical valve increase a woman's risk during pregnancy the most. Then high-risk left-sided obstructive disease, pulmonary heart disease, high-risk aortopathy, and coronary artery disease also increase a woman's risk.

Modified World Health Organization Classification

Thorne and colleagues proposed the World Health Organization (WHO) classification for cardiac complications in 2006.[17] The multidisciplinary workgroup classifying pregnant cardiac patients into 4 risk categories. WHO classification I is not considered higher risk than the general population. WHO classification II causes a small increased risk of maternal mortality and morbidity. In WHO classification III patients, there is a significant increased maternal mortality and morbidity. Mechanical valves, systemic right ventricle patients, and Fontan palliated single ventricle patients are classified as WHO classification III. In WHO classification IV, pregnancy is not recommended. Patients with severe left ventricular systolic dysfunction, severe left-sided obstructive disease, pulmonary hypertension, or severely dilated aorta fall into this category.

ZAHARA

Similar to the original CARPREG in 2010, ZAHARA created a risk scoring system but included more women with CHD.[18] Mechanical valve prothesis during pregnancy categorizes patients in the highest risk group with a 70% chance of complication during pregnancy. Other risk factors that increase a patient's risk with ZAHARA include left heart obstructive disease with peak gradients greater than 50 mm Hg, cardiac medications before pregnancy, and history of arrhythmias. Moderate or severe mitral or tricuspid valve regurgitation, NYHA functional class III to IV, and history of cyanotic disease may also increase a woman's risk of complications.

Comparison of Risk Stratification Systems

When the original CARPREG, ZAHARA, and the modified WHO (mWHO) Classification were compared in different populations. The mWHO classification is consistently the most accurate at predicting high-risk patients.[19,20] Recently registries and multicenter studies have added more disease-specific data to relatively sparse literature.[21] ROPAC is one of the largest multinational registries for pregnancy and heart disease. It was established in 2007 and now has almost 6000 pregnancies enrolled with a high ACHD population (57%).[22]

HIGH-RISK HEART DISEASE DURING PREGNANCY
Mechanical Valves

All of the risk stratification scoring systems classify mechanical valves as high risk during pregnancy.[15–18] Most of the complications involve anticoagulation of the mechanical valve. Women with mechanical valves are at a higher risk of thrombosis during pregnancy and require adequate anticoagulation. Warfarin is the most reliable form of anticoagulation to prevent valve thrombus in women but has the highest risk of fetal malformations and miscarriage. The rate of fetal malformations seems to be dose dependent. Patients on less than 5 mg daily have fewer neonatal adverse events. Low-molecular-weight heparin dosing is less reliable during pregnancy and needs to be based off of factor Xa levels.[10] ROPAC reviewed 134 women with mechanical valves.[23] The maternal mortality was 1.5%, which was significantly higher than patients without prosthetic valves. Although 58% of women with mechanical valves had an uneventful pregnancy, 4% of women had a valve thrombosis during the first trimester when they were being transitioned off warfarin to heparin or low-molecular-weight heparin. Almost a quarter of patients experienced a hemorrhagic event. Warfarin during the first trimester showed higher rate of miscarriage.[23] If a woman is on warfarin during her third trimester, she should be transitioned to unfractionated heparin infusion before delivery. If there is preterm delivery while the woman is anticoagulated on warfarin, the neonate may need to be reversed with vitamin K or fresh frozen plasma. There still need to be better consensus recommendations on the safest anticoagulation for both mother and baby.[10]

Severe Left-Sided Obstructive Disease

Stenotic heart disease may not tolerate the hemodynamic changes of pregnancy as well as regurgitant valve disease. All of the risk stratification systems list severe left-sided obstructive disease as high risk or contraindicated for pregnancy.[15–18] ROPAC described almost 100 women with moderate-to-severe aortic valve disease.[24] Twenty percent of patients required hospitalization during pregnancy for cardiac concerns. Most women had severe aortic stenosis and 7% developed asymptomatic heart failure and another 26% developed symptomatic heart failure. They did not describe any mortality in this cohort.

Fontan Palliated Single Ventricles

Fontan palliated single ventricle patients are at high risk (mWHO Class III) during pregnancy.[17] These women were born with one hypoplastic ventricle and underwent multiple surgeries throughout early childhood to separate the systemic and pulmonary circulations. The Fontan procedure is in the final step in palliation. After the Fontan palliation, the systemic veins drain directly into the pulmonary arteries and the systemic ventricle pumps directly to the body.[25] Most women will survive into adulthood and reach childbearing age.[26] As adults, these women may develop recurrent heart failure, arrhythmias, increased risk for thromboembolic events, Fontan-associated liver disease, and cyanosis due to fenestrations or collateral vessels. Many women will need heart transplantation for long-term survival as an adult.[27]

Recently, there have been a few retrospective studies that look at both the maternal and neonatal outcomes in single ventricle patients. Caudwell and colleagues described the British experience including 54.8% miscarriage rate, one (1.9%) intrauterine death, 3.2% neonatal death, and only 42.7% live births.[28] Most of the live births were preterm and small for gestational age. Because Fontan palliated patients have a limited cardiac reserve, it is difficult for them to augment their cardiac output during pregnancy for adequate fetal growth.[29] Most common maternal complications were postpartum hemorrhage (42.6%), heart failure (13.5%), and arrhythmias (11.6%) in the British experience.[28] A larger multiinternational retrospective study investigated antithrombotic therapy in this population during pregnancy,[30] which was associated with high rates of bleeding (35%) and life treating bleeding (13%). The bleeding occurred both antepartum (45%) and post partum (42%). Aspirin and prophylactic heparin had lower rates of bleeding compared with other forms of anticoagulation. Garcia Ropero and colleagues have the largest systemic review of Fontan pregnancy.[31] They reviewed 255 pregnancies in 133 women. Pregnancy loss (69%) was the most common outcome of the pregnancy. They reported 8.4% supraventricular arrhythmias and 3.9% heart failure. Most of the infants were delivered preterm, only 20% of infants were small for gestational age, and there were 5% neonatal deaths. None of the recent retrospective studies or registries have looked at late outcomes of women and whether pregnancy decreases long-term transplant-free survival.

Pregnancy may expose women to more blood products and ultimately decrease their chance of qualifying for a heart transplantation.[32]

Although Fontan palliated patients are not contraindicated to proceed with pregnancy, it is important that these high-risk patients are managed in comprehensive adult congenital referral centers in combination with maternal fetal medicine.[33] If patients have residual shunts, they should have air filters on all intravenous lines, which prevent paradoxic embolus or stroke. Positive pressure ventilation should be avoided if possible because it decreases their preload and flow through the Fontan and Glenn baffles.[34] Wolfe and colleagues recommend monitoring women with Fontan palliation on pulse oximetry and telemetry. In the initial postpartum period, their group recommends monitoring in the cardiac intensive care unit for the first 24 hours after delivery and in the hospital for at least 72 hours.[33]

Systemic Right Ventricles

Systemic right ventricle patients have a morphologic right ventricle that pumps blood to the body. If these patients survive to childbearing age, they either have congenital corrected transposition of the great arteries or D-transposition of the great arteries that have undergone an atrial switch procedure as a child.[6] As systemic right ventricle patients age, they have higher rates of atrial arrhythmias, heart block, and systemic ventricular failure. The mWHO classification categorizes these patients as high risk but not contraindicated for pregnancy (mWHO III).[17] The ROPAC registry looked at systemic right ventricle including patients with transposition of the great arteries status after an atrial switch procedure and congenitally corrected transposition of the great arteries.[35] There was no mortality in these 162 women, but maternal morbidity included 9.8% heart failure, 3.1% atrial arrhythmias, and 3.7% ventricular tachycardia. Almost 50% of women required caesarean section. Neonatal outcomes included 20.9% prematurity and 17.8% small for gestational age and less than 1% fetal loss. Significant predictors of poor outcomes were systemic right ventricular systolic function less than 40% and clinical signs of heart failure. Similar to Fontan palliated patients, systemic right ventricles may eventually need a heart transplant, and pregnancy may expose these women to more blood products, making them poor transplant candidates in the future.

Pulmonary Arterial Hypertension Associated with Congenital Heart Disease

Severe pulmonary hypertension is a modified WHO classification IV and a contraindication for pregnancy.[17] In the past, mortality in this population was reported to be very high, between 30% and 56%. Most demonstrate progressive right heart failure.[36] Newer data are more promising. Ladouceur and colleagues reported the French cohort of 28 pregnancies, which reported lower (5%) maternal mortality, but most of the infants were delivered preterm (78%) by caesarean section (67%).[37] Li and colleagues described 93 women with pulmonary hypertension related to CHD. Similar to the French study there was a reality low mortality of only 6% but 35% experienced heart failure and 11% had a pulmonary hypertensive crisis.[38] About half of the patients in this cohort were on medications to treat pulmonary hypertension. The largest study is from the ROPAC registry, which demonstrated 3% mortality, and death could occur up to a week post partum.[39] Similar to the cyanotic Fontan palliated patient, if the patient has an intravenous line, he/she should have air filters to prevent paradoxic embolus.[34]

Aortic Dilation

CARPREG II and mWHO classify severe aortic dilation as high-risk lesion, and pregnancy may be contraindicated depending on the size.[16,17] Aortic dilation that falls into mWHO classification IV is seen in Marfan patients with aorta greater than 4.5 cm and bicuspid aortic valve patient with aorta size greater than 5.0 cm. In 2021, ROPAC described almost 200 women with thoracic aortic disease including patients with Marfan syndrome, bicuspid aortic valve, Turner syndrome, and vascular Ehlers-Danlos syndrome.[40] Only 4 patients (2%) had aortic dissection during pregnancy and 3 patients had Marfan syndrome. There was a high cesarean section rate of 63%. Imaging of the aorta with regional medical imaging or computed tomography scan is recommended before pregnancy.

SUMMARY

Women with CHD should be evaluated and cared during pregnancy in an ACHD referral center in collaboration with maternal fetal medicine to try to optimize care for both mother and baby. Most women with CHD will do well during pregnancy without significant cardiac or neonatal complications. High-risk types of CHD increase a woman's risk for preterm delivery, intrauterine growth restriction, arrhythmias, heart failure. and rarely death. Before pregnancy, a woman's medications should be evaluated to make sure they are not contraindicated in pregnancy and discuss a weaning plan if needed. A woman should be offered genetic counseling before pregnancy to discuss the risk that her infant will have CHD. Fetal echocardiograms during the second trimester and pulse oximetry screening for critical CHD should help identify infants with CHD before discharge from the nursery.

Best Practices

Women with congenital heart disease who become pregnant have a higher risk of obstetric and newborn morbidities. Preconceptual counseling and risk stratification is imperative, and a multidisciplinary treatment plan during the pregnancy can improve obstetric, neonatal and maternal outcomes.

REFERENCES

1. Gilboa SM, Devine OJ, Kucik JE, et al. Congenital heart defects in the United States: estimating the magnitude of the affect population in 2010. Circulation 2016;134(2):101–9.
2. Canobbio MM, Warnes CA, Aboulhosn J, et al. Management of pregnancy in patients with complex congenital heart disease: a scientific statement for healthcare professionals from the American Heart Association. Circulation 2017;135:e50–87.
3. Bhatt AB, DeFaria Yeh D. Pregnancy and adult congenital heart disease. Cardiol Clin 2015;33(4):611–23.
4. Salam AM, Ertekin E, van Hagen IM, et al. Atrial fibrillation or flutter during pregnancy in patients with structural heart disease: data from the ROPAC (Registry on Pregnancy and Cardiac Disease). JACC Clin Electrophysiol 2015;1(4):284–92.
5. Ertekin E, van Hagen IM, Salam AM, et al. Ventricular tachyarrhythmia during pregnancy in women with heart disease: data from the ROPAC, a registry from the European Society of Cardiology. Int J Cardiol 2016;220:131–6.
6. Stout KK, Daniels CJ, Aboulhosn JA, et al. 2018 AHA/ACC Guideline for management of adults with congenital heart disease: executive summary. Circulation 2019;139:e637–97.

7. Ruys TPE, Maggioni A, Johnson MR, et al. Cardiac medication during pregnancy, data from ROPAC. Int J Cardiol 2014;177(1):124–8.

8. Rolnik DL, Nicolaides KH, Poon LC. Prevention of preeclampsia with aspirin. Am J Obstet Gynecol 2020. S0002-9378(20)30873-5.

9. Battarbee AN, Sinkey RG, Harper LM, et al. Chronic hypertension in pregnancy. Am J Obstet Gynecol 2020;222(6):532–41.

10. Nishimura RA, Warnes CA. Anticoagulation during pregnancy in women with prosthetic valves: evidence, guidelines and unanswered questions. Heart 2015; 101:430–5.

11. Sachdeva R, Valente AM, Armstrong AK, et al. ACC/AHA/ASE/HRS/ISACHD/ SCAI/SCCT/SCMR/SOPE 2020 Appropriate use criteria for multimodality imaging during the follow up care of patients with congenital heart disease: a report of the American College of Cardiology solution set oversight committee and appropriate use criteria task force, American heart association, American society of echocardiography, Heart rhythm society, International Society for Adult Congenital Heart Disease, Society of cardiovascular angiography and interventions, Society of cardiovascular computed tomography, Society for cardiovascular magnetic resonance, and society of pediatric echocardiography. J Am Coll Cardiol 2020;75(6):657–703.

12. Pierpont ME, Brueckner M, Chung WK, et al. Genetic basis for congenital heart disease revisited. A scientific statement from the American Heart Association. Circulation 2018;138:e653–711.

13. Chitra N, Vijayalakshmi IB. Fetal echocardiography for early detection of congenital heart diseases. J Echocardiogr 2017;15:13–7.

14. Martin GR, Ewer AW, Gaviglio A, et al. Updated Strategies for pulse oximetry screening for critical congenital heart disease. Pediatrics 2020;146:1–10.

15. Sui SC, Sermer M, Colman JM, et al. Prospective multicenter study of pregnancy outcomes in women with cardiac disease. Circulation 2001;104(5):515–21.

16. Silversides CK, Grewal J, Mason J, et al. Pregnancy outcomes in women with heart disease. The CARPREG II Study. J Am Coll Cardiol 2018;71(21):2419–30.

17. Thorne S, MacGregor A, Nelson-Piercy C. Risks of contraception and pregnancy in heart disease. Heart 2006;92(10):1520–5.

18. Drenthen W, Boersma E, Balci A, et al. Predictors of pregnancy complications in women with congenital heart disease. Eur Heart J 2010;31(17):2124–32.

19. Kim YY, Goldberg LA, Awh K, et al. Accuracy of risk prediction scores in pregnant women with congenital heart disease. Congenit Heart Dis 2019;14(3):470–8.

20. Balci A, Sollie-Szarynska KM, van der Bijl AG, et al. Prospective validation and assessment of cardiovascular and offspring risk models for pregnant women with congenital heart disease. Heart 2014;100(17):1373–81.

21. Krieger EV, Stout KK. Progress: the ROPAC multinational registry advances our understanding of an important outcome in pregnant women with heart disease. Heart 2014;100(3):188–9.

22. Roos-Hesselink J, Baris L, Johnson M, et al. Pregnancy outcomes in women with cardiovascular disease: evolving trends over 10 years in the ESC Registry of pregnancy and cardiac disease (ROPAC). Eur Heart J 2019;40(47):3848–55.

23. Van Hagen IM, Roos-Hesselink JW, Ruys TP, et al. Pregnancy in women with a mechanical heart valve: data of the European society of Cardiology registry of pregnancy and cardiac disease (ROPAC). Circulation 2015;132(2):132–42.

24. Orwat S, Diller GP, van Hagen IM, et al. Risk of pregnancy in moderate and severe aortic stenosis: from the multinational ROPAC registry. J Am Coll Cardiol 2016;68(16):1727–37.

25. Rychik J, Atz AM, Celermajer DS, et al. Evaluation and management of child and adult with Fontan circulation: a scientific statement from the American heart association. Circulation 2019;140(6):e234–84.
26. D'Udekem Y, Iyengar AJ, Galati JC, et al. Redefining expectations of long-term survival after the Fontan procedure: twenty-five years of follow-up from the entire population of Australia and New Zealand. Circulation 2014;130(11 Suppl1): S32–8.
27. Book WM, Gerardin J, Saraf A, et al. Clinical phenotypes of fontan failure: implications for management. Congenit Heart Dis 2016;11(4):296–308.
28. Cauldwell M, Steer PJ, Bonner S, et al. Retrospective UK multicenter study of the pregnancy outcomes of women with a Fontan repair. Heart 2018;104(5):401–6.
29. Afshar Y, Tan W, Jones WM, et al. Maternal Fontan procedure for gestational- age neonate: a 10-year retrospective study. Am J Obstet Gynecol 2019;1(3):100036.
30. Ginnius A, Zentner D, Valente AM, et al. Bleeding and thrombotic risk in pregnant women with Fontan physiology. Heart 2020;107(17):1390–7.
31. Garcia Ropero A, Baskar S, Roos Hasselink JW, et al. Pregnancy in women with a fontan circulation: a systemic review of literature. Circ Cardiovasc Qual Outcomes 2018;11(5):e004575.
32. Stout KK, Broberg CS, Book WM, et al. Chronic heart failure in congenital heart disese. A scientific statement from the American Heart Association. Circulation 2016;133:770–801.
33. Wolfe NK, Sabol BA, Kelly JC, et al. Management of Fontan circulation in pregnancy: a multidisciplinary approach to care. Am J Obstet Gynecol 2021;3(1): 100257.
34. Gerardin JF, Earing MG. Preoperative evaluation of adult congenital heart disease for non-cardiac surgery. Curr Cardiol Rep 2018;20(9):76.
35. Tutarel O, Baris L, Budts W, et al. Pregnancy outcomes in women with a systemic right ventricle and transposition of the great arteries results from the ESC-EORP Registry of Pregnancy and Cardiac disease (ROPAC). Heart 2021;0:1–7.
36. Ntiloudi D, Giannakoulas G. Pregnancy still contraindicated in pulmonary arterial hypertension related to congenital heart disease: true or False? Eur J Prev Cardiol 2019;26(10):1064–9.
37. Ladouceur M, Benoit L, Radojevic J, et al. Pregnancy outcomes in patients with pulmonary arterial hypertension associated with congenital heart disease. Heart 2017;103(4):287–92.
38. Li Q, Dimopoulos K, Liu T, et al. Peripartum outcomes in a large population of women with pulmonary hypertension associated with congenital heart disease. Eur J Prev Cardiol 2019;26(10):1067–76.
39. Sliwa K, van Hagen IM, Budts W, et al. Pulmonary hypertension and pregnancy outcomes: data from the pregnancy and cardiac disease (ROPAC) of the European society of Cardiology. Eur J Heart Fail 2016;18(9):1119–28.
40. Campens L, Baris L, Scott NS, et al. Pregnancy outcome in thoracic aortic disease data from Registry of pregnancy and cardiac disease. Heart 2021; 107(21):1704–9.

Advances in Understanding the Mechanism of Transitional Neonatal Hypoglycemia and Implications for Management

Diana L. Stanescu, MD, Charles A. Stanley, MD*

KEYWORDS

- Hyperinsulinism • Transitional hypoglycemia • High-risk newborn • KATP channel
- Hypoxia inducible factor • Congenital hyperinsulinism • Pancreatic islets

KEY POINTS

- Transitional neonatal hypoglycemia is a form of hyperinsulinism
- Fetal/early neonatal hyperinsulinism is caused by a lowering of the glucose threshold for insulin release
- The low fetal/early neonatal glucose threshold is caused by decreased trafficking of KATP channels to the surface of the beta-cell plasma membrane
- The hypoxic environment of fetal life is a signal controlling decreased KATP channel trafficking
- Knowledge of the mechanisms of transitional hypoglycemia in normal and persistent hypoglycemia in high-risk newborns provides an important basis for improving management of all forms of neonatal hypoglycemia

INTRODUCTION

"Everybody talks about the weather, but nobody ever does anything about it." Charles Dudley Warner (often misattributed to Mark Twain)

Controversies About Neonatal Hypoglycemia

In a 1973 state-of-the-art review on hypoglycemia in children, endocrinology experts from Washington University School of Medicine in St Louis, MO, USA (1) observed that

Division of Endocrinology, Department of Pediatrics, The Childrens Hospital of Philadelphia, University of Pennsylvania Perelman School of Medicine, 34th Street & Civic Center Boulevard, Philadelphia, PA 19104, USA
* Corresponding author.
E-mail address: stanleyc@chop.edu

Clin Perinatol 49 (2022) 55–72
https://doi.org/10.1016/j.clp.2021.11.007
0095-5108/22/© 2021 Elsevier Inc. All rights reserved.
perinatology.theclinics.com

the mechanisms responsible for transient hypoglycemia in normal newborns were unknown, (2) observed that there was no a priori reason to assume that glucose-dependent tissues (such as the brain) were "more tolerant of low glucose supply than those of the adult," and (3) recommended that it should be appropriate to use the same standards for treatment of hypoglycemia in neonates as in older children.[1] These observations generated vociferous objections from international experts in neonatology who (1) countered that the current neonatal practice was to consider as hypoglycemia only plasma glucose levels less than 35 mg/dL in normal-birth-weight newborns or less than 25 mg/dL in low-birth-weight infants, (2) countered that these values had a scientific basis in statistical surveys of normal- and low-birth-weight newborns, and (3) expressed concern that using higher glucose levels to define hypoglycemia would expose vast numbers of neonates to risks of unnecessary interventions.[2,3]

This controversy about neonatal hypoglycemia has continued to frustrate both sides down to the present with little change.[4–6] In part, this reflects obvious differences in viewpoint between specialists, caring for small groups of babies at very high risk of hypoglycemic brain damage from rare congenital disorders, and neonatologists, responsible for large numbers of mostly low-risk newborn babies. An additional frequently expressed concern is the potential for excessive risks to practitioners from medicolegal suits.[5] However, at the root of the controversy has been our continued dearth of knowledge about the underlying mechanisms of neonatal hypoglycemia, especially in normal newborns, and also in high-risk groups, such as babies with birth asphyxia or intrauterine growth retardation. Rather than rehashing fruitless arguments about numerical "definitions" of neonatal hypoglycemia, this report outlines our current understanding of the physiologic and pathophysiological mechanisms of neonatal hypoglycemia, including both the common transitional hypoglycemia of normal newborns and the less frequent, but important, persistent hypoglycemia seen in high-risk groups (**Fig. 1**). Our review focuses on emerging information about the central role of pancreatic islet insulin regulation in the fetal-newborn transition, the possibility of shared mechanisms between transitional and persistent forms of neonatal hypoglycemia, as well as implications for important future improvements in management and treatment.

"Defining" NEONATAL HYPOGLYCEMIA: THE NUMERICAL ALBATROSS AROUND OUR NECKS

"There are three kinds of lies: lies, damned lies, and statistics." Source unknown (often misattributed to Mark Twain)

As noted above, controversy about neonatal hypoglycemia originated around the so-called statistical definition of hypoglycemia, representing the mean minus 2 SD of glucose values in newborns during the first days following birth: plasma glucose levels less than 35 mg/dL in normal infants and less than 25 mg/dL in low-birth-weight infants. The use of such a statistical definition has been soundly criticized for, among other things, not being equivalent to "physiologically normal" and, therefore, was replaced about 2 decades ago with a so-called operational definition of neonatal hypoglycemia, glucose levels less than 47 mg/dL.[7] However, as pointed out in the Endocrinology Society hypoglycemia guidelines for adults, no single plasma glucose value can be used to "define" a glucose concentration value that causes symptoms or brain damage, because the thresholds for hypoglycemia symptoms due to neuroendocrine responses and cognitive impairment due to neuroglycopenia occur across a range of plasma glucose levels (**Fig. 2**).[8,9] Moreover, the glucose

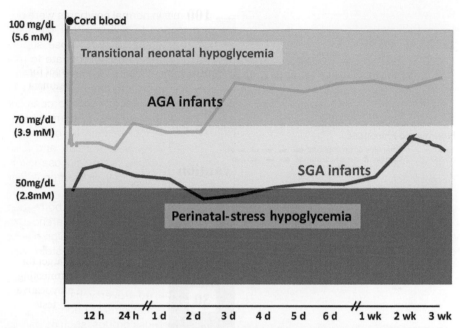

Fig. 1. Mean plasma glucose levels after birth. Mean plasma glucose from 206 determinations in 179 full-sized infants (appropriate for gestational age (AGA)) and from 442 determinations in 104 low-birth-weight infants ("SGA") between birth and 28 days of life. Note discontinuous timescale. Cord blood levels are similar to maternal glucose levels. Mean glucose levels in AGA infants fall into range for neurogenic symptoms during first 2 days and then increase into normal range of older children and adults; mean glucose levels become lower in SGA infants and remain low for several weeks. Colored areas as in **Fig. 2**. (*Adapted from* Cornblath M, Reisner SH. Blood glucose in the neonate and its clinical significance. N Engl J Med 1965;273(7):378-81).

thresholds for neuroendocrine responses to hypoglycemia are subject to modification by changes in availability of alternative brain fuels (especially the ketones beta-hydroxybutyrate [BOHB] and acetoacetate) as well as blunted by previous episodes of hypoglycemia (hypoglycemia-associated autonomic failure).[10]

An alternative approach that has become popular among neonatologists is to attempt to "define" neonatal hypoglycemia based on studies associating neonatal plasma glucose levels with long-term neurodevelopmental outcomes. Several such studies have recently been reported, but all share obvious limitations, including being merely association studies that cannot be linked to specific episodes or specific glucose concentrations in the newborn period and the fact that the ability to detect neurodevelopmental deficits changes with age of assessment.[11,12]

It has been argued that detection of symptoms of hypoglycemia in newborn infants is too difficult/impossible for assessing glucose thresholds for symptoms in the manner used in adults and older children, illustrated in **Fig. 2**. Attempts to bypass this using various technologies in newborns (eg, by electroencephalographic monitoring) have proven unsuccessful.[13] On the other hand, observations in hypoglycemic newborns suggest that it might be possible to develop methods to acutely relate plasma glucose levels to changes in newborn behavior similar to the methods used to examine responses to induced hypoglycemia in adults. One example is the

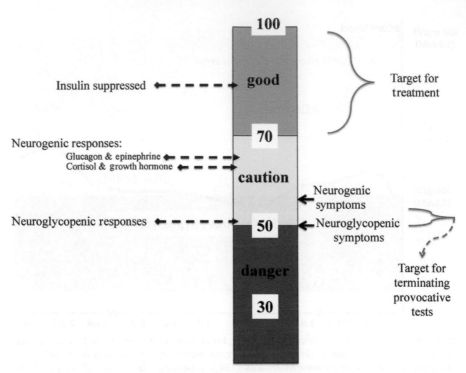

Fig. 2. Interpreting glucose levels and glucose treatment targets. Glucose thresholds are shown for suppression of insulin secretion, neurogenic (neuroendocrine hormone-mediated) responses, and neuroglycopenic (impaired cognition) responses. Colors show normal range (*green*), range for symptoms due to activation of sympathetic nervous system (*yellow*), and range for impaired neuronal function (*red*).[8]

comment by the authors of a study of glycemic responses to epinephrine injection in 1- to 2-day-old newborns in 1954 that following the increase in plasma glucose levels from 40 to 50 up to 70 to 100 mg/dL, the babies appeared more "comfortable, relaxed, stopped crying, and fell asleep."[14]

DISCRIMINATING THE ETIOLOGY OF HYPOGLYCEMIA IN NEONATES
Transitional hypoglycemia in normal newborns, persistent hypoglycemia in high-risk newborns, genetic hypoglycemia disorders

Before the publication of the 1973 review of pediatric hypoglycemia disorders described in the Introduction section, the field of pediatric hypoglycemia disorders had been dominated by "Idiopathic Hypoglycemia of Infancy," a pseudo-diagnostic category described by MacQuarrie[15] in 1954. By 1973, experience with the growing number of possible hypoglycemia disorders in infants and children had demonstrated the importance of defining the underlying mechanism for hypoglycemia to determine the most appropriate specific method of treatment (pharmacologic, surgical, nutritional, etc.).[1] The method that has been proved to be most useful for identifying the mechanism of hypoglycemia has been an evaluation of the metabolic and hormone responses to fasting (**Fig. 3**).[6] When this "fasting systems" approach has been applied to newborns with persistent hypoglycemia associated with high-risk factors (birth asphyxia, IUGR, erythroblastosis fetalis, eclampsia or maternal hypertension,

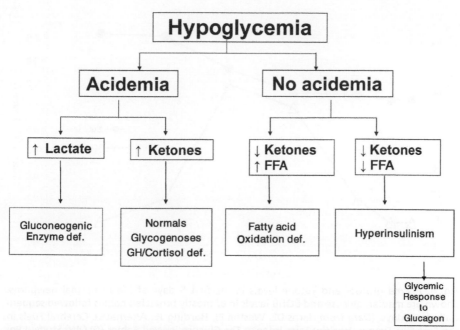

Fig. 3. Hypoglycemia diagnosis based on plasma metabolic fuel responses. Measurement of major fuels (lactate as a gluconeogenic substrate, FFA from adipose tissue lipolysis, and beta-hydroxybutyrate as the major ketone from hepatic ketogenesis) at the time of hypoglycemia segregates major groups of disorder: gluconeogenesis defects, ketotic hypoglycemia disorders, fatty acid oxidation defects, and hyperinsulinism or its mimickers. Supplemental glucagon stimulation test can support the diagnosis of hyperinsulinism. FFA, free fatty acids; GH/cortisol def, growth hormone and/or cortisol deficiency. (*Adapted from* Thornton PS, Stanley CA, De Leon DD, et al. Recommendations from the Pediatric Endocrine Society for Evaluation and Management of Persistent Hypoglycemia in Neonates, Infants, and Children. J Pediatr 2015;167(2):238–45.)

maternal diabetes), hyperinsulinism has been demonstrated to be the causative mechanism by features, including increased glucose utilization, inappropriate suppression of ketogenesis and lipolysis, and inappropriately large glycemic response to glucagon or epinephrine.[16,17] Two corollaries of this observation are (1) that the persistent form of neonatal hypoglycemia in high-risk infants can appropriately be termed perinatal stress-induced hyperinsulinism (or prolonged neonatal hyperinsulinism) and (2) that its treatment should be chosen to be specific for insulin-induced hypoglycemia (eg, diazoxide), rather than nonspecific, ineffective ones (eg, glucocorticoids).

In a similar manner, available evidence indicates that transitional hypoglycemia in normal newborns is also caused by hyperinsulinism, including suppressed ketogenesis and inappropriately large glycemic response to glucagon or epinephrine.[18] This transitional hyperinsulinism in normal newborns seems to reflect persistence of the fetal pattern of a lower glucose threshold for suppression of insulin release by pancreatic beta-cells, which is essential for maintaining fetal growth. The recent Glucose in Well Babies (GLOW) study from New Zealand showed that the transitional period of neonatal hypoglycemia was completed by the fourth day of life in normal, breast-fed infants.[19] As shown in **Fig. 4**, mean plasma glucose concentrations were 59 ± 11 mg/dL for the first 48 hours and then increased between 48 and 72 hours

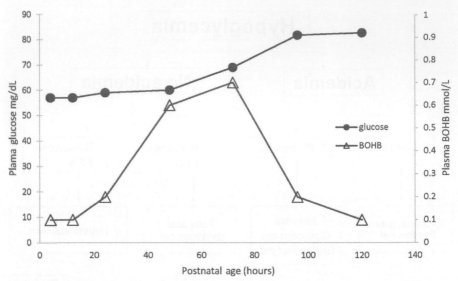

Fig. 4. Plasma glucose and ketone levels in the first 5 days of life in normal newborns. Shown are median glucose and BOHB levels in 67 mostly breastfed babies followed sequentially for 5 days. (*Data from* Harris DL, Weston PJ, Harding JE. Alternative Cerebral Fuels in the First Five Days in Healthy Term Infants: The Glucose in Well Babies (GLOW) Study. J Pediatr 2021;231:81-86).

to stabilize at 83 mg/dL (the same basal plasma glucose level of normal children and adults). A follow-up report of cerebral fuel levels in these GLOW study neonates showed that the period of transitional hypoglycemia actually consists of *2 phases*. In the first phase, plasma ketones (BOHB) were suppressed during the first 24 to 36 hours after birth (mean 0.1–0.2 mM); they then increased during the second phase between 36 and 72 hours (mean BOHB 0.7 mM at 72 hours) and finally declined again to basal levels by 96 to 120 hours (mean 0.2–0.1 mM) once plasma glucose levels had reached 70 to 100 mg/dL, the normal range for extrauterine life.[20] During the first phase, the low plasma BOHB was unrelated to glucose levels, consistent with insulin-induced hypoglycemia, and confirmed that ketones do not compensate for low plasma glucose levels on the first 1 to 2 days of life. During the second phase, plasma BOHB was mildly increased even as plasma glucose levels increased and began to show a more normal inverse relationship to glucose, consistent with a ketotic form of hypoglycemia. Thus, in breast-fed newborns, transitional neonatal hypoglycemia is composed of 2 distinct phases: (1) the initial phase between birth and 48 hours represents hypoglycemia due to persistence of the fetal pattern of hyperinsulinism and (2) the second phase from 48 to 96 hours, in contrast, represents a mildly ketonemic fasting state, reflecting resolution of hyperinsulinism. The ongoing hypoglycemia in this phase likely reflects the nutrient-limited state of these breast-fed infants before maternal milk production has increased to fully meet the nutritional needs of the baby.

EVIDENCE THAT THE MECHANISM OF TRANSITIONAL NEONATAL HYPOGLYCEMIA (HYPERINSULINISM) IS A LOWER GLUCOSE THRESHOLD FOR PANCREATIC BETA-CELL INSULIN SECRETION

In their review of hypoglycemia disorders in children, in 1973, Pagliara and colleagues[21] speculated on the potential mechanisms for transitional hypoglycemia in normal newborns. The investigators focused chiefly on possible developmental delays in activity of hepatic enzymes of gluconeogenesis or glycogenolysis, most likely because these were the sites of most of the hypoglycemic disorders in children that were known at that time. However, as noted earlier, a review of available clinical evidence by the Pediatric Endocrine Society committee on hypoglycemia concluded that transitional hypoglycemia is a form of hyperinsulinism caused by a lower glucose threshold for glucose-stimulated insulin release in the fetus and immediate newborn period.[18] The following sections briefly review older descriptions of beta-cell function in the fetal/neonatal period but focus on our recent studies of isolated pancreatic islets from fetal and newborn rats, which demonstrate that hyperinsulinism is the cause of neonatal hypoglycemia and implicate impaired KATP channel trafficking in response to fetal hypoxemia as the underlying mechanism.

○ Previous studies of fetal and newborn insulin secretion have focused primarily on the observation that human and rodent fetal islets have increased insulin response to low concentrations of glucose, but have poor maximum insulin response to stimulation with high glucose concentrations.[22,23] The low glucose threshold for insulin secretion has been suggested to possibly reflect expression of genes normally "forbidden" from expression in beta-cells, such as hexokinase-1 or MCT1, linked to the process of beta-cell replication or differentiation.[22,24] The poor insulin response to high glucose of fetal islets has been suggested to reflect impairments in glycolysis,[25] the mitochondrial oxidation pathway,[26] or distal steps in calcium-mediated insulin release of fetal islets.[27] Owing to the lack of a specific target to explain the developmental changes in insulin regulation from these previous studies, we recently initiated studies described later to define the threshold for glucose-stimulated insulin secretion (GSIS) in the early postnatal period and determine the site of transition.

○ Recent studies of insulin regulation in the fetal-neonatal transition (Yang J, et al. Endocrinology, 2021[28]) state the following:

1. *The glucose threshold for GSIS is lower in fetal and newborn rats.*[28] Experiments were carried out using freshly isolated perfused islets from fetal and newborn rats to determine the threshold for GSIS using stepwise ramp stimulation with glucose levels from 0 to 25 mM (**Fig. 5**). Islets from embryos on the last day of gestation (E22) and pups on postnatal day P1 responded to the lowest concentration of glucose (3 mM) with insulin release nearly half of the maximal response to 25 mM glucose; this contrasts with mature islets from 2-week-old and adult rats, which released insulin only above a threshold of 5 mM glucose and a 4- to 5-fold greater response at 25 mM glucose. The glucose threshold for insulin release increased steadily over the first week of life, closely paralleling the time course of hypoglycemia in early postnatal rat pups from days P1 through P7. This is consistent with the important role of the threshold for GSIS in determining the concentration of glucose in the circulation.

2. The low glucose threshold of fetal and neonatal islets reflects differences in the pathway of insulin secretion distal to glycolysis at the level of the beta-cell KATP channel.[28] To localize the site in the pathway of GSIS responsible for the low glucose threshold in fetal and early neonatal rats, experiments were carried out comparing P1 and P14 islet thresholds for amino acid stimulation of insulin secretion via oxidation of glutamate by the mitochondrial enzyme glutamate dehydrogenase (GDH) (**Fig. 6**). Compared with mature P14 islets, P1 islets had a lower threshold for stimulation of insulin secretion

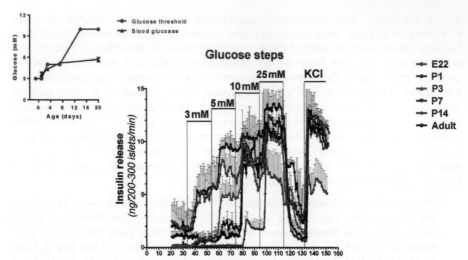

Fig. 5. Developmental shift in glucose threshold for insulin release in fetal and early neonatal rats. Freshly isolated islets were perfused with a stepwise ramp stimulation by glucose from 3 to 25 mM, followed by maximal insulin release with KCl. Glucose thresholds were defined by the lowest glucose concentration stimulating insulin release greater than baseline release by glucose-free perfusion. Shown are rates of insulin release (mean ± standard deviation of 3–4 replicate experiments). The inset compares the time course of changes in mean plasma glucose concentration and mean glucose threshold for islet insulin release. (*Adapted from* Yang J, Hammoud B, Li C, et al. Decreased KATP channel activity contributes to the low glucose threshold for insulin secretion of rat neonatal islets. Endocrinology 2021.)

by BCH, a nonmetabolizable allosteric activator of GDH oxidation of glutamate (1 mM vs 3 mM); this indicates that the lower glucose threshold for insulin release in fetal/neonatal islets is determined at a site downstream of glycolysis and distal to mitochondrial ATP generation.

    To further localize the site of the low threshold for glucose-stimulated insulin release in early neonatal islets, we examined the response of insulin secretion to the insulin secretagogue, tolbutamide, an inhibitor of KATP channel activity (see **Fig. 6**). Compared with P14 islets, islets from P1 mice showed markedly lower insulin responses at all concentrations of tolbutamide, even though insulin responses to maximum depolarization with KCl were similar. This impairment in KATP channel function suggested either that KATP channel activity was reduced in P1 islets or that the number of channels on the surface of the beta-cell plasma membrane may be smaller in P1 islets than in P14 islets.

3. The low glucose threshold for stimulation of insulin secretion in the fetal and early neonatal period is caused by reduced trafficking of KATP channels to the surface of the beta-cell plasma membrane.[28] Single dispersed beta-cells were used to measure the density of glyburide-sensitive K^+ channels in P3 and P14 rats. The proportion of beta-cells with low glyburide-sensitive K^+ current was significantly greater in islets from P3 compared with P14 pups, indicating reduced density of KATP channels on the plasma membrane (**Fig. 7**). The pathway of KATP channel trafficking from the Golgi to the plasma membrane surface is diagrammed in **Fig. 8**. Previous reports have shown that

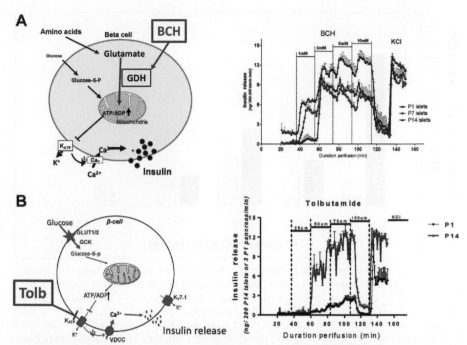

Fig. 6. Developmental shift in insulin response to stimulation of insulin secretion by GDH and tolbutamide. (*A*) Lower threshold for insulin release in response to BCH in early neonatal rat islets implies control site is distal to mitochondrial ATP production. Shown are insulin responses of freshly isolated islets to stepwise ramp stimulation of GDH (glutamate dehydrogenase) by the leucine analog, BCH (mean ± SD of 3–4 replicate experiments). The threshold for response to BCH increases from 1 mM on P1 up to 3 mM on P14. (*B*) Impaired insulin response to inhibition of KATP channel by tolbutamide ramp in P1 versus P14 islets. (*Adapted from* Yang J, Hammoud B, Li C, et al. Decreased KATP channel activity contrlbutes to the low glucose threshold for insulin secretion of rat neonatal islets. Endocrinology 2021.)

activation of this trafficking pathway to increase KATP channels on the plasma membrane surface by leptin or low glucose decreases insulin secretion.[29,30] In contrast, inhibition of trafficking in the PHPT1 knockout mouse model causes severe neonatal hyperinsulinemic hypoglycemia.[31]

The consequence of reduced KATP channels on the surface of beta-cell plasma membrane is a flattening of the insulin-glucose response curve (**Fig. 9**). In normal control humans, insulin secretion rapidly increases as plasma glucose levels are increased. Patients with monogenic diabetes type 2 (MODY2) due to heterozygous inactivating mutations of GCK (glucokinase, the beta-cell glucose sensor) have an increased glucose threshold for insulin secretion and a rightward shift in the insulin-glucose response curve; this results in mild baseline hyperglycemia, but a normal maximum capacity for insulin release. In contrast, patients with MODY1, due to inactivating mutations of the HNF4A transcription factor, show flattening of the insulin-glucose response; this leads to hyperinsulinism in early infancy and then to diabetes in early adulthood.[32] Recent findings indicate that beta-cells in these patients

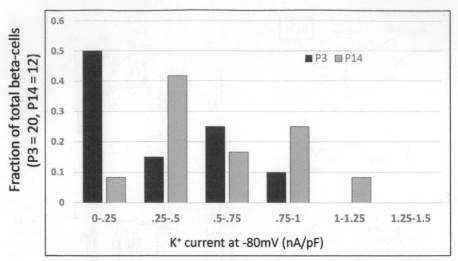

Fig. 7. Lower plasma membrane surface KATP channels in P3 versus P14 beta-cells. Glyburide-sensitive KATP channel K+ currents were measured in patch-clamped dispersed beta-cells (n = 20 P3 cells, n = 12 P14 cells). Plotted is the distribution of cells with different ranges of K+ currents (Mann-Whitney test comparing 2 groups: P3 versus P14: *P* = .032). (*Adapted from* Yang J, Hammoud B, Li C, et al. Decreased KATP channel activity contributes to the low glucose threshold for insulin secretion of rat neonatal islets. Endocrinology 2021.)

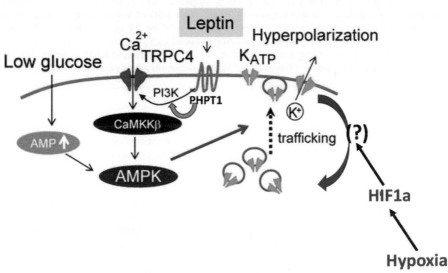

Fig. 8. Modulation of GSIS by altered KATP channel trafficking to beta-cell membrane surface. Leptin or low glucose increases the threshold for GSIS by increasing KATP channel trafficking (Park, PNAS 2013; Shyng, JBC 2013). Inhibition of the pathway of leptin-stimulated KATP channel trafficking in PHPT1-KO mice impairs KATP channel trafficking leading to severe neonatal hyperinsulinism (Srivastava, Diabetes 2018). Hypoxia, via HIF1a, also impairs KATP channel trafficking at an unknown step to cause lowering of glucose threshold for GSIS in the fetal and early neonatal periods.

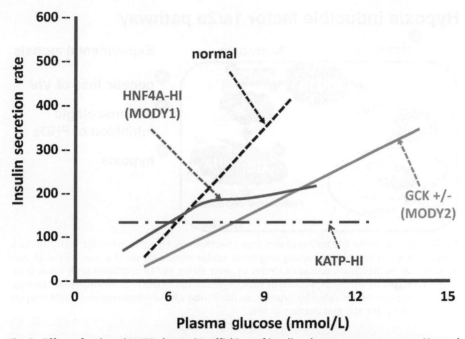

Fig. 9. Effect of reduced KATP channel trafficking of insulin-glucose response curve. Normal humans show a rapid increase in insulin secretion as plasma glucose increases (*black*); carriers of glucokinase-inactivating mutations (MODY2) have a right-shifted curve with high basal glucose but near-normal maximum response to high glucose (*green*); carriers of inactivating mutations of HNF4A and impaired KATP channel gene expression show flatter insulin-glucose response curve leading to hyperinsulinemic-hypoglycemia in early infancy, but diabetes in early adult life (*blue*); absence of KATP channels in infants with KATP-HI further flattens the insulin-glucose response curve and severe baseline hypoglycemia, as well as impaired glucose tolerance (*red*). (*Modified from* Polonsky KS. Lilly Lecture 1994. The beta-cell in diabetes: from molecular genetics to clinical research. Diabetes 1995;44(6):705–17.)

have decreased expression of the 2 channel subunits and reduced levels of KATP channels.[33] In parallel, patients with KATP-HI (KATP form of Hyperinsulinism) due to genetic mutations causing complete inactivation of KATP channels have more severe flattening of the insulin-glucose response curve, resulting in severe hyperinsulinism at birth.[34] These patients also manifest glucose intolerance later in adolescence or adult life. Our finding of reduced KATP channel trafficking in fetal and early neonatal rat beta-cells is, thus, consistent with previous observations that fetal beta-cells respond to low concentrations of glucose, but have limited responsiveness to high glucose levels (cf. the insulin-glucose response profiles of E22 versus adult islets shown in **Fig 5**).

4. Hypoxia may be the signal for reduced KATP channel trafficking in fetal beta-cells leading to transitional and perinatal-stress-induced hyperinsulinism in newborn infants.

Hypoxia is an obvious potential signal controlling the low glucose threshold for GSIS in fetal/neonatal beta-cells: the fetus is in a hypoxic environment before delivery and perinatal hypoxia is the major factor causing perinatal-stress-induced hyperinsulinism.

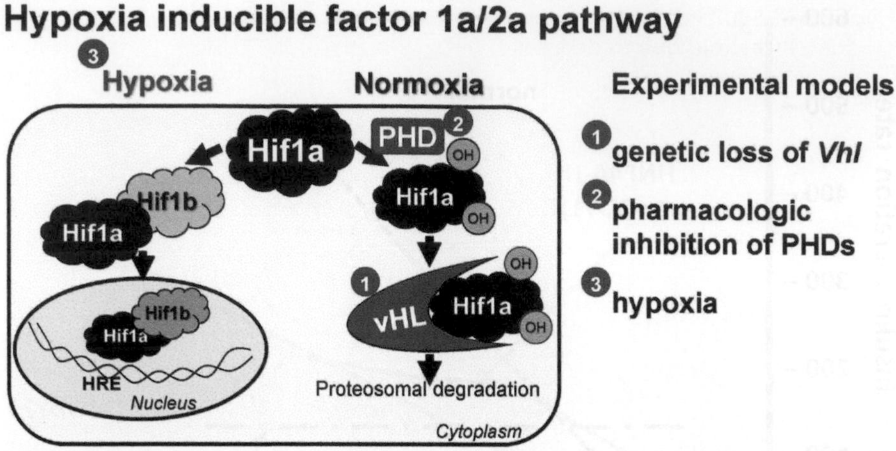

Hypoxia inducible factor 1a/2a pathway

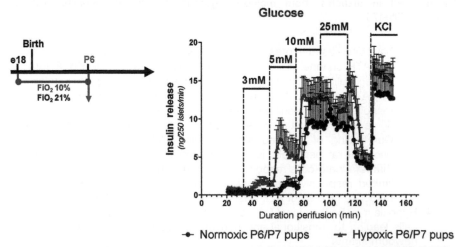

Fig. 10. Hypoxia inducible pathway and sites of activation. Hypoxia inducible factor HIF1a is constitutively expressed but rapidly degraded under normoxia via the von Hippel-Lindau proteosomal degradation pathway. Under hypoxic stress, HIF1a combines with other transcription factors to induce expression of various mediators of the hypoxic response. The hypoxia response can be activated by hypoxia, by inhibition of prolyl hydroxylases (PHD) enzyme activity, and by genetic inactivation of vHL.

The effects of hypoxia are signaled by the hypoxia inducible factor 1a (HIF1), a constitutively expressed transcription factor whose level is suppressed under normoxic conditions by rapid degradation via prolyl hydroxylation and the von Hippel-Lindau (vHL) ubiquitination pathway (**Fig. 10**). The downstream effects of HIF1a can be induced by several methods: a hypoxic environment, inhibitors of prolyl hydroxylase, or genetic

Fig. 11. Hypoxia in the perinatal period causes persistence of fetal low glucose threshold for insulin release. Exposure to hypoxia from E18 to P6 lowers the glucose threshold for GSIS in freshly isolated islets from P6/P7 newborn rat pups. (*Data from* Yang J, Hammoud B, Ridler A, et al. Postnatal activation of hypoxia pathway disrupts β-cell functional maturation.)

Hypoxia in adult islets: Culturing islets for 24 or 48 hrs leads to a decrease in glucose threshold due to decrease in KATP-channel trafficking

A   B

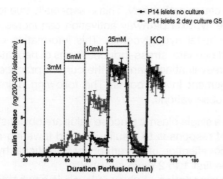

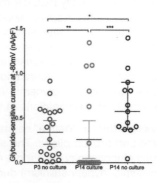

Fig. 12. Hypoxia in adult islets lowers the glucose threshold for GSIS. Culturing isolated islets from adult rats for 24 or 48 hours leads to a decrease in glucose threshold due to decrease in KATP channel trafficking. * is p = 0.032 ** is p = 0.01 *** is p = 0.003. (*Data from* Yang J, Hammoud B, Ridler A, et al. Postnatal activation of hypoxia pathway disrupts β-cell functional maturation.)

ablation of vHL. As shown in **Fig. 11**, islets from mouse pups exposed to a low-oxygen environment in utero from embryonic day E18 and after delivery through P6 have a lower glucose threshold compared with control normoxic P6 islets. Similarly, as shown in **Fig. 12**, mature P14 islets cultured for 24 to 48 hours, presumed to have hypoxic interiors due to lack of blood flow, also have a lower threshold for GSIS and markedly increased proportion of beta-cells with reduced trafficking of KATP channels.[35] Simulation of HIF1 pathway by a prolyl hydroxylase inhibitor also lowers the glucose threshold for GSIS in neonatal rats (data not shown). In addition, it has been reported that constitutive activation of HIF1A in mice with knockout of vHL results in lethal postnatal hypoglycemia.[36] The precise mechanism by which hypoxia regulates surface expression of beta-cell KATP channels requires further study. However, these observations indicate that hypoxia activation of the HIF1A pathway causes a lower threshold for GSIS, potentially through decreased KATP channel trafficking, in both newborns with transitional neonatal hypoglycemia and in those with perinatal stress-induced hyperinsulinism, as well as in mature adult pancreatic beta-cells.

SUMMARY AND IMPLICATIONS FOR IMPROVING MANAGEMENT OF NEONATAL HYPOGLYCEMIA

The results of the aforementioned studies of isolated fetal and neonatal rat islets confirm the conclusion of the Pediatric Endocrine Society Committee on Hypoglycemia, based on clinical observations, and demonstrate that the prime mover in transitional hypoglycemia in normal newborns and in persistent hypoglycemia in high-risk newborns is the pancreatic beta-cell. Studies of isolated rat islets indicate that the threshold for GSIS is lower in the fetus and early neonatal period, leading to a transitional period of hyperinsulinemic hypoglycemia. Based on results of the recent GLOW study, this seems to last for the first 24 to 48 hours after birth in normal newborns. The mechanism underlying this lower glucose threshold seems to be decreased trafficking of KATP channels to the plasma membrane surface of beta-cells, which is signaled, at least in part, by the hypoxic conditions of fetal life. This is likely a positive adaptation for the fetus that ensures secretion of adequate insulin secretion to maintain growth. However, it is potentially maladaptive after birth if the degree of postnatal hyperinsulinemic hypoglycemia is severe enough to cause brain injury. This is especially true for cases with various perinatal stress, where hypoxia pathway activation can increase both the severity and persistence of postnatal hypoglycemia. This information on the mechanism of both the transitional and perinatal stress-induced forms of neonatal hypoglycemia provides a foundation for reevaluating many of the current practices and guidelines for hypoglycemia management in newborns. The following points outline some of the implications of these observations.

1. Previous efforts to "define" neonatal as a single plasma glucose value are obviously flawed and too simplistic. The scale of responses to insulin-induced lowering of plasma glucose may be a more realistic reflection of the effects of transitional hypoglycemia (hyperinsulinism) during the first 1 to 2 days after birth.
2. Multiple factors should influence the interpretation of glucose levels in newborns, including plasma levels of ketones, postnatal age, physical findings (eg, small for gestational age (SGA), large for gestational age (LGA), Beckwith-Wiedemann features), family history of hypoglycemia/diabetes, etc. For example, low plasma glucose levels with low ketones at 72 hours of age suggests the likelihood of a persistent hyperinsulinism disorder due to perinatal stress or a genetic form of congenital hyperinsulinism. In contrast, low plasma glucose with elevated levels of ketones at 72 hours of age in a breast-fed infant suggests maternal milk production may be not yet sufficient.
3. Because the cause of transitional neonatal hypoglycemia clearly resides in the beta-cell, it seems unlikely that, as noted by Pagliara and colleagues[1] in 1973, other glucose-dependent tissues of the fetus and newborn infant, including the brain, would be more tolerant to low glucose supply than those of older children and adults. The risk of brain injury due to hypoglycemia is especially high in hyperinsulinism, because the capacity to provide ketones as an alternative fuel for the brain is blocked. The common assumption that ketones can compensate for low glucose levels in newborns, quoted in the American Academy of Pediatrics neonatal guideline,[5] should be abandoned in view of both the present demonstration of transitional hyperinsulinism and the results of the GLOW study showing that ketones remain suppressed during hypoglycemia in the first 24 to 36 hours after birth in normal newborns; ketones remain suppressed for longer in neonates with perinatal stress hyperinsulinism and congenital hyperinsulinism disorders.
4. The fact that hyperinsulinism underlies all 3 major causes of neonatal hypoglycemia, (transitional hypoglycemia, perinatal stress hyperinsulinism, and congenital hyperinsulinism) suggests that glucagon may be useful for both acute and short-term treatment of neonatal hypoglycemia. With the availability of newer stable preparations of glucagon, minidoses of glucagon might be an alternative for managing mild episodes of neonatal hypoglycemia to the recently introduced oral dextrose gel.[37,38]
5. As the period of transitional neonatal hyperinsulinism with hypoketonemia seems to be limited to the first 36 to 48 hours of life in normal newborns, routine bedside monitoring of plasma ketones in addition to plasma glucose may facilitate identification of infants likely to have a persistent hyperinsulinemic hypoglycemia disorder,

such as perinatal stress hyperinsulinism or congenital hyperinsulinism. Newborns with both low ketone and low glucose levels beyond 24 to 48 hours of age should be considered at very high risk of having a persistent hyperinsulinism disorder. In contrast, combined monitoring of glucose and ketones may make it possible to exclude these serious disorders as early as the second day of life and avoid unnecessary delays in discharge from the nursery.

Best Practices

WHAT IS THE CURRENT PRACTICE FOR TRANSITIONAL NEONATAL HYPOGLYCEMIA IN NORMAL NEWBORNS AND PERI-NATAL STRESS HYPERINSULINISM IN HIGH-RISK NEWBORNS? This report outlines recent evidence confirming that hyperinsulinemic hypoglycemia is the underlying cause of these common neonatal disorders, as well as, the rarer genetic disorders of insulin secretion.

BEST PRACTICE OBJECTIVE: The detection and management of hypoglycemia in normal, high-risk, and neonates with persistent hypoglycemia disorders. The two equally important goals are to (1) prevent potential seizures and/or permanent brain injury and to (2) identify infants with persistent hypoglycemia disorders prior to being discharged home.

WHAT CHANGES IN CURRENT PRACTICE ARE LIKELY TO IMPROVE OUTCOMES? Increased focus on detection of newborns with persistent forms of hypoglycemia prior to discharge is necessary to reduce their currently high risk of permanent brain injury and improve their long-term outcomes. IS THERE A CLINICAL ALGORITHM? The Pediatric Endocrine Society Recommendations outline algorithms for identification of at-risk infants with on-going persistent hypoglycemia. These are based on testing ability to maintain normal levels of plasma glucose during short periods of fasting prior to discharge (sometimes called the "skip a feed test"). The evidence outlined in this report clearly demonstrates that hypoglycemia in normal newborns and in high-risk neonates are forms of hyperinsulinemic hypoglycemia induced by the normal hypoxic conditions in utero and aggravated by peri-partum stresses; i.e. transitional hyperinsulinism in normal newborns and prolonged hyperinsulinism in at-risk infants (birth asphyxia, SGA, LGA, infant of diabetic mother, maternal toxemia). Because suppression of ketones is the hallmark of hyperinsulinism, bedside monitoring of ketones in addition to glucose, especially during the pre-discharge fasting test, can improve the detection of both prolonged hyperinsulinism in high-risk infants and persistent hyperinsulinism in babies with genetic disorders of insulin regulation.

MAJOR RECOMMENDATIONS
1. Rather than using a single value of glucose to "define" hypoglycemia in neonates, consider employing the scale shown in Fig 2 for interpreting plasma glucose concentrations.
2. Include frequent monitoring of ketones (beta-hydroxybutyrate), in addition to glucose, for detecting persistent or prolonged forms of hypoglycemia (i.e., hyperinsulinism), for all infants prior to discharge home.
3. Consider the use of glucagon as a simple, rapid method in acute management of hypoglycemia in newborns who are likely to have hyperinsulinism – this applies to nearly all newborns, including transitional hyperinsulinism in normal newborns, prolonged hyperinsulinism in at-risk neonates, and persistent hyperinsulinism in genetic disorders of insulin secretion).

RATING FOR THE STRENGTH OF THE EVIDENCE: The above recommendations can be rated as "suggestions" based on the mechanism of the three major forms of neonatal hypoglycemia: transitional hyperinsulinism in normal newborns, prolonged hyperinsulinism in at-risk groups, and persistent hyperinsulinism in the many genetic disorders of insulin secretion.

BIBLIOGRAPHIC SOURCES: Thornton PS, Stanley CA, De Leon DD, et al. Recommendations from the Pediatric Endocrine Society for Evaluation and Management of Persistent Hypoglycemia in Neonates, Infants, and Children. J Pediatr 2015, 167:238-45. (Ref #6)Stanley CA, Rozance PJ, Thornton PS, et al. Re-evaluating "transitional neonatal hypoglycemia": mechanism and implications for management. J Pediatr 2015, 166:1520-5 (Ref #18)Yang J, Hammoud B, Ridler A, et al. Postnatal activation of hypoxia pathway disrupts β-cell functional maturation (in preparation 2021) (Ref #35)Yang J, Hammoud B, Li C, et al. Decreased KATP channel activity contributes to the low glucose threshold for insulin secretion of rat neonatal islets. Endocrinology 2021, 162:1-14 (Ref #28)Harris DL, Weston PJ, Harding JE. Alternative Cerebral Fuels in the First Five Days in Healthy Term Infants: The Glucose in Well Babies (GLOW) Study. J Pediatr 2021, 231:81-86 (Ref #20).

DISCLOSURE

D.E.S. was supported by American Diabetes Association Junior Faculty Development Award (1-16-JDF086). C.A.S. was supported by National Institutes of Health grant R37-DK056268.

REFERENCES

1. Pagliara AS, Karl IE, Haymond M, et al. Hypoglycemia in infancy and childhood. I. J Pediatr 1973;82:365–79.
2. Cornblath M, Pildes RS, Schwartz R. Hypoglycemia in infancy and childhood. J Pediatr 1973;83(4):692–3.
3. Raivio K, Hallman N. Hypoglycemia in infancy and childhood. J Pediatr 1973; 83(4):693–7.
4. Adamkin DH, Polin RA. Imperfect advice: neonatal hypoglycemia. J Pediatr 2016; 176:195–6.
5. Committee on Fetus and Newborn, Adamkin DH. Postnatal glucose homeostasis in late-preterm and term infants. Pediatrics 2011;127(3):575–9.
6. Thornton PS, Stanley CA, De Leon DD, et al. Recommendations from the Pediatric Endocrine Society for Evaluation and Management of Persistent hypoglycemia in neonates, infants, and children. J Pediatr 2015;167(2):238–45.
7. Cornblath M, Hawdon JM, Williams AF, et al. Controversies regarding definition of neonatal hypoglycemia: suggested operational thresholds. Pediatrics 2000; 105(5):1141–5.
8. Cryer PE. The barrier of hypoglycemia in diabetes. Diabetes 2008;57(12): 3169–76.
9. Cryer PE, Axelrod L, Grossman AB, et al. Evaluation and management of adult hypoglycemic disorders: an endocrine Society clinical practice guideline. J Clin Endocrinol Metab 2009;94(3):709–28.
10. Cryer PE. Mechanisms of hypoglycemia-associated autonomic failure in diabetes. N Engl J Med 2013;369(4):362–72.
11. Kaiser JR, Bai S, Gibson N, et al. Association between transient newborn hypoglycemia and fourth-grade achievement test proficiency: a population-based study. JAMA Pediatr 2015;169(10):913–21.
12. McKinlay CJD, Alsweiler JM, Anstice NS, et al. Association of neonatal glycemia with neurodevelopmental outcomes at 4.5 Years. JAMA Pediatr 2017;171(10): 972–83.
13. Harris DL, Weston PJ, Williams CE, et al. Cot-side electroencephalography monitoring is not clinically useful in the detection of mild neonatal hypoglycemia. J Pediatr 2011;159(5):755–60.
14. Desmond MM, Hild JR, Gast JH. The glycemic response of the newborn infant to epinephrine administration: a preliminary report. J Pediatr 1950;37(3):341–50.
15. McQuarrie I. Idiopathic spontaneously occurring hypoglycemia in infants; clinical significance of problem and treatment. AMA Am J Dis Child 1954;87(4):399–428.

16. Collins JE, Leonard JV, Teale D, et al. Hyperinsulinaemic hypoglycaemia in small for dates babies. Arch Dis Child 1990;65(10):1118–20.

17. Hoe FM, Thornton PS, Wanner LA, et al. Clinical features and insulin regulation in infants with a syndrome of prolonged neonatal hyperinsulinism. J Pediatr 2006; 148(2):207–12.

18. Stanley CA, Rozance PJ, Thornton PS, et al. Re-evaluating "transitional neonatal hypoglycemia": mechanism and implications for management. J Pediatr 2015; 166(6):1520–5.

19. Harris DL, Weston PJ, Gamble GD, et al. Glucose profiles in healthy term infants in the first 5 days: the glucose in well babies (GLOW) Study. J Pediatr 2020;223: 34–41.

20. Harris DL, Weston PJ, Harding JE. Alternative cerebral fuels in the first five days in healthy term infants: the glucose in well babies (GLOW) Study. J Pediatr 2021; 231:81–6.

21. Pagliara AS, Karl IE, Haymond M, et al. Hypoglycemia in infancy and childhood. II. J Pediatr 1973;82(4):558–77.

22. Blum B, Hrvatin S, Schuetz C, et al. Functional beta-cell maturation is marked by an increased glucose threshold and by expression of urocortin 3. Nat Biotechnol 2012;30(3):261–4.

23. Hrvatin S, O'Donnell CW, Deng F, et al. Differentiated human stem cells resemble fetal, not adult, beta cells. Proc Natl Acad Sci U S A 2014;111(8):3038–43.

24. Thorrez L, Laudadio I, Van Deun K, et al. Tissue-specific disallowance of house-keeping genes: the other face of cell differentiation. Genome Res 2011;21(1): 95–105.

25. Weinhaus AJ, Poronnik P, Cook DI, et al. Insulin secretagogues, but not glucose, stimulate an increase in [Ca2+]i in the fetal rat beta-cell. Diabetes 1995;44(1): 118–24.

26. Rorsman P, Arkhammar P, Bokvist K, et al. Failure of glucose to elicit a normal secretory response in fetal pancreatic beta cells results from glucose insensitivity of the ATP-regulated K+ channels. Proc Natl Acad Sci U S A 1989;86(12): 4505–9.

27. Huang C, Walker EM, Dadi PK, et al. Synaptotagmin 4 regulates pancreatic beta cell maturation by modulating the Ca(2+) sensitivity of insulin secretion vesicles. Dev Cell 2018;45(3):347–61.

28. Yang J, Hammoud B, Li C, et al. Decreased KATP channel activity contributes to the low glucose threshold for insulin secretion of rat neonatal islets. Endocrinology 2021;162(9):bqab121.

29. Chen PC, Kryukova YN, Shyng SL. Leptin regulates KATP channel trafficking in pancreatic beta-cells by a signaling mechanism involving AMP-activated protein kinase (AMPK) and cAMP-dependent protein kinase (PKA). J Biol Chem 2013; 288(47):34098–109.

30. Park SH, Ryu SY, Yu WJ, et al. Leptin promotes K(ATP) channel trafficking by AMPK signaling in pancreatic beta-cells. Proc Natl Acad Sci U S A 2013; 110(31):12673–8.

31. Srivastava S, Li Z, Soomro I, et al. Regulation of KATP channel trafficking in pancreatic beta-cells by protein histidine phosphorylation. Diabetes 2018;67(5): 849–60.

32. Polonsky KS. Lilly Lecture 1994. The beta-cell in diabetes: from molecular genetics to clinical research. Diabetes 1995;44(6):705–17.

33. Haliyur R, Tong X, Sanyoura M, et al. Human islets expressing HNF1A variant have defective beta cell transcriptional regulatory networks. J Clin Invest 2019; 129(1):246–51.
34. Stanley CA. Perspective on the genetics and diagnosis of congenital hyperinsulinism disorders. J Clin Endocrinol Metab 2016;101(3):815–26.
35. Yang J, Hammoud B, Ridler A, et al. Postnatal activation of hypoxia pathway disrupts β-cell functional maturation (in preparation 2021).
36. Puri S, Garcia-Nunez A, Hebrok M, et al. Elimination of von Hippel-Lindau function perturbs pancreas endocrine homeostasis in mice. PLoS One 2013;8(8): e72213.
37. Harris DL, Weston PJ, Signal M, et al. Dextrose gel for neonatal hypoglycaemia (the Sugar Babies Study): a randomised, double-blind, placebo-controlled trial. Lancet 2013;382(9910):2077–83.
38. Cornblath M, Reisner SH. Blood glucose in the neonate and its clinical significance. N Engl J Med 1965;273(7):378–81.

Coronavirus Disease 2019 Infection in Newborns

Jeffrey M. Perlman, MB, ChB[a],*, Christine Salvatore, MD[b]

KEYWORDS

- SARS-CoV-2 • COVID-19 • Vertical transmission • Maternal vaccination
- Preterm birth • Breast milk • Syncytiotrophoblast

KEY POINTS

- Newborns with positive severe acute respiratory syndrome coronavirus 2 (SARS-CoV-2) test results appear to have minimal burden of illness that is directly associated with a viral infection.
- A symptomatic SARS-CoV-2–infected mother increases the risk for preterm and medically induced preterm birth.
- There is an important association of societal and health disparity and positive SARS-CoV-2 infection.
- In population studies, there is a consistent association of SARS-CoV-2 infection and a reduction in preterm birth rates.
- Messenger RNA-based coronavirus disease 2019 vaccines in pregnant women lead to maternal antibody production and transplacental transfer of passive immunity to the neonate.

INTRODUCTION

The coronavirus disease 2019 (COVID-19) pandemic owing to the novel severe acute respiratory syndrome coronavirus 2 (SARS-CoV-2) has spread worldwide with serious consequences on global public health during the past 1.5 years. During this time, it has become apparent that adults with comorbidities have the highest risk for severe disease and death; meanwhile, it became clearer that children, even though not immune from acquiring the infection, had a less severe presentation and outcome compared with adults. Seroprevalence from some reports seems similar to adults, but the observed cases are less, indicating most likely that children are asymptomatic or very mildly ill to draw medical attention and to be tested.[1–4]

a Division of Newborn, Weill Cornell Medicine, 1283 York Avenue, New York, NY 10065, USA;
b Division of Pediatric Infectious Diseases, Weill Cornell Medicine- New York Presbyterian Hospital, 505 East 70th Street, New York, NY 10065, USA
* Corresponding author.
E-mail address: Jmp2007@med.cornell.edu

Clin Perinatol 49 (2022) 73–92
https://doi.org/10.1016/j.clp.2021.11.005
0095-5108/22/© 2021 Elsevier Inc. All rights reserved.
perinatology.theclinics.com

As of April 2021, the American Academy of Pediatrics (AAP) reported that the cumulative percentage of children positive for SARS-CoV-2 was 13.6% of total cases, but only 0.1% to 1.9% needed hospitalization, with a death rate of 0% to 0.03% depending on the reporting state.[5] Although the natural course is uneventful in most pediatric cases, a very small percentage can develop, about 2 to 4 weeks after the acute COVID-19 infection, a hyperinflammatory state, which is now known as multisystem inflammatory syndrome in children.[6]

In March 2020, little was known about the possible consequences of SARS-CoV-2 infection in pregnant women and fetuses, and there was scant information regarding vertical transmission, neonatal outcomes, and optimal management of the mother-newborn dyad. Respiratory viruses uncommonly result in intrauterine transmission of infection to fetuses, and because SARS-CoV-2 is a respiratory virus, intrauterine transmission was anticipated to be low. On the other hand, the most appropriate perinatal management of the newborns was unknown. Many worldwide societies initially advised, as preferred management to decrease the risk of perinatal transmission, isolation of the newborns immediately after delivery, formula or expressed breast-milk feeding, and no contact, if possible, with the mother for 14 days or at least 7 days from symptoms onset.[7–9] Over the months, several studies showed that the proportion of newborns who tested positive for COVID-19 in the perinatal period was low, from 0% to 6.9% depending on the study.[10–13] Two studies from New York City demonstrated that transmission of COVID-19 appears unlikely to occur despite newborns rooming-in with the mother immediately after birth and breastfeeding, if associated with adequate parental education of safe infection control practices, such as surgical mask wearing at all times and frequent hand and breast hygiene.[10,14] Nevertheless, there are still open questions about newborns when exposed to COVID-19, as they are a particularly vulnerable population with unique challenges in their management.

POSSIBLE METHODS OF MATERNAL TRANSMISSION TO NEWBORNS

There are 3 potential methods of transmission:
- Intrauterine transmission through occult maternal viremia and hematogenous spread to the fetus through the placenta or through ingestion of viral particles present in the amniotic fluid (AF). The extent of this mechanism appears to be rare with only a few case reports in literature.
- Intrapartum transmission through contact with maternal-infected secretions, either respiratory droplets or vaginal secretions, at time of birth.
- Postnatal transmission through contact with infected secretions from any infected caregiver, who could be parents, medical staff, or other household member. As SARS-CoV-2 is a respiratory virus, this seems to be the most prevalent mechanism of transmission to newborns.[15,16]

Most neonates born to asymptomatic COVID-positive mothers are triaged to a regular nursery.[10,14,17] Neonates born to symptomatic mothers are more likely to be admitted to a neonatal intensive care unit (NICU) perhaps as a consequence of premature delivery secondary to the severity of maternal symptoms (see later discussion). For in utero transmission to occur, the virus must be present in maternal blood and be able to cross the placenta to infect the fetus.[18] The presence of angiotensin-converting enzyme 2 (ACE2), the SARS-CoV-2 receptor, in maternal-fetal interface cells, including stromal cells and perivascular cells of decidua, cytotrophoblast, and syncytiotrophoblast (ST) in placenta, as well as specific cell types of human fetal heart, liver, and lung suggests transplacental passage and fetal infection may be possible.[19]

Intrapartum infection can occur through exposure of the infant to infectious virus in maternal blood or secretions during the birth process. Evaluation of a newborn at risk for SARS-CoV-2 particularly with maternal symptoms and/or positive maternal nasopharyngeal (NP) swab should include detection of virus by polymerase chain reaction (PCR) in umbilical cord blood, AF, neonatal blood, NP swab within 24 hours, repeated at 48 hours and 7 days, and from stool and urine. In addition, a placental swab from the fetal side for viral detection should be obtained. In addition, where appropriate, cord blood should be obtained for immunoglobulin G (IgG) and IgM antibodies. In this regard, a classification defining confirmed, probable, or possible infection has been proposed by Shah and colleagues[20] (**Box 1**).

EPIDEMIOLOGIC STUDIES AND POTENTIAL TRANSPLACENTAL VERTICAL TRANSMISSION

Edlow and colleagues[21] undertook a cohort study among pregnant women to quantify SARS-CoV-2 viral load in maternal and neonatal biofluids and incidence of fetoplacental infection. Participants included 127 pregnant women of whom 64 tested positive for SARS-CoV-2 and 63 tested negative. Of the 64 positive women, 23 (36%) were asymptomatic, 22 (34%) had mild disease, 7 (11%) had moderate disease, 10 (16%) had severe disease, and 2 (3%) had critical disease. Among 107 women, there was no detectable viremia in maternal or cord blood and no evidence of vertical transmission. Among 77 neonates tested in whom SARS-CoV-2 antibodies were quantified in cord blood, one had detectable IgM to nucleocapsid. Among 88 placentas tested, SARS-CoV-2 RNA was not detected in any. In antibody analyses, among 37 women with SARS-CoV-2 infection, antireceptor binding domain IgG was detected in 24 women (65%) and antinucleocapsid was detected in 26 women (7%). Nonoverlapping placental expression of SARS-CoV-2 receptors ACE2 and transmembrane

---

Box 1
Classification of confirmed, , probable and possible infection in symptomatic and asymptomatic newborns[20]

Symptomatic newborns
1. For confirmed infection in symptomatic newborns, there should be detection of the virus by PCR in umbilical cord blood or neonatal blood collected within first 12 hours of birth or AF collected before rupture of membrane.
2. For probable infection, there should be detection of the virus by PCR in NP swab at birth (collected after cleaning baby) and placental swab from fetal side of placenta in a newborn born via CS before rupture of membrane.
3. Possible infection would include no detection of the virus by PCR in NP swab at birth (collected after cleaning baby) but the presence of anti–SARS-CoV-2 IgM antibodies in umbilical cord blood or neonatal blood collected within first 12 hours of birth.

Asymptomatic newborns
4. Confirmed infection would include detection of the virus by PCR in cord blood, or neonatal blood collected within first 12 hours of birth.
5. Probable infection would include detection of the virus by PCR in AF collected before rupture of membrane but no detection in umbilical cord blood or neonatal blood collected within first 12 hours of birth.
6. Possible infection would include the presence of anti–SARS-CoV-2 IgM in umbilical cord blood or detection of the virus by PCR in placental tissue but no detection of the virus by PCR in umbilical cord blood or neonatal blood collected within first 12 hours of birth or AF.

serine protease 2 (TMPRSS2) was noted. In summary, there was no evidence of placental infection or definitive vertical transmission of SARS-CoV-2. Transplacental transfer of anti–SARS-CoV-2 antibodies was inefficient.

Bahadur and colleagues[22] questioned whether there was antenatal or intrapartum vertical transmission from mother to baby after SAR-SCoV-2 infection during pregnancy. From 75 studies, 18 newborns were SARS-CoV-2–positive. A first reverse transcriptase (RT) -PCR diagnostic test was done in 449 babies, and a second diagnostic test was done in 82 babies. Positive results in the first RT-PCR were seen in 14 (3.1%) newborns. Three babies with negative first RT-PCR became positive on the second RT-PCR on days 6 or 7. Testing of AF for SARS-CoV-2 was observed in a few cases. These findings indicate a strong likelihood that intrapartum vertical transmission of SARS-CoV-2 from mother to baby, although rare, is possible.

Single case reports highlighting the transplacental vertical passage of SARS-CoV-2 from maternal to the fetal compartment are as described in **Table 1**.

The authors describe a series of cases (n = 15) that highlight the potential small risk for the transplacental passage of the virus (see **Table 1**). There were 4 confirmed cases of transplacental passage of SARS-CoV-2,[23–26] one case of probable infection 27[27–32] 7 possible cases 28-33[33] and 2 cases of infection proximal to delivery.[34,35]

These few cases of early-onset neonatal SARS-CoV-2 infection indicate that intrapartum vertical transmission of SARS-CoV-2 from mother to baby, although rare, occurs. Infected infants with SARS-CoV-2 may be symptomatic or asymptomatic. Signs include early fever as well as respiratory and neurologic symptoms. Improving access to molecular testing of AF, cord blood, urine, stool, and breast milk, as well as cord blood antibody testing should be a priority to enable investigators to further describe the epidemiology of congenital and neonatal disease in the setting of maternal SARS-CoV-2 infection.

CORONAVIRUS DISEASE 2019 DIAGNOSIS AND IMPACT ON MOTHER AND NEWBORN

Villar and colleagues[36] reported on the extent of SARS-CoV-2 (COVID-19) in pregnancy and the risk of adverse maternal and neonatal outcomes compared with pregnant individuals without COVID-19. Seven hundred six pregnant women with COVID-19 and 1424 pregnant women without COVID-19 were enrolled in a multinational cohort study. Women with a COVID-19 diagnosis were at significantly higher risk for (a) preeclampsia (PEC)/eclampsia (relative risk [RR] 1.76), (b) intensive care unit admission (RR, 5.04), (c) maternal mortality (RR, 22.3), (d) preterm birth (PTB; RR, 1.59), (e) medically indicated PTB (RR, 1.97), (f) severe neonatal morbidity index (RR, 2.66), and (h) severe perinatal morbidity and mortality index (RR, 2.14). Fever and shortness of breath for any duration were associated with increased risk of severe maternal complications (RR, 2.56) and neonatal complications (RR, 4.97). Asymptomatic women remained at higher risk only for maternal morbidity (RR, 1.24) and PEC (RR, 1.63). Among positively tested women, 13% of their neonates tested positive. Cesarean section (CS) delivery (RR, 2.15) but not breastfeeding (RR, 1.10) was associated with increased risk for neonatal test positivity.

Angelidou and colleagues[37] identified 255 neonates born to 250 mothers with positive SARS-CoV-2 test results. This included 79 (32%) symptomatic and 170 (68%) asymptomatic mothers. Worsening COVID-19 illness prompted delivery in 23 mothers (9%), of which 20 (87.0%) were via CS. Six neonates (2.2%) presented with positive SARS-CoV-2 test results within the first week of life. Of the 6 neonates, 2 neonates presented with respiratory distress and were delivered preterm, 1 neonate had nasal

Table 1
Case series describing transplacental (vertical) severe acute respiratory syndrome coronavirus 2 infection

Case No.	Author	Description
1	Vivanti et al,[23] 2020	A 23-yr-old gravida 1, para 0 mother who presented with respiratory symptoms and was SARS-CoV-2–positive. Delivery was via CS with SARS-CoV-2–positive AF. The placenta demonstrated a very high viral load as well as histologic and immune histochemical findings consistent with placental inflammation. A male neonate was delivered at 35 5/7 wk GA with a birth weight (BW) of 2540 g. Apgar scores were 4, 2, and 7 at 1, 5, and 10 min, respectively. Delivery room resuscitation included bag mask positive pressure ventilation and intubation. The baby was extubated after ~6 h. NP and rectal swabs obtained on DOL 1, 3, and 18 were all positive for the S and E SARS-CoV-2 genes. In addition, blood and bronchial lavage fluid obtained before extubation was positive for SARS-CoV-2. On DOL 3, the neonate suddenly presented with irritability, poor feeding, axial hypertonia, and opisthotonos. Cerebrospinal fluid (CSF) was negative for SARS-CoV-2, bacteria, fungi, herpes simplex virus 1 and 2. The infant gradually improved over subsequent days and was discharged on DOL 18. MRI on DOL 11 demonstrated bilateral gliosis of the deep periventricular and subcortical white matter.
2	Kirtsman et al,[24] 2020	A 40-yr-old gravida 2, para 1 mother who presented with myalgia, decreased appetite, fatigue, dry cough, and temperature of 39°C in the 24 h before delivery. An NP swab was positive for SARS-CoV-2. Delivery was via CS with artificial rupture of membranes at delivery with clear AF. A male neonate of BW 2930 g was delivered vigorous. The Apgar scores were 9 and 9 at 1 and 5 min, respectively. Placental tissue was positive from the maternal and fetal side, the parenchyma and chorion for SARS-CoV-2 gene targets. Vaginal secretions and NP swabs obtained on DOL 1, 2, and 7 were all positive for SARS-CoV-2 gene targets. Neonatal plasma tested positive on day 4, and stool tested positive on day 7. Breast milk was also positive on DOL 2 but not on DOL 7. The neonate was discharge on DOL 4.
3	Von Kohorn et al,[25] 2020	A 34-wk GA 2414-g male neonate was born to a mother with a history of cough for a week; diagnosed 14 h before delivery with positive NP swab for SARS-CoV-2 infection. Delivery was via CS. AF was clear. Apgar scores were 7 and 9 at 1 and 5 min, respectively. The physical examination was normal. The infant continued to be asymptomatic and was discharged on DOL 8 and

(continued on next page)

Table 1 (*continued*)		
Case No.	Author	Description
		remained healthy through the first months of life. The cord blood, NP swabs on DOL 2, 4, 7, and urine were positive for SARS-CoV-2. Placental tissue was negative SARS-CoV-2 gene targets and cord serum, and plasma was seronegative for IgM and IgG antibodies.
4	Lorenz et al,[26] 2020	A healthy 40 3/7-wk GA female newborn born to a mother who an elevated temperature (maximum 38.1°C) during labor coupled with a history of mild respiratory infection and loss of smell and taste. She tested positive for SARS-CoV-2. Apgar scores were 9 and 9 at 1 and 5 min, respectively. At 24 h, the newborn developed refractory fever (38.6°C), appeared lethargic, and progressed to encephalitic symptoms (ie, hyperexcitable, high-pitched crying) over the next 30 h. She was transferred to a tertiary center NICU. The newborn's NP and rectal swabs tested positive for SARS-CoV-2. Bacterial cultures of CSF and blood were sterile. CSF tested negative for SARS-CoV-2. A cranial ultrasound scan was unremarkable. The initial chest radiograph was normal; however, the newborn developed respiratory distress at about 80 h of life and needed continuous positive airway pressure and oxygen therapy until DOL 6. At DOL 10, severe staccato-like coughing emerged, and another chest radiograph was consistent with bilateral pneumonia. The newborn's NP and rectal swaps remained positive for SARS-CoV-2 through 14 d after birth. The patient was discharged free of symptoms on DOL 14.
5	Sisman et al,[27] 2020	A 34-wk gestation 3280-g female infant born to a 37-yr-old gravida 4, para 3 woman. She was admitted for evaluation of preterm labor. Her NP swab was positive for SARS-CoV-2. Labor was augmented with oxytocin on the third day after hospitalization following premature preterm rupture of membranes 8 h before delivery. The AF was clear. Delivery was vaginal. Apgar scores were 7 and 9 at 1 and 5 min of life, respectively. There was no respiratory distress. The infant's NP swab was positive by RT-PCR for SARS-CoV-2 at 24 and 48 h of life. The infant developed fever and respiratory distress, that is, mild subcostal retractions, tachypnea on DOL 2. Blood and CSF bacterial cultures, and surface, blood, and CSF for herpes simplex virus DNA PCR were obtained. All cultures were negative. Respiratory signs resolved within 3 d, and the infant was weaned to room air by DOL 5. NP RT-PCR for SARS-CoV-2 remained

(continued on next page)

Table 1 (*continued*)		
Case No.	**Author**	**Description**
		positive on DOL 14. SARS-CoV-2 virus was detected in the placental tissue. The infant was discharged home on DOL 21.
6	Patanè et al,[28] 2020	Two cases. The first represents a mother who presented at 37 6/7 wk GA who presented with a fever and a cough and had a positive NP swab for COVID. Delivery was vaginal. The BW was 2660 g. Apgar scores were 9 and 10 at 1 and 5 min, respectively. No skin-to-skin contact was permitted; however, rooming-in and breastfeeding with a mask were allowed. The newborn had a positive result for COVID-19 from NP swabs obtained immediately after birth, and at DOL 1 and 7. The neonate remained asymptomatic and was discharged from the hospital at 10 DOL after being hospitalized for observation.
		The second case represents a mother who presented at 35 1/7 wk of gestation with a fever, cough, and a positive COVID-19 NP swab test. Delivery was via CS secondary to a non-reassuring fetal status. The newborn was female with a BW of 2686 g. Apgar scores were 9 and 10 at 1 and 5 min, respectively. She was admitted to the NICU. A neonatal NP swab obtained at birth was negative for SARS-CoV-2, but a follow-up NP swab obtained on DOL 7 was positive. No contact between the mother and the neonate during that period occurred. The neonate was discharged on DOL 20 after hospitalization for routine late preterm care.
		The placentas of these 2 women demonstrated SARS-CoV-2 antigens seen in the villous ST on the fetal side of the placenta in both cases.
7	Alamar et al,[29] 2020	A 32-yr-old gravida 2, para 0 female who presented at 35 6/7 wk GA with vaginal bleeding. She reported fever, mild chills, fatigue, dysgeusia, and anosmia beginning 1 d before arrival. A 2630-g female neonate was delivered via emergent CS due to bleeding. The Apgar scores were 9 and 9 at 1 and 5 min, respectively. The newborn was asymptomatic. The maternal pharyngeal screen for SARS-CoV-2 was positive on postpartum day 1. The infant's NP PCR for SARS-CoV-2 was positive on DOL 1, 2, and 7. The mother and infant remained afebrile, asymptomatic, and hemodynamically stable throughout the hospitalization. In situ hybridization for SARS-CoV-2 RNA revealed a strong signal in the villous ST but not in villous stromal cells, Hofbauer cells, or villous endothelium.

(*continued on next page*)

Table 1 (continued)		
Case No.	**Author**	**Description**
8	Alzamora et al,[30] 2020	A 41-yr-old gravida 3, para 2 who presented with a 4-d history of malaise, low-grade fever, and progressive shortness of breath. An NP swab was positive for COVID-19. The patient progressed to respiratory failure requiring mechanical ventilation on day 5 of disease onset. Delivery was via CS. The neonatal NP RT-PCR swab on DOL 1 was positive for SARS-CoV-2. Maternal IgM and IgG were positive on postpartum day 4 (day 9 after symptom onset); neonatal immunoglobulins were negative.
9	Parsa et al,[31] 2020	A 41-yr-old mother who presented with signs and symptoms of acute respiratory illness, including shortness of breath and cough. RT-PCR on the mother was positive, and she was diagnosed with COVID-19 pneumonia. Delivery was via emergency CS. A term 3500-g female infant was delivered with Apgar scores of 9 and 10 at 1 and 5 min, respectively. The RT-PCR results of the AF and neonate (<24 h after birth) were positive for COVID-19. She was admitted to the NICU and received routine care. She developed a fever on DOL 10; all tests were negative. NP swabs were negative on DOL 11 and 14. She was discharged on DOL 28 in good condition.
10	Lima-Rogel et al,[32] 2021	A term 3450-g male infant born to a 19-yr-old asymptomatic mother via CS secondary to fetal bradycardia. The mother roomed in with another mother-baby pair, both positive for SARS-CoV-2. On DOL 2, the neonate developed tachypnea with distress, and a chest radiograph suggested pneumonia. On DOL 3, both the mother and the newborn RT-PCR were positive for SARS-CoV-2; the mother remained asymptomatic. The neonate required mechanical ventilation and was transferred to a tertiary level neonatal unit on day 5. He was extubated on DOL 8. An RT-PCR test for SARS-CoV-2 was negative on DOL 8, and he was discharged DOL 21.
11	Zamaniyan et al,[33] 2020	A 22-y-old mother who presented with respiratory symptoms, myalgia, and fever with positive testing for SARS-CoV-2. After 3 d, she underwent a CS and delivered a 30 5/7-wk 2350-g female infant with Apgar scores of 9 and 9 at 1 and 5 min, respectively. The infant exhibited initial fever and was treated with antibiotics. She recovered and was without issues by DOL 8. Cultures from the AF and from the NP at DOL 1 and 7 were positive for SARS-CoV-2.

(continued on next page)

| Table 1 |
| *(continued)* |

Case No.	Author	Description
12	Dong et al,[57] 2020	A 29-yr-old gravida 1, para 0 mother who presented 1 mo before delivery at 34 2/7 wk gestation suspected of being exposed to SARS-CoV-2. Over the next month, her NP swabs were repeatedly SARS-CoV-2–positive. Vaginal swab 1 day before delivery was negative for SARS-CoV-2. Delivery was via CS. Apgar scores were 9 and 10 at 1 and 5 min, respectively. The BW was 3120 g. The neonate was asymptomatic. At 2 h of age, both IgG and IgM levels as well as cytokines, interleukin-6 (IL-6), and IL-10 were elevated. Five NP RT-PCR swabs from 2 h to 16 d of age were negative. Her IgM and IgG levels were still elevated a month later. Discharge was on DOL 30.
13	Hascoët et al,[34] 2020	A mother presented with COVID-19 infection with positive RT-PCR results 6 wk before delivery. She exhibited fever and profound asthenia for 10 d. The mother was considered cleared with negative NP and stool SARS-CoV-2 RT-PCR before delivery. Labor was uncomplicated, and delivery was vaginal. A 39-wk healthy-appearing female infant was delivered. The baby was initially fed with expressed milk and then directly breastfed. RT-PCR testing of the breast milk yielded negative results. NP swabs yielded negative results on DOL 3; however, testing of the baby's stool yielded positive results on day 1. IgG antibodies were detected in the mother and newborn, and IgM antibodies in the mother only. The infant was seen in clinic 45 d following delivery and 12 wk from maternal symptoms and positive PCR. Physical examination was normal. IgG antibodies detection remained positive; however, IgM antibodies were negative.
14	Bandyopadhyay et al,[35] 2021	A 37 2/7 wk female newborn born to a 24-yr-old mother who developed a low-grade fever. Her RT-PCR pharyngeal swab for SARS-CoV-2 at the time was positive. Repeat RT-PCR pharyngeal swab 2 wk later was again positive. A repeat RT-PCR test done 2 d before delivery was negative. Delivery was vaginal. The BW was 2590 g. Apgar scores were 8 and 9 at 1 and 5 min, respectively. The newborn was formula fed. An NP swab specimen collected immediately from the newborn (16 h) after birth was positive; qualitative infant serum IgG antibody test was positive for SARS-CoV-2 infection with a concurrent negative qualitative IgM antibody test. Repeat NP swabs obtained on DOL 2 and 3 were negative. The newborn remained in the NICU for 9 d.

congestion, and 3 neonates were asymptomatic. Adjusting for maternal symptoms, delivery mode, and rooming-in practice, mothers with high social vulnerability index (≥90th percentile) were more likely to have neonates with positive SARS-CoV-2 test results (adjusted odds ratio [OR], 4.95) (P = .008). Newborns with positive SARS-CoV-2 test results appeared to have minimal burden of illness that was directly associated with a viral infection. Those born in the context of delivery prompted by worsening maternal COVID-19 symptoms were more likely to be PTB, which led to a need for resuscitation in the delivery room, more respiratory morbidity, and longer length of stay.

Gale and colleagues[38] carried out a prospective UK population-based cohort study of 66 inpatient newborns with confirmed SARS-CoV-2 infection in the first 28 days of life (DOL; incidence 5.6 [95% confidence interval [CI], 4.3–7.1] per 10,000 live births), of whom 28 (42%) had severe neonatal SARS-CoV-2 infection (incidence 2.4 [1.6–3.4] per 10,000 live births). Of these newborns, 16 (24%) were born preterm. (a) Thirty-six (55%) babies were from white ethnic groups (SARS-CoV-2 infection incidence 4.6 [3.2–6.4] per 10,000 live births), (b) 14 (21%) babies were from Asian ethnic groups (15.2 [8.3–25.5] per 10,000 live births), (c) 8 (12%) babies were from black ethnic groups (18.0 [7.8–35.5] per 10,000 live births), and (d) 7 (11%) babies were from mixed or other ethnic groups (5.6 [2.2–11.5] per 10,000 live births). One (2%) newborn died of a cause unrelated to SARS-CoV-2 infection.

Norman and colleagues[39] evaluated neonatal outcomes in relation to maternal SARS-CoV-2 test positivity during pregnancy in Sweden. Of 88,159 infants, 2323 (2.6%) were delivered by mothers who tested positive for SARS-CoV-2. There was an association of maternal SARS-CoV-2 infection with newborns' admission for neonatal care (11.7% versus 8.4%; OR, 1.47; 95% CI, 1.26–1.70) and any neonatal respiratory disorder (2.8% vs 2.0%; OR, 1.42; 95% CI, 1.07–1.90). There was a higher rate of preterm delivery (near term) among infected mothers: 8.8% versus 5.5% in the SARS-CoV-2–positive group versus the comparison group, respectively. There were no differences in neonatal mortality, length of hospital stay, or breastfeeding rates.

Mullins and colleagues[40] reported the outcome of SARS-CoV-2–infected pregnancies from a collaboration between investigators of 2 registries, the UK and Global Pregnancy and Neonatal outcomes in COVID-19 (PAN-COVID) study and the AAP Section on Neonatal-Perinatal Medicine (SONPM) National Perinatal COVID-19 Registry. Analysis of data from the PAN-COVID registry included pregnancies with suspected or confirmed maternal SARS-CoV-2 infection at any stage in pregnancy, and the AAP-SONPM National Perinatal COVID-19 registry included pregnancies with positive maternal testing for SARS-CoV-2 from 14 days before delivery to 3 days after delivery. The outcome on 4005 pregnant women with suspected or confirmed SARS-CoV-2 infection (n = 1606 from PAN-COVID and n = 2399 from AAP-SONPM) was available. For obstetric outcomes in those with confirmed infection in PAN-COVID and AAP-SONPM, respectively, maternal death occurred in 0.5% and 0.2% of cases, early neonatal death occurred in 0.3% and 0.3% of cases, and stillbirth occurred in 0.6% and 0.4% of cases, respectively. Preterm delivery (<37 weeks' gestation) was noted in 16.1% of women with confirmed infection in PAN-COVID and in 15.7% of women in AAP-SONPM. The rates of a small-for-gestational-age (SGA) neonate were 9.7% in those with confirmed infection and 9.6% in AAP-SONPM. The findings from the UK and US registries of pregnancies with SARS-CoV-2 infection were remarkably concordant.

The above studies indicate that a symptomatic SARS-CoV-2–infected mother increases the risk for preterm and medically induced PTB.[36] An asymptomatic COVID-19–positive mother was not associated with an increased risk of neonatal morbidity. Two studies in this section highlight an important association of societal and health disparity and positive SARS-CoV-2 infection. Thus, mothers with a high social vulnerability index ($\geq$90th percentile) were more likely to have neonates with positive SARS-CoV-2 test results.[37] In a second study, a high proportion of newborns from black, Asian, or minority ethnic groups was more likely to have newborns with positive SARS-CoV-2 infection.[38] Newborns with positive SARS-CoV-2 test results appear to have minimal burden of illness that is directly associated with a viral infection but rather through the impact of preterm delivery, undertaken because of the mother's worsening illness.[37] Preterm delivery affected a higher proportion of women than expected based on historical and contemporaneous national data.[40] The proportions of pregnancies affected by stillbirth, SGA infant, or early neonatal death were comparable to those in historical and contemporaneous UK and US data. The reported incidence of positive neonatal SARS-CoV-2 PCR test ranges from 0.56% to 2%.[37-40] Finally, neonatal mortality as a result of SARS-CoV-2 is extremely rare.

FURTHER EVIDENCE TO SUPPORT A RELATIONSHIP BETWEEN SEVERE ACUTE RESPIRATORY SYNDROME CORONAVIRUS 2 AND PREMATURE BIRTHS

The question of whether SARS-CoV-2 infection is associated with increased or decreased likelihood of premature births is important to delineate. From the preceding section, the evidence suggests that premature birth is more likely to occur in the setting of symptomatic mothers. Conversely, a reduction in premature birth rates has been suggested from population studies that may reflect a change in social behavior that occurred during the pandemic.

In the below discussion, the authors present several population studies that have addressed this very relevant question.

Simpson and colleagues[41] evaluated 67,747 births during the pandemic period (March to September 2020) and compared the outcomes to 348,633 births delivered during a comparable historical period (2015–2019) in Canada. No differences in the overall risk of PTB, stillbirth, or other perinatal outcomes during the first 6 months of the COVID-19 pandemic were noted. However, a small reduction in PTB less than 32 weeks' gestational age (GA) in the 2 groups (1.3% versus 1.2%; OR, 0.89; 95% CI, 0.80–0.99), which persisted after multivariable adjustment (OR, 0.91; 95% CI, 0.85–0.98) was observed.

Philip and colleagues[42] evaluated regional trends of very low birth weight (VLBW) (<1500 g) and extremely low birth weight (ELBW) infants (<1000 g) in 1 designated health area of Ireland over 2 decades (January to April 2001–2019) versus a similar time period in 2020. The regional historical VLBW rate per 1000 live births was 8.18 (95% CI, 7.21–9.29), which was reduced to 2.17 per 1000 live births during the first 4 months of 2020, reflecting a rate ratio of 3.77 (95% CI, 1.21–11.75) (P = .02), representing a 73% reduction of VLBW. There were no ELBW infants admitted to the regional NICU during the 4 months in 2020. When the data were extended through June 30, these observations persisted.

Hedermann and colleagues[43] explored the impact of COVID-19 lockdown on PTBs using a nationwide register conducted on all 31,180 live singleton newborns born between March 12 and April 14 during 2015 to 2020 in Denmark. There were 5162 singleton and 1566 premature births during the lockdown in 2020. The distribution of GA was significantly different (P = .004) during the lockdown period versus the previous 5 years. This reflected a significantly lower rate of extremely premature newborns (<28 weeks) delivered during the lockdown versus the corresponding mean rate for the same dates in the previous years (OR, 0.09; 95% CI, 0.01–0.40, P<.001) (90% reduction).

Harvey and colleagues[44] used Tennessee birth records from 2015 to 2020 and restricted analyses to March 22 to April 30 for each year to reduce the effect of seasonality. There were 49,845 births during the study period. The PTB rate (<37 weeks) during the 2020 stay-at-home order was lower than rates in previous years (10.2% vs 11.3%; $P = .003$). Specifically, late preterm (35–36 6/7 weeks' gestation) birth rates were also lower (5.8% vs 6.5%; $P = .03$). There was no difference in GA less than 32 weeks ($P = .27$). There was a higher rate of assisted ventilation during the pandemic versus the comparison period (4.5% vs 3.2%) ($P<.001$), respectively. This extended to premature infants less than 37 weeks, that is, 17.9 versus 12.3% ($P<.001$), respectively. After accounting for maternal age, education, race/ethnicity, diabetes, and hypertension, the ratio for PTB in 2020 compared with 2015 to 2019 was 0.86 (95% CI, 0.79–0.93).

Pasternak and colleagues[45] compared the risk for PTB and stillbirth among births from April 1 through May 31, 2020 with births from all April through May in the years 2015 to 2019 in Sweden. There was no association between being born in 2020 versus 2015 to 2019 and risk for extremely PTB (adjusted OR, 0.92; CI, 0.66–1.28), very PTB (adjusted OR, 1.09; CI, 0.85–1.40), or stillbirth (adjusted OR, 0.78; CI, 0.57–1.06). This nationwide study did not find any associations between being born during a period in 2020 and the risk for any of the PTB categories or stillbirth.

The authors reviewed data from their institution (New York Presbyterian Hospital) where PTB rates were compared for different GA categories for years 2017 to 2019 versus 2020. There was no difference in the number of births for the ELBW and VLBW infants but a significant reduction for the near term (34–36 6/7 week) newborn (**Table 2**).

There was a consistent association of SARS-CoV-2 infection and a reduction in PTB rates in 5 of the 6 studies reviewed. In 2 studies,[42,43] there was a striking reduction in VLBW infants less than 28 weeks and/or less than 1500 g ranging from 73% to 90%. A third study demonstrated a smaller reduction (11%) in the number of VLBW infants <32 weeks.[41] One study demonstrated a 14% reduction noted in the late preterm infant, an effect that was similar to the authors' observations.[44] Why the reduction in PTB delivery rates? The COVID-19 pandemic lockdown drastically changed lives in many ways, including a change in the working environment (work from home where possible), reducing physical interactions with a focus on hygiene (frequent hand washing, social distancing, and wearing a mask). These changes may have influenced the overall inflammatory state of pregnant women.

MATERNAL SEVERE ACUTE RESPIRATORY SYNDROME CORONAVIRUS 2 INFECTION, MATERNAL VACCINATION, AND ANTIBODY PRODUCTION IN CORD BLOOD AND BREAST MILK

It remains unclear whether the maternal immune response to infection protects the fetus (**Table 3**). Moreover, the impact of maternal vaccination on maternal and

Table 2
Number of neonates admitted per year (2017–2020) as a function of gestational age

Gestational Age, wk	2017	2018	2019	2020
<27	16	9	18	18
≥27–30 6/7	41	41	32	44
31–33 6/7	68	77	84	70
34–36 6/7	174	173	195	127[a]

[a] $P<.05$ comparing 2020 to prior years.

Table 3
Studies that evaluated the impact of severe acute respiratory syndrome coronavirus 2 infection as well as maternal vaccination on immunoglobulin G , immunoglobulin M, and immunoglobulin A antibody concentrations and the impact of severe acute respiratory syndrome coronavirus 2 infection on breast milk

Author	Study Description
Flannery et al,[46] 2021	1471 mother/newborn dyads were studied to assess the association between maternal and neonatal SARS-CoV-2–specific antibody concentrations. SARS-CoV-2 IgG and/or IgM antibodies were detected in 83 of 1471 women (6%) at the time of delivery, and IgG was detected in cord blood from 72 of 83 newborns (87%). IgM was not detected in any cord blood specimen, and antibodies were not detected in any infant born to a seronegative mother. Placental transfer ratios >1.0 were observed among women with asymptomatic SARS-CoV-2 infections as well as those with mild, moderate, and severe COVID-19. Cord blood antibody concentrations correlated with maternal antibody concentrations and with duration between onset of infection and delivery. The findings indicate the potential for maternally derived SARS-CoV-2–specific antibodies to provide neonatal protection from coronavirus disease 2019.
Perl et al,[47] 2021	Study included 84 breastfeeding mothers who provided 504 breast milk samples in Israel. All participants received 2 doses of the Pfizer-BioNTech vaccine 21 d apart. Breast milk samples were collected before administration of the vaccine and then once weekly for 6 wk starting at week 2 after the first dose. Robust secretion of SARS-CoV-2–specific IgA and IgG antibodies was found in breast milk for 6 wk after vaccination. IgA secretion was evident as early as 2 wk after the first vaccine when 61.8% of samples tested positive, increasing to 86.1% at week 4 (1 wk after the second vaccine). Anti–SARS-CoV-2–specific IgG antibodies remained low for the first 3 wk, which increased to 91.7% of samples tested positive at week 4, increasing to 97% at weeks 5 and 6. Antibodies found in breast milk showed strong neutralizing effects, suggesting a potential protective effect against infection in the infant.
Collier et al,[48] 2021	This was an evaluation of the immunogenicity of COVID-19 mRNA vaccines in pregnant and lactating women, including against emerging SARS-CoV-2 variants of concern. This prospective cohort study enrolled 103 women (30 pregnant, 16 lactating, and 57 neither pregnant nor lactating) who received a COVID-19 vaccine and 28 women (22 pregnant and 6 nonpregnant unvaccinated) with confirmed SARS-CoV-2 infection. The women received either the mRNA-1273 (Moderna) or the BNT162b2 (Pfizer-BioNTech) COVID-19 vaccines. After the second vaccine dose, fever was reported in 4 pregnant women (14%), 7 lactating women (44%), and 27 nonpregnant women (52%). Binding, neutralizing, and functional nonneutralizing antibody responses as well as CD4 and CD8 T-cell responses were present in all the women following vaccination. Binding and neutralizing antibodies were also observed in infant cord blood and breast milk. Binding and neutralizing antibody titers against the SARS-CoV-2 B.1.1.7 and B.1.351 variants of concern were reduced, but T-cell responses were preserved against viral variants. COVID-19 mRNA vaccine administration was immunogenic in pregnant women, and vaccine-elicited antibodies were transferred to infant cord blood and breast

(continued on next page)

Table 3 (continued)	
Author	**Study Description**
	milk. Importantly, pregnant and nonpregnant women who were vaccinated developed cross-reactive antibody responses and T-cell responses against SARS-CoV-2 variants of concern.
Prabhu et al,[49] 2021	This was an evaluation of the impact of mRNA vaccine administered to 122 pregnant women of whom 55 had received one and 67 who received both vaccine doses. This included 85 who received the Pfizer-BioNTech vaccine, and 37 who received the Moderna vaccine. All women tested negative for SARS-CoV-2 infection using RT-PCR on NP swabs; all women and neonates were asymptomatic at birth and until time of discharge. Of the women tested at birth, 87 (71%) produced an IgG response, 19 (16%) produced both IgM and IgG response, and 16 (13%) had no detectable antibody response; the latter were within 4 wk of initial vaccine dose. The number of women who mounted an antibody response and conferred passive immunity to their neonates increased as a function of the number of weeks elapsed. All women and cord blood samples, except for one, had detectable IgG antibodies by 4 wk after the first vaccine dose. The earliest detection of antibodies in women occurred 5 d postvaccine dose 1, and the earliest detection of antibodies in cord blood occurred 16 d postvaccine dose 1. Forty-four percent of cord blood samples from women who received only 1 vaccine dose had detectable IgG, whereas 99% from women who received both vaccine doses had detectable IgG in cord blood. Maternal IgG levels increased significantly week by week, starting 2 wk after the first vaccine dose as well as between the first and second weeks after the second vaccine dose. Maternal IgG levels were linearly correlated with cord blood IgG levels ($r = 0.50$, $P<.0001$).
Chambers et al,[50] 2020	This was a study of women who tested positive by RT-PCR tests to determine whether there is transmission of infectious virus to the infant through breast milk. Breast milk samples were self-collected and mailed to the study center. In some cases, women also provided stored samples collected before enrollment. Only women who tested positive by RT-PCR tests were included. In addition, conditions of Holder pasteurization commonly used in human milk banks were mimicked by adding SARS-CoV-2 (200 × median tissue culture infectious dose 50%) to breast milk samples from 2 different control donors who provided milk samples before the onset of the pandemic. There were 18 women who provided between 1 and 12 samples, with a total of 64 samples collected at varying time points before and after the positive SARS-CoV-2 RT-PCR test result. All but 1 woman had symptomatic disease. One breast milk sample had detectable SARS-CoV-2 RNA. The positive sample was collected on the day of symptom onset; however, an additional sample taken 2 d before symptom onset and 2 samples collected 12 and 41 d later tested negative for viral RNA. The breastfed infant was not tested. No replication-competent virus was detectable in any sample, including the sample that tested positive for viral RNA. Following Holder pasteurization, viral RNA was not detected by RT-PCR in the 2 samples that had been spiked with replication-competent SARS-CoV-2, nor was culturable virus detected. However, virus was detected by culture in nonpasteurized aliquots of the same 2 milk-virus mixtures. These findings are reassuring given the known benefits of breastfeeding and human milk provided through milk banks.

neonatal antibody production remains unclear. Flannery and colleagues[46] studied 1471 mother/newborn dyads. SARS-CoV-2 IgG and/or IgM antibodies were detected in 83 of 1471 women (6%) at the time of delivery, and IgG was detected in cord blood from 72 of 83 newborns (87%). IgM was not detected in any cord blood specimen. Placental transfer ratios more than 1.0 were observed among all women whether asymptomatic or with severity of infection. Cord blood antibody concentrations correlated with maternal antibody concentrations and with duration between onset of infection and delivery.

Perl and colleagues[47] studied 84 breast-feeding mothers who had received 2 doses of the Pfizer-BioNTech vaccine 21 days apart. Robust secretion of SARS-CoV-2–specific IgA and IgG antibodies was found in breast milk for 6 weeks after vaccination. IgA secretion was evident as early as 2 weeks after the first vaccine, increasing to 86.1% at week 4. Specific IgG antibodies increased to 97% at weeks 5 and 6. In addition, antibodies found in breast milk showed strong neutralizing effects, suggesting a protective effect against infection in the infant.

Collier and colleagues[48] evaluated the immunogenicity of COVID-19 messenger RNA (mRNA) vaccines (either Moderna or Pfizer-BioNTech) in 30 pregnant women, 16 lactating women, 57 nonpregnant women, and 28 women (22 pregnant and 6 nonpregnant unvaccinated women) with confirmed SARS-CoV-2 infection. Binding, neutralizing, and functional nonneutralizing antibody responses as well as CD4 and CD8 T-cell responses were present in all the women following vaccination. Binding and neutralizing antibodies were also observed in infant cord blood and breast milk. T-cell responses were preserved against viral variants. COVID-19 mRNA vaccine administration was immunogenic in pregnant women, and vaccine-elicited antibodies were transferred to infant cord blood and breast milk. Importantly, pregnant and nonpregnant women who were vaccinated developed cross-reactive antibody responses and T-cell responses against SARS-CoV-2 variants of concern.

Prabhu and colleagues[49] evaluated the impact of mRNA vaccine administered to 122 SARS-CoV-2–negative pregnant women (85 who received the Pfizer-BioNTech and 37 who received the Moderna vaccine). Of the women tested at birth, 87 (71%) women produced an IgG response, 19 (16%) women produced both IgM and IgG response, and 16 (13%) women had no detectable antibody response. Women who mounted an antibody response and conferred passive immunity to their neonates increased as a function of the number of weeks since vaccination. The earliest detection of antibodies in women occurred 5 days post–initial vaccine dose, and the earliest detection of antibodies in cord blood was 16 days after the initial vaccine dose. Importantly, 99% of women who received both vaccine doses had detectable IgG in cord blood. Maternal IgG levels were linearly correlated with cord blood IgG levels.

A separate question is whether there is transmission of infectious virus to the newborn through breast milk. Chambers and colleagues[50] studied symptomatic women (n = 18) who tested positive by RT-PCR testing. In addition, conditions of Holder pasteurization commonly used in human milk banks were mimicked by adding SARS-CoV-2 to breast milk samples from 2 different control donors who provided milk samples before onset of the pandemic. No replication-competent virus was detectable in any of the 64 samples. Following Holder pasteurization, viral RNA was not detected by RT-PCR in the 2 samples that had been spiked with replication-competent SARS-CoV-2. However, virus was detected by culture in nonpasteurized aliquots of the same 2 milk-virus mixtures.

mRNA-based COVID-19 vaccines in pregnant women lead to maternal antibody production, and this can occur as early as 5 days after the first vaccination dose and transplacental transfer of passive immunity to the neonate as early as 16 days after the first vaccination dose. The increasing levels of maternal IgG over time and the increasing placental IgG transfer ratio over time suggest that timing between vaccination and birth (as shown by Perl and colleagues[47] and Prabhu and colleagues[49]) is likely to be an important factor to consider in vaccination strategies of pregnant women. The variability in antibody transfer and lack of transfer in 13% of cases in the study[49] highlight the importance of additional studies to understand factors that influence transplacental transfer of IgG antibodies as well as the protective nature of these antibodies.

PLACENTA FINDINGS IN SEVERE ACUTE RESPIRATORY SYNDROME CORONAVIRUS2–POSITIVE MOTHERS

Several studies have evaluated the placentas of mothers who were SARS-CoV-2–positive. The pathologic findings appear to reflect whether the mother was asymptomatic or symptomatic.

Jaiswal and colleagues[51] described the histopathologic alterations in the placenta of 27 SARS-CoV-2–positive singleton pregnancies with no symptoms or mild COVID-19-related symptoms and an equal number of SARS-CoV-2–negative singleton pregnancies. Features of maternal vascular malperfusion were significantly higher in the placentas of COVID-19-positive pregnancies. The percentage of spontaneously delivered women was comparable in the 2 groups. Schwartz and Morotti[52] summarized the spectrum of pathology findings from pregnant women with COVID-19 based on the infection status of their infants. Placentas from infected maternal-neonatal dyads were characterized by the finding of mononuclear cell inflammation of the intervillous space (chronic histiocytic intervillositis), coupled with ST necrosis. Hecht and colleagues[53] examined 19 SARS-CoV-2–positive exposed placentas for histopathologic findings and for expression of ACE2 and TMPRSS2 by immunohistochemistry. ACE2 membranous expression was observed in the ST of the chorionic villi and was predominantly in a polarized pattern with expression highest on the stromal side of the ST. Cytotrophoblast and extravillous trophoblast expressed ACE2. TMPRSS2 expression was only present weakly in the villous endothelium and rarely in the ST.

Hosier and colleagues[54] analyzed the placenta for the presence of SARS-CoV-2. SARS-CoV-2, which localized predominantly to ST cells at the maternal-fetal interface of the placenta. Histologic examination of the placenta revealed a dense macrophage infiltrate. Argueta and colleagues[55] investigated the impact of SARS-CoV-2 infection on the placenta from a cohort of women who had tested positive for SARS-CoV-2 at delivery. Three placentas with high virus content were obtained from mothers who presented with severe COVID-19 and whose pregnancies resulted in adverse outcomes, including intrauterine fetal demise, stillbirth, and a preterm delivered baby admitted to the NICU. Infection was restricted to ST cells that envelope the fetal chorionic villi and are in direct contact with maternal blood. The infected placentas displayed massive infiltration of maternal immune cells, including macrophages into intervillous spaces, potentially contributing to inflammation of the tissue.

ST cells that envelope the fetal chorionic villi are in direct contact with maternal blood and are particularly vulnerable to SARS-CoV-2. Infection in many studies was restricted to the ST cell with subsequent necrosis. Placentas from infected maternal-neonatal dyads display massive infiltration of maternal immune cells, including macrophages into intervillous spaces. Massive infiltration of maternal immune cells coupled with ST necrosis appears to heighten the risk for maternal-fetal viral transmission. ACE2 membranous expression was observed in the ST of the chorionic villi predominantly in a polarized pattern with expression highest on the stromal side of the ST.

SUMMARY

Maternal SARS-CoV-2 infection can present with or without symptoms at the time of birth. The reported incidence of positive neonatal SARS-CoV-2 PCR test ranges from 0.56% to 6.9%. Symptomatic mothers are likely to be associated with PTB. By contrast, population studies demonstrate a consistent association of SARS-CoV-2 infection and a reduction in PTB rate. Newborns with positive SARS-CoV-2 test results appeared to have minimal burden of illness that is directly associated with a viral infection. Finally, maternal vaccination in pregnant women leads to maternal antibody production with passive transfer to their fetuses, which increases as a function of time.

CLINICS CARE POINTS

- Asymptomatic COVID 19 positive mothers need not be separated from their newborn baby after delivery.
- Breast-feeding is safe if associated with adequate parental education of safe infection control practices.
- COVID-19 vaccination is recommended for women who are pregnant or breastfeeding.
- Women who are pregnant may receive a booster vaccine shot.

DISCLOSURE

The authors have no commercial or financial conflicts of interest to disclose.

REFERENCES

1. Castagnoli R, Votto M, Licari A, et al. Severe acute respiratory syndrome coronavirus 2 (SARS-CoV-2) infection in children and adolescents. A systematic review. JAMA Pediatr 2020;174(9):882–9.
2. Viner R, Mytton O, Bonell C, et al. Susceptibility to SARS-CoV-2 infection among children and adolescents compared with adults. A systematic review and meta-analysis. JAMA Pediatr 2021;175(2):143–56.
3. Parri N, Lenge M, Buonsenso D. Children with Covid-19 in pediatric emergency departments in Italy. N Engl J Med 2020;383:187–90.
4. Mehta N, Mytton O, Mullins E, et al. SARS-CoV-2 (COVID-19): what do we know about children? A systematic review. Clin Infect Dis 2020;71(9):2469–79.
5. Services.AAP.org. Children and COVID-19: state-level data report. 2021. Available at: https://services.aap.org/en/pages/2019-novel-coronavirus-covid-19-infections/children-and-covid-19-state-level-data-report/. July 8, 2021.
6. Dufort E, Koumans E, Chow E, et al. Multisystem inflammatory syndrome in children in New York State. N Engl J Med 2020;383:347–58.
7. Puopolo KM, Hudak ML, Kimberlin DW, et al. Management of infants born to mothers with COVID-19. AAP; 2020. Available at: https://www.tn.gov/content/dam/tn/health/documents/cedep/novel-coronavirus/AAP_COVID-19-Initial-Newborn-Guidance.pdf. July 8, 2021.
8. Wang L, Shi Y, Xiao T, et al. Chinese expert consensus on the perinatal and neonatal management for the prevention and control of the 2019 novel coronavirus infection (first edition). Ann Transl Med 2020;8(3):47–2020.
9. Evaluation and management considerations for neonates at risk for COVID-19. CDC.gov. 2020. Available at: https://www.cdc.gov/coronavirus/2019-ncov/hcp/caring-for-newborns.html. May 31, 2020.

10. Salvatore CM, Han J, Acker K, et al. Neonatal management and outcomes during the COVID-19 pandemic. Lancet Child Adolesc Health 2020;4(10):721–7.
11. Shalish W, Lakshminrusimha S, Manzoni P, et al. COVID-19 and neonatal respiratory care: current evidence and practical approach. Am J Perinatol 2020;37(08): 780–91.
12. Knight M, Bunch K, Vousden N, et al. Characteristics and outcomes of pregnant women admitted to hospital with confirmed SARS-CoV-2 infection in UK: national population based cohort study. BMJ 2020;369:m2107.
13. Martinez-Perez O, Vouga M, Cruz Melguizo S, et al. Association between mode of delivery among pregnant women with COVID-19 and maternal and neonatal outcomes in Spain. JAMA 2020;324(3):296–9.
14. Dumitriu D, Emeruwa U, Hanft E, et al. Outcomes of neonates born to mothers with severe acute respiratory syndrome coronavirus 2 infection at a large medical center in New York City. JAMA Pediatr 2021;175(2):157–67.
15. Han MS, Seong MW, Heo EY, et al. Sequential analysis of viral load in a neonate and her mother infected with severe acute respiratory syndrome coronavirus 2. Clin Infect Dis 2020;71(16):2236–9.
16. Slaats MALJ, Versteylen M, Gast KB, et al. Case report of a neonate with high viral SARSCoV-2 loads and long-term virus shedding. J Infect Public Health 2020; 13(12):1878–84.
17. Perlman J, Oxford C, Chang C, Salvatore C, Di Pace J. Delivery Room Preparedness and Early Neonatal Outcomes During COVID19 Pandemic in New York City [published online ahead of print, 2020 May 14]. Pediatrics 2020;e20201567. https://doi.org/10.1542/peds.2020-1567.
18. Siberry GK, Reddy UM, Mofenson LM. SARS-COV-2 maternal-child transmission: can it occur before delivery and how do we prove it? Pediatr Infect Dis J 2020; 39(9):e263–4.
19. Li M, Chen L, Zhang J, et al. The SARS-CoV-2 receptor ACE2 expression of maternal-fetal interface and fetal organs by single-cell transcriptome study. PLoS One 2020;15(4):e0230295.
20. Shah PS, Diambomba Y, Acharya G, et al. Classification system and case definition for SARS-CoV-2 infection in pregnant women, fetuses, and neonates. Acta Obstet Gynecol Scand 2020;99(5):565–8.
21. Edlow AG, Li JZ, Collier AY, et al. Assessment of maternal and neonatal SARS-CoV-2 viral load, transplacental antibody transfer, and placental pathology in pregnancies during the COVID-19 pandemic. JAMA Netw Open 2020;3(12): e2030455.
22. Bahadur G, Bhat M, Acharya S, et al. Retrospective observational RT-PCR analyses on 688 babies born to 843 SARS-CoV-2 positive mothers, placental analyses and diagnostic analyses limitations suggest vertical transmission is possible. Facts Views Vis Obgyn 2021;13(1):53–66.
23. Vivanti AJ, Vauloup-Fellous C, Prevot S, et al. Transplacental transmission of SARS-CoV-2 infection. Nat Commun 2020;11(1):3572.
24. Kirtsman M, Diambomba Y, Poutanen SM, et al. Probable congenital SARS-CoV-2 infection in a neonate born to a woman with active SARS-CoV-2 infection. CMAJ 2020;192(24):E647–50.
25. Von Kohorn I, Stein SR, Shikani BT, et al. In utero severe acute respiratory syndrome coronavirus 2 infection. J Pediatr Infect Dis Soc 2020;9(6):769–71.
26. Lorenz N, Treptow A, Schmidt S, et al. Neonatal early-onset infection with SARS-CoV-2 in a newborn presenting with encephalitic symptoms. Pediatr Infect Dis J 2020;39(8):e212.

27. Sisman J, Jaleel MA, Moreno W, et al. Intrauterine transmission of SARS-COV-2 infection in a preterm infant. Pediatr Infect Dis J 2020;39(9):e265–7.
28. Patanè L, Morotti D, Giunta MR, et al. Vertical transmission of coronavirus disease 2019: severe acute respiratory syndrome coronavirus 2 RNA on the fetal side of the placenta in pregnancies with coronavirus disease 2019-positive mothers and neonates at birth. Am J Obstet Gynecol MFM 2020;2(3):100145.
29. Alamar I, Abu-Arja MH, Heyman T, et al. A possible case of vertical transmission of severe acute respiratory syndrome coronavirus 2 (SARS-CoV-2) in a newborn with positive placental in situ hybridization of SARS-CoV-2 RNA. J Pediatr Infect Dis Soc 2020;9(5):636–9.
30. Alzamora MC, Paredes T, Caceres D, et al. Severe COVID-19 during pregnancy and possible vertical transmission. Am J Perinatol 2020;37(8):861–5.
31. Parsa Y, Shokri N, Jahedbozorgan T, et al. Possible vertical transmission of COVID-19 to the newborn; a case report. Arch Acad Emerg Med 2020;9(1):e5.
32. Lima-Rogel V, Villegas-Silva R, Coronado-Zarco A, et al. Perinatal COVID-19: a case report, literature review, and proposal of a national system for case record. Bol Med Hosp Infant Mex 2021;78(1):34–40.
33. Zamaniyan M, Ebadi A, Aghajanpoor S, et al. Preterm delivery, maternal death, and vertical transmission in a pregnant woman with COVID-19 infection. Prenat Diagn 2020;40(13):1759–61.
34. Hascoët JM, Jellimann JM, Hartard C, et al. Case series of COVID-19 asymptomatic newborns with possible intrapartum transmission of SARS-CoV-2. Front Pediatr 2020;8:568979.
35. Bandyopadhyay T, Sharma A, Kumari P, et al. Possible early vertical transmission of COVID-19 from an infected pregnant female to her neonate: a case report. J Trop Pediatr 2021;67(1):fmaa094.
36. Villar J, Ariff S, Gunier RB, et al. Maternal and neonatal morbidity and mortality among pregnant women with and without COVID-19 infection: the INTERCOVID Multinational Cohort Study. JAMA Pediatr 2021;175(8):817–26.
37. Angelidou A, Sullivan K, Melvin PR, et al. Association of maternal perinatal SARS-CoV-2 infection with neonatal outcomes during the COVID-19 pandemic in Massachusetts. JAMA Netw Open 2021;4(4):e217523.
38. Gale C, Quigley MA, Placzek A, et al. Characteristics and outcomes of neonatal SARS-CoV-2 infection in the UK: a prospective national cohort study using active surveillance. Lancet Child Adolesc Health 2021;5(2):113–21.
39. Norman M, Navér L, Söderling J, et al. Association of maternal SARS-CoV-2 infection in pregnancy with neonatal outcomes. JAMA 2021;325(20):2076–86.
40. Mullins E, Hudak ML, Banerjee J, et al. Pregnancy and neonatal outcomes of COVID-19: coreporting of common outcomes from PAN-COVID and AAP-SONPM registries. Ultrasound Obstet Gynecol 2021;57(4):573–81.
41. Simpson AN, Snelgrove JW, Sutradhar R, et al. Perinatal outcomes during the COVID-19 pandemic in Ontario, Canada. JAMA Netw Open 2021;4(5):e2110104.
42. Philip RK, Purtill H, Reidy E, et al. Unprecedented reduction in births of very low birthweight (VLBW) and extremely low birthweight (ELBW) infants during the COVID-19 lockdown in Ireland: a 'natural experiment' allowing analysis of data from the prior two decades. BMJ Glob Health 2020;5(9):e003075.
43. Hedermann G, Hedley PL, Bækvad-Hansen M, et al. Danish premature birth rates during the COVID-19 lockdown. Arch Dis Child Fetal Neonatal Ed 2021;106(1):93–5.

44. Harvey EM, McNeer E, McDonald MF, et al. Association of preterm birth rate with COVID-19 statewide stay-at-home orders in Tennessee. JAMA Pediatr 2021; 175(6):635–7.
45. Pasternak B, Neovius M, Söderling J, et al. Preterm birth and stillbirth during the COVID-19 pandemic in Sweden: a nationwide cohort study. Ann Intern Med 2021;174(6):873–5.
46. Flannery DD, Gouma S, Dhudasia MB, et al. Assessment of maternal and neonatal cord blood SARS-CoV-2 antibodies and placental transfer ratios. JAMA Pediatr 2021;175(6):594–600.
47. Perl SH, Uzan-Yulzari A, Klainer H, et al. SARS-CoV-2-specific antibodies in breast milk after COVID-19 vaccination of breastfeeding women. JAMA 2021; 325(19):2013–4.
48. Collier AY, McMahan K, Yu J, et al. Immunogenicity of COVID-19 mRNA vaccines in pregnant and lactating women. JAMA 2021;325(23):2370–80.
49. Prabhu M, Murphy EA, Sukhu AC, et al. Antibody response to coronavirus disease 2019 (COVID-19) messenger RNA vaccination in pregnant women and transplacental passage into cord blood. Obstet Gynecol 2021;138(2):278–80.
50. Chambers C, Krogstad P, Bertrand K, et al. Evaluation for SARS-CoV-2 in breast milk from 18 infected women. JAMA 2020;324(13):1347–8.
51. Jaiswal N, Puri M, Agarwal K, et al. COVID-19 as an independent risk factor for subclinical placental dysfunction. Eur J Obstet Gynecol Reprod Biol 2021; 259:7–11.
52. Schwartz DA, Morotti D. Placental pathology of COVID-19 with and without fetal and neonatal infection: trophoblast necrosis and chronic histiocytic intervillositis as risk factors for transplacental transmission of SARS-CoV-2. Viruses 2020; 12(11):1308.
53. Hecht JL, Quade B, Deshpande V, et al. SARS-CoV-2 can infect the placenta and is not associated with specific placental histopathology: a series of 19 placentas from COVID-19-positive mothers. Mod Pathol 2020;33(11):2092–103.
54. Hosier H, Farhadian SF, Morotti RA, et al. SARS-CoV-2 infection of the placenta. J Clin Invest 2020;130(9):4947–53.
55. Argueta LB, Lacko LA, Bram Y, et al. SARS-CoV-2 infects syncytiotrophoblast and activates inflammatory responses in the placenta. bioRxiv 2021. https://doi.org/10.1101/2021.06.01.446676.

Black Babies Matter

James W. Collins Jr, MD, MPH[a],*, Richard J. David, MD[b]

KEYWORDS

- Infant mortality • Preterm birth • Racial disparity • Racial discrimination
- Social class • African–American

KEY POINTS

- African–American women's lifelong exposure to structural and interpersonal racial discrimination are risk factors for preterm birth and consequent infant mortality.
- Paternal class status is associated with adverse birth outcome independent of maternal race and class status.
- Race and class inequities are intertwined and are the root causes of the African–American (compared with White) women's birth outcome disadvantage.

INTRODUCTION

Despite dramatic reductions in overall infant mortality rates (<365 day, IMR) since the 1960s, the African–American: non-Latinx White infant mortality rate ratio increased from 1.6 to 2.2.[1] For decades United States policymakers, highlighted by Healthy People 2010 and 2020 objectives, have been unable to eliminate this appalling racial inequity.[2] Preterm birth (<37 weeks, PTB) and low birth weight (<2500 g, LBW) are the leading causes of death for African–American infants. Reflecting advances in neonatal intensive care, our ability to save the life of extremely preterm infants has increased remarkably over recent decades. However, in both races the PTB rates are increasing.[3] In 2018%, 13.8% of all African–American births were preterm compared with 9.1% of White births.[3] Moreover, African–American infants are more than twice as likely to be born less than 34 weeks compared with White infants, 5.8% versus 2.9%, respectively.[4]

To understand the racial disparity in adverse birth outcome, we need to focus beyond the biomedical level. It is been estimated that only 10% of population health differences are attributable to health care.[5] Prenatal care accounts for a relatively small component of the African–American women's pregnancy outcome

a Neonatal Intensive Care Unit, Division of Neonatology, Ann & Robert H. Lurie Children's Hospital of Chicago, Northwestern University Feinberg School of Medicine, Box 45, 225 E. Chicago Avenue, Chicago, IL 60611, USA; b Division of Neonatology, Stroger Hospital of Cook County, University of Illinois at Chicago College of Medicine, 1969 Ogden Avenue, Chicago, IL 60612, USA
* Corresponding author.
E-mail address: jcollins@northwestern.edu

Clin Perinatol 49 (2022) 93–101
https://doi.org/10.1016/j.clp.2021.11.017
0095-5108/22/© 2021 Elsevier Inc. All rights reserved.

disadvantage. In the US, race is a social classification that precisely captures the impact of racism. As such, upstream factors closely related to racism impact African–American women's reproductive health and account for the bulk of birth outcome disparities.[6]

When millions of people witnessed the extrajudicial execution of George Floyd, an unarmed, handcuffed African–American male accused of passing a counterfeit twenty-dollar bill, in a calm, matter-of-fact manner by the knee of a White policeman pressing on his neck, something snapped in America. For many Whites who oppose racism and may even have made efforts to dismantle discriminatory policies, this striking image drove home a truth, one that African–Americans have been aware of for centuries. The ideal of equality has inspired generations, but for people of color, it has remained just that, an ideal, and one that is poorly reflected in their daily lives.[7]

The objective of this essay is to examine the impact of the historical context of racism in the US on the African–American women's pregnancy outcome disadvantage. In the process, we propose a paradigm to address the racial health inequity in adverse birth outcome by considering the interplay of racism and social class.

DISCUSSION
African–American Citizenship in the United States

During African–Americans approximately 400 years in the US, 62% (1619–1865) has been spent in chattel slavery. This created the slave health deficit in the African–American population. During the subsequent 100 years (1865–1965), African–Americans had no citizenship rights and the slave health deficit was uncorrected. Since the 1960s, there have been major struggles to transition from segregation and discrimination to the integration of African–Americans. There have been ongoing disparate health status and birth outcomes between the races with institutional racism and bias in effect.

African–Americans are three times more likely to be killed by police than non-Latinx Whites and 1.3 times more likely to be unarmed.[8] Using 2013 to 2018 data from the Mapping Police Violence and 2018 CDC birth certificates of singleton births to African–American and White women from 49 states with sufficient PTB data (all but Wyoming), Wang and colleagues found that states with more police killings of unarmed African–Americans had wider racial PTB disparities than states with fewer killings.[9] The findings persisted when police killing rates were taken into consideration.[9]

Discriminatory behavior of police officers reflects structural racism and state culture, which are proxies of upstream causes of health inequities due to differential access to health-promoting environments. Police killings are also likely to have spillover effects contributing to the list of chronic stressors across the life-course of African–American women, leading to adverse birth outcomes.

The investigation of immigrant Black women and their US-born descendants highlights the importance of these upstream processes. The rates of LBW and very low birth weight (<1500 g, VLBW) infants among sub-Saharan African-born Black and Caribbean-born Black women are less than that of US-born Black women and approximates that of US-born White women.[10,11] We discovered that the birth weight of the US-born daughters of European-born White women increased across a generation.[12] The opposite occurred among the US-born daughters of African and Caribbean-born Black women.[12] In contrast to foreign-born Black women, US-born Black women navigate structural and personally mediated racial discrimination throughout their lives.

Structural Racial Discrimination

Redlining is the practice of denying or charging more for services such as insurance, banking, access to health care, or employment to residents in often racially-determined areas. The term refers to the practice of marking a red line on a map to delineate the area whereby banks would not invest. In large part reflecting the historical legacy and contemporary practice of redlining, the geographic separation African–Americans and Whites is almost complete in the vast majority of metropolitan areas. Most disturbing, the races are exposed to the extremes of residential environment with a disproportionately high percentage of African–American women residing in impoverished neighborhoods during their pregnancies with high rates of handgun violence.[13,14]

The limited available data provide evidence that redlining is a structural determinant of PTB risk.[15,16] Using the Illinois vital records and Home Mortgage Disclosure Act data, we found that PTB rates were higher among African–American women who resided in redlined areas than nonredlined neighborhoods in Chicago.[15] Moreover, PTB rates were elevated in redlined, high-proportion African–American areas than nonredlined high-proportion African–American areas.[15] Similarly, Krieger reported an association between historical redlining and PTB among singleton births in New York City.[16]

Neighborhood poverty during pregnancy is a well-established risk factor for adverse birth outcome regardless of race, however, reflecting the higher prevalence of impoverishment among African–American (compared with White) women the percentage of adverse birth outcome attributable to urban impoverishment is dramatically greater among African–American women.[13,17–19] Violent crime is increasingly recognized as an element of the residential environment and it has been associated with increased rates of adverse birth outcome independent of neighborhood income.[14,20] Using a 5-year dataset of birth files (2010–2014) from Chicago, IL with appended census income and police crime report data, Matoba and colleagues[14] found that women who resided in the highest (compared with the lowest) violence tertile neighborhoods during their pregnancies had nearly a twofold greater risk of PTB independent of individual-level factors.

The limited published literature shows that exposure to neighborhood poverty during early life (fetal, infancy, childhood) is an additional risk factor poor birth outcome. Using the Illinois transgenerational birth-file (TGBF) with appended US census income information, we found that African–American women with a lifelong residence in impoverished areas had extremely high rates of PTB and small-for-gestational age (birth weight < 10th percentile, SGA), highlighting the birth outcome consequence of lifelong exposure to disadvantaged neighborhoods.[21,22] Interestingly, African–American women with early-life residence in impoverished neighborhoods who subsequently experience low, modest, or high upward economic mobility by adulthood had lower rates of adverse birth outcome than those who remained impoverished at the time of delivery.[21,22] A similar pattern occurred among African–American with an early-life exposure to modest impoverishment who experienced upward economic mobility.[21] Contextual factors closely linked to accessibility to health-promoting environments seem to explain these findings as the associations persisted after controlling for adulthood individual-level characteristics such as maternal education, prenatal care usage, and cigarette smoking.

The developmental origins of health and disease hypothesis focus on aberrant fetal programming for adulthood disease via epigenetic modifications. Fetal undernutrition is the leading explanation. With respect to the US-born Black women's pregnancy outcome, we suspect that aspects of their social environment subject them to influences during fetal life that results in their slowed growth *in utero* and programs them to have preterm or SGA infants during adulthood. Consistent with the fetal programming conceptual model, African–American women's upward economic mobility is not associated with a decreased risk of PTB among those mothers born at LBW.[21]

Personally Mediated Racial Discrimination

An established literature shows that African–American women's exposure to interpersonal racism is a risk factor for adverse birth outcome.[23–26] We found that African–American women who delivered preterm infants were more likely to experience interpersonal racial discrimination during their lifetime than African–American women who deliverer term infants.[23] The adverse effect of perceived discrimination was strongest among women aged 20 to 29 years, and generally considered as an optimal childbearing decade. The relationship between exposure to interpersonal racial discrimination and PTB seems to be modified by coping behaviors.[24,26] Bravemen and colleagues[25] investigated 2202 African–American and 8122 White women with singleton live-births in California during 2011 to 2014 and found that 37% of African–American versus 6% of White women reported chronic worry about racial discrimination. Most striking, chronic worry about racial discrimination was associated with a twofold greater risk of PTB among African–American women. Interestingly, the racial disparity in PTB was attenuated and became nonsignificant when adjusted for chronic worry about racial discrimination.[25] The underlying mechanism seems to be related to stress and/or the physiologic responses to chronic stressors which accumulate over the life-course of US-born Black women, resulting in an enhanced inflammatory response, comprised fetal development, and poor pregnancy outcomes.[27–29]

Social Class

Despite leading the world in advances in neonatal care, the first-year mortality rate of White Americans exceeds that of 27 developed nations.[6] Moreover, the PTB rate of White women in the US is higher than that of European women White women.[30] Similar to race, class inequity is a fundamental characteristic of American society and a strong predictor of birth outcome.[6,31] The stress and anxiety associated with fear of unemployment, loss of medical insurance, homelessness, and food shortage creates psychological stress that becomes embodied, just as surely as the free-floating anxiety attributed to fear of racial discrimination. For a sizable proportion of the US population, socioeconomic status and related stresses have only worsened over recent decades with the widening gulf between the wealthiest and working-class families. Understanding the high rates of White infant mortality requires an appreciation of inequity based on social class.[6]

In both races, women's lower class status is an established risk factor for adverse birth outcome.[19,32–34] Braveman and colleagues[32] compared infant mortality rates for American women according to the level of education attainment, a strong measure for socioeconomic status. They found that the infant mortality rate for women with less than 12 years of education was 2.4-times higher than for college graduates among White women, and 1.4-times higher among African–American women. In an investigation of singleton births in Chicago, we found that upper-class born White women's deterioration in class status was associated with a twofold greater risk of infant mortality independent of selected biologic, medical, and behavioral variables.[19] While both studies illustrate the birth outcome inequity attributable to women's social position, it is important to keep the impact of race and class in perspective: the infant mortality rate of African–American college graduates, although significantly less than that of African–American women who do not complete high school, is still higher than the infant mortality rate of White women with less than 12 years of education.

Maternal and child health research has routinely investigated the impact of social class as defined by mother's characteristics. However, a prior study found that differences in paternal acknowledgment on infant's birth certificates accounted for a larger proportion of both the Black:White and US-born Black: foreign-born Black women's disparities in PTB rates than maternal education.[35] Most pertinent, the socioeconomic and cultural landscape of African–American fatherhood strongly suggests that the role of paternal socioeconomic position (SEP) is particularly salient to the racial disparity in adverse birth outcome.[36] High school and college graduation rates for African–American men are less than that of African–American women by a wide margin.[37] The joblessness in the African–American community has been a pivotal factor in declining marriage rates.[37] Similarly, the disproportionate role of incarceration among African–American men reduces their economic and marital prospects.[38]

The contribution of men's class status beyond that captured by marital status to adverse birth outcome is gaining greater investigational attention.[39–44] Blumenshine and colleagues[39] used California vital records linked to population-based questionnaire data with the mother as the reporter of paternal education and found that acknowledged father's low education level correlated with increased PTB rates independent of maternal education. In an investigation of national vital records, Ekeke and colleagues[44] reported that rates of PTB and LBW among US-born and foreign-born Black women decreased as paternal educational attainment increased. Using Oaxaca decomposition analyses, we showed that approximately 15% of the maternal nativity (country of birth) disparity in PTB rates among infants with acknowledged fathers was explained by paternal education. In stark contrast, only about 4% of the maternal nativity disparity in PTB rates among infants with acknowledged fathers was explained by maternal education.[44]

In a series of investigations in which men's lifelong class status was objectively defined by their neighborhood income during early-life and adulthood, we demonstrated an association between paternal SEP and adverse birth outcome.[39–43] Father's lifelong low (compared with high) class status was a risk factor for early (<34 weeks) PTB regardless of maternal age, marital status, education, and race/ethnicity.[42] Reflecting the greater percentage of African–American births to low SEP men, approximately 40% of LBW deliveries to African–American women's seems to be attributable to their partners early-life, adulthood, or lifelong low SEP, a proportion more than four times that observed in White women.[39] A causal relationship is plausible. We found that White and African–American women's selected pregnancy-related risk factors (ie, inadequate prenatal care, suboptimal weight gain, and cigarette smoking) accounted for a significant percentage of the excess early PTB rates among low (compared with high) SEP fathers.[43]

Public Health Implications: Go to the Roots of the Problem

While other affluent industrialized countries don't have a pervasive racial infant health inequity as the US, they do have social classes. Yet, their infant mortality rates are lower than that of the US. Most importantly and perhaps less well known is the US dismal international ranking in expenditures on social supports designed to mitigate the consequents of economic stress.

The US has a higher level of income inequality than most other developed countries, with a Gini coefficient of 0.39. That places the US 34th among the 40 Organization for Economic Co-operation and Development (OECD) countries for equality.[45] Not surprisingly, this income gap correlates with infant mortality.[46] Closely related, US has a threefold higher poverty rate than in many OECD countries. Social policies and laws that safeguard workers' jobs, offer parental leave, and subsidize child-care are all weaker in the US than in other comparable nations.[47] US expenditures for support of young families (child allowance, maternity and paternity leave, early childhood education) are approximately one-third that of the OECD countries with comparable per capita income.

In their classic 2005 *Health Affairs* article about race, class and health, Kawachi and colleagues[48] noted that one of the main functions of racism in the US has been to divide people with common class interests. They wrote: "One of the less studied elements of our view is the harm done to White working-class Americans by the use of racism. It is possible to trace accounts of how racism was used to weaken unionization efforts in the United States or to mislead white Americans about social policy in building a conservative political bloc in the South and elsewhere." That was the infamous "Southern strategy" by means of which the Republican Party gained political dominance throughout the former slave states.

As we recently noted in an editorial in the *Archives of Disease in Childhood*, "The American focus on racial identity is a product of the unique history of race politics in North America. The historic role played by chattel slavery in the foundation of the country's economy in the centuries prior to 1863—and the ongoing racial discrimination in economic opportunity since then—are unique among the wealthy countries that make up the OECD. Clearly, other wealthy countries have their own historical baggage from colonialism and less than fair treatment of immigrants of color, but no other country was founded on the expropriation and near extermination of one ethnic group and the enslavement of another. Because of this history, racial identity tends to overshadow class identity in the American psyche."[49]

The "divide-and-conquer" strategy described by Kawachi and colleagues,[48] by weakening the political power of nonelites, results in a disadvantage for most Americans in terms of health-promoting social policy. However, this strategy has provided an advantage for the upper stratum of corporate America. Capital accumulation is facilitated by reduced expenditures on social programs, providing a competitive edge against international rivals, despite massive military expenditures by the US. Thus, the U.S. government has assumed the mantle of "leader of the free world" despite having the poorest health indicators. The ideological dimension of this leadership has historically used racial bias to hinder the promotion of social policies that do not enhance the market, such as national health insurance.[50,51]

SUMMARY

Since race and class inequities came into existence together, "conjoined twins" in the words of Ibram X. Kendi.[52] They will need to be dismantled together. We encourage health professionals to understand these intertwined inequities and how they underlie the African–American women's birth outcome disadvantage. This includes expanding medical school curricula which include historical background and address racial bias in the clinical setting. As clinicians in neonatal intensive care units, we can make a meaningful difference in parents' lives during this time of crisis by relating to them with understanding and respect. However, it is our role as members of society that we are called on to help eliminate unjust systems. The oppression produced by these systems underlies the social and economic inequities that are the root cause of the racial disparity in adverse birth outcome. If we truly hope to see the racial disparity in pregnancy, birth, and infancy outcomes disappear, being a good physician is simply not enough.[7]

Best Practices

- We encourage clinicians and policy makers to address the social and economic inequities that are the root cause of birth outcome disparities.

DISCLOSURE

Funding was provided by the March of Dimes Foundation (Grants 12-FY09-159 and 21-FY16-111, to JWC)

REFERENCES

1. Available at: https://www.cdc.gov/mmwr/preview/mmwrhtml/mm6301a9.htm accessed May 19, 2021.
2. Centers for Disease Control and Prevention. Healthy people 2010: overview 2011. Available at: https://www.cdc.gov/nchs/data/hpdata2010/hp2010_final_review_overview.pdf. Accessed September 19, 2020.
3. Available at: www.marchofdimes.org/peristats/tools/reportcard.aspx Accessed May 19, 2021
4. Martin JA, Hamilton BE, Osterman MJK, et al. Births: final data for 2013. Natl Vital Stat Rep 2015;64(1):1–65. Division of vital statistics.
5. Schroeder SA. American health improvement depends upon addressing class disparities. Prev Med 2016;92:6–15.
6. David RJ, Collins JW. Layers of inequity: power, policy and health. Am J Public Health 2014;104:S8–10.
7. David R, Collins J. Why does racial inequity in health persist. J Perinatol 2021;41: 346–450.
8. Sinyangwe S, Mckesson D, Prichnett B. Mapping police violence 2020. Available at: http://mappingpoliceviolence.org. Accessed May 19, 2021.
9. Yang N, Collins J, Burris H. States with more killings of unarmed black people have larger black-white preterm birth disparities. J Perinatol 2021;41:358–9.
10. David RJ, Collins JW. Differing birth weights among infants of U.S.-born blacks, African-born blacks, and U.S.-born whites. N Engl J Med 1997;337:1209–14.
11. Pallotto EK, Collins JW, David RJ. The enigma of maternal race and infant birth weight: a population-based study of U.S.-born black and Caribbean-born black women. Am J Epidemiol 2000;151:1080–5.
12. Collins JW, Wu SY, David RJ. Differing intergenerational birth weights among the descendants of U.S.-born and foreign-born whites and African-Americans in Illinois. Am J Epidemiol 2002;155:210–6.
13. Collins JW, Wambach J, David RJ, et al. Women's lifelong exposure to neighborhood poverty and low birth weight: a population-based study. Matern Child Health J 2009;13:326–33.
14. Matoba N, Reina M, Prachand N, et al. Neighborhood gun violence and birth outcomes in Chicago. Matern Child Health J 2019;23:1251–9.
15. Matoba N, Suprenant S, Rankin K, et al. Mortgage discrimination and preterm birth among African American women: an exploratory study. Health Place 2019;59:102193.
16. Krieger N, Van Wye G, Huynh M, et al. Structural racism, historical redlining, and risk of preterm birth in New York city, 2013-2017. Am J Public Health 2020;110: 1046–53.

17. Pearl M, Braveman P, Abrams B. The relationship of neighborhood socioeconomic characteristics to birthweight among 5 ethnic groups in California. Am J Public Health 2001;91:1808–14.
18. Collins JW Jr, David RJ, Rankin KM, et al. Transgenerational effect of neighborhood poverty on low birth weight among African Americans in Cook County, Illinois. Am J Epidemiol 2009;169:712–7.
19. Collins J, Colgan J, DeSisto C, et al. Affluent-Born White Mother's descending neighborhood income and infant mortality: a population-based study. Matern Child Health J 2018;22:1484–91.
20. Messer LC, Kaufman JS, Dole N, et al. Violent crime exposure classification and adverse birth outcomes: a geographically-defined cohort study. Int J Health Geogr 2006;5:22.
21. Collins JW, Rankin KM, David R. African-American women's upward economic mobility and preterm birth: the effect of fetal programming. Am J Public Health 2011;101:714–9.
22. Collins J, Marina A, Rankin K. African-American women's upward economic mobility and small for gestational age births: a population-based study. Matern Child Health J 2018;22:1183–9.
23. Collins JW Jr, David RJ, Handler A, et al. Very low birthweight in African American infants: the role of maternal exposure to interpersonal racial discrimination. Am J Public Health 2004;94:2132–8.
24. Slaughter-Acey JC, Sealy-Jefferson S, Helmkamp L, et al. Racism in the form of micro aggressions and the risk of preterm birth among black women. Ann Epidemiol 2016;26:7–13.
25. Braveman P, Heck K, Egerter S, et al. Worry about racial discrimination: a missing piece of the puzzle of Black-White disparities in preterm birth? PLoS One 2017; 12:e0186151.
26. Rankin KM, David RJ, Collins JW. African-American women's exposure to interpersonal racial discrimination in public settings and preterm birth: the effect of coping mechanisms. Ethn Dis 2011;21:370–5.
27. Hogue CJ, Bremner JD. Stress model for research into preterm delivery among black women. Am J Obstet Gynecol 2005;192:S47–55.
28. Coussons-Read ME, Okun ML, Nettles CD. Psychosocial stress increases inflammatory markers and alters cytokine production across pregnancy. Brain Behav Immun 2007;21:343–50.
29. Matoba N, Mestan K, Collins J. Understanding racial disparities in preterm birth through the placenta. Clin Ther 2021;43:287–96.
30. Beck S, Wojdyla D, Say L, et al. The worldwide incidence of preterm birth: a systematic review of maternal mortality and morbidity. Bull World Health Organ 2010; 88:31–8.
31. Isaacs SL, Schroeder SA. Class – the ignored determinant of the nation's health. N Engl J Med 2004;351:1137–42.
32. Braveman PA, Cubbin C, Egerter S, et al. Socioeconomic disparities in health in the United States: what the patterns tell us. Am J Public Health 2010;100: S186–96.
33. Meyer J, Warren N, Reisine S. Job control, substantive complexity, and risk for low birth weight and preterm delivery: an analysis from a state birth registry. Am J Indust Med 2007;50:664–75.
34. Collins J, Rankin K, David R. Downward economic mobility and preterm birth: an exploratory study of Chicago-born upper class white mothers. Matern Child Health J 2015;19:1601–7.

35. DeSisto C, Hirai A, Collins J, et al. Deconstructing a disparity: Explaining excess preterm birth among U.S.-born black women. Ann Epidemiol 2018;28:225–30.
36. Mincy R. Black males left behind. Washington, DC: The Urban Institute Press; 2006.
37. Jewel KS. The survival African-American family: the institutional impact of U.S. social policy. Connecticut: Praeger; 2003.
38. Maurer M, King R. Uneven justice: states rates of incarceration by race and ethnicity. The sentencing project, research and advocacy for reform. Washington, DC: The Sentencing Project; 2007.
39. Blumenshine P, Egerter M, Braveman P. Father's education: an independent marker of risk for preterm birth. Matern Child Health J 2011;15:60–7.
40. Collins J, Rankin K, David R. Paternal lifelong socioeconomic position and low birth weight rates: relevance to the African-American women's birth outcome disadvantage. Matern Child Health J 2016;20:1759–66.
41. Enstad S, DeSisto C, Rankin K, et al. Father's lifetime socioeconomic status, small for gestational age, and infant mortality: a population-based study. Ethn Dis 2019; 29:9–16.
42. Collins J, Rankin K, Desisto C, et al. Early and late preterm birth rates among US-Born urban women: the effect of men's lifelong class status. Matern Child Health J 2019;23:1621–6.
43. Collins J, DeSisto C, Weiss A, et al. Excess early (< 34 Weeks) preterm rates among non-acknowledged and acknowledged low socioeconomic position fathers: the role of women's selected pregnancy-related risk factors. Matern Child Health J 2020;24:612–9.
44. Ekeke P, Rankin K, DeSisto C, et al. The excess preterm birth rate among US-born (compared to foreign-born) black women: the role of father's education. Matern Child Health J 2021. https://doi.org/10.1007/s10995-020-03117-9.
45. Available at: https://data.oecd.org/inequality/income-inequality.htm Accessed May 19, 2021.
46. Muntaner C, Lynch JW, Hillemeier M, et al. Economic inequality, working-class power, social capital, and cause-specific mortality in wealthy countries. Int J Health Serv 2002;32:629 56.
47. Tikkanen RS, Eric C, Schneider EC. Social spending to improve population health — does the United States spend as wisely as other countries? N Engl J Med 2020;382:885–7.
48. Kawachi I, Daniels N, Robinson DE. Health disparities by race and class: why both matter. Health Aff 2005;24:343–52.
49. David R. Inequity at birth and population health. Inequity at birth and population health. Arch Dis Child 2019;104:929–30.
50. Gilmore GE. Defying dixie: the radical roots of civil rights, 1919-1950. New York: W.W. Norton & Co; 2008.
51. McGhee H. The sum of us: what racism costs everyone and how we can prosper together. New York: Penguin Random House; 2021.
52. Kendi IX. How to be and antiracist. New York: One World Publishers; 2019.

Pulmonary Vasodilator Therapy in Persistent Pulmonary Hypertension of the Newborn

Megha Sharma, MD[a], Emily Callan, MD[b],
G. Ganesh Konduri, MD[b],*

KEYWORDS

- Hypoxic respiratory failure • Inhaled nitric oxide • Bronchopulmonary dysplasia
- Cyclic GMP • Prostaglandins

KEY POINTS

- Up to one-third of newborns with PPHN do not respond to inhaled nitric oxide (iNO).
- Advances in understanding PPHN pathobiology in animal models have provided the basis for alternative therapeutic targets in iNO nonresponders.
- Efficacy of other vasodilators is limited to observational studies.
- Randomized clinical trials from resource-constrained settings without access to iNO/ECMO support the use of some alternate vasodilators. Benefit of such therapies in the infants already on iNO remains unclear.
- Conduct of traditional randomized trials in PPHN is challenging due to the low incidence of PPHN and low enrollment into trials.

INTRODUCTION

Persistent pulmonary hypertension of the newborn (PPHN) is a clinical syndrome characterized by sustained elevation of pulmonary vascular resistance (PVR) after birth, resulting in extrapulmonary right-to-left shunting and severe hypoxemia. PPHN affects approximately 2 infants per 1000 live births and the highest incidence occurs in late preterm infants (34–36 weeks of gestational age) at 5.4 per 1000 live births compared with term infants at 1.6 per 1000 live births.[1] Inhaled nitric oxide (iNO), a potent pulmonary vasodilator, had a transformational impact on the management of infants with

Conflicts of interest: Authors have no relevant financial conflicts of interest to disclose.
[a] Division of Neonatology, Department of Pediatrics, Arkansas Children's Hospital, University of Arkansas for Medical Sciences, Little Rock, AR, USA; [b] Division of Neonatology, Department of Pediatrics, Medical College of Wisconsin, Children's Research Institute, Children's Wisconsin, Wauwatosa, WI, USA
* Corresponding author. 999 North 92nd Street, CCC Suite C410, Wauwatosa, WI 53226.
E-mail address: gkonduri@mcw.edu

Clin Perinatol 49 (2022) 103–125
https://doi.org/10.1016/j.clp.2021.11.010
0095-5108/22/© 2021 Elsevier Inc. All rights reserved.
perinatology.theclinics.com

PPHN. However, up to 30% of PPHN infants fail to respond to iNO and face increased risk of complications, including the need for extracorporeal membrane oxygenation (ECMO) to survive.[2] Improved knowledge of the pathobiology of PPHN combined with the critical need to improve outcomes in iNO nonresponsive infants has led to the development and clinical application of alternative vasodilators. However, the lack of high-quality evidence in this area presents a clinical dilemma and therapeutic challenge to the bedside clinician. This review focuses on optimizing the response to iNO and the use of alternative pulmonary vasodilators in the management of PPHN. We will summarize the literature on the use of other pulmonary vasodilators, suggest a management approach based on our experience and outcomes, and discuss challenges involved in future randomized clinical trials in this field.

BACKGROUND

PPHN is often a complication of many lung diseases and systemic disorders that lead to elevated PVR.[1,2] The fetal pulmonary circulation is characterized by elevated PVR and low pulmonary blood flow.[3,4] At birth, PVR decreases exponentially with a subsequent rise in lung blood flow to facilitate gas exchange during postnatal life.[3,4] This transition at birth in response to oxygen and other birth-related stimuli involves structural reorganization of the pulmonary vessel walls, recruitment of intraacinar arteries, and gradual vascular remodeling.[4–6] Elevated PVR in infants suffering from PPHN can be a consequence of a plethora of neonatal disorders that lead to vasoconstriction, medial hypertrophy of the pulmonary arteries (PAs), or decreased blood vessel density due to the failure of angiogenesis. The conditions that lead to high PVR are listed in **Box 1**.

Endogenous vascular signals

The endothelial cells (ECs) and smooth muscle cells (SMCs) in the pulmonary blood vessels together mediate the transitional changes in lung vasculature at birth. The endothelium plays a key role in generating vasodilators and limiting vasoconstrictors,[6–8] thus mediating an immediate, local alteration of vascular tone[6] (**Fig. 1**). NO, the key

---

Box 1
Etiology of PPHN in neonates

Maladaptation of pulmonary vasculature (abnormal, "reactive" pulmonary vasoconstriction)
- Parenchymal lung diseases, such as meconium aspiration syndrome (MAS), respiratory distress syndrome (RDS), and pneumonia
- In response to systemic disorders, such as hypothermia, sepsis, fetal hypoxia/distress, hypercapnia, acidosis, and hyper-viscosity
- Toxic/pharmacologic exposure in utero (maternal SSRI(selective serotonin reuptake inhibitor) use)

Maldevelopment of pulmonary vasculature (remodeling of pulmonary vasculature)
- In utero closure of ductus arteriosus (maternal cyclooxygenase inhibitor use)
- Sustained pulmonary over-circulation in congenital heart disease with large left-to-right shunts
- Intrauterine growth restriction
- Genetic/chromosomal anomalies (Trisomy 21, alveolar-capillary dysplasia, surfactant protein deficiency)

Underdevelopment of pulmonary vasculature (hypoplastic pulmonary vessels; ↓cross-sectional area)
- Congenital diaphragmatic hernia
- Pulmonary hypoplasia (premature prolonged rupture of membranes, oligohydramnios and anhydramnios, space-occupying lesions in the chest).

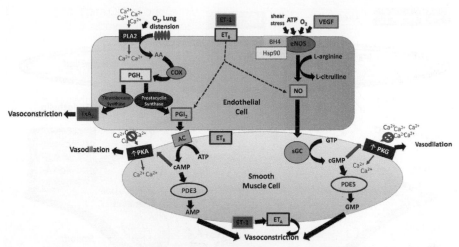

Fig. 1. Mechanisms of endothelium-dependent pulmonary vasodilation and vasoconstriction. Oxygen, lung distension, shear stress, ATP, & VEGF activate endothelial nitric oxide synthase (eNOS) and cyclooxygenase directly or indirectly. Release of NO and prostacyclin (PGI2) leads to activation of soluble guanylate cyclase (sGC) and adenylate cyclase (AC), respectively, in vascular smooth muscle cells (SMC) with generation of cGMP and cAMP, respectively. Activation of the corresponding protein kinases G and A (PKG and PKA) by cyclic nucleotides leads to decreased calcium influx and subsequent SMC relaxation. Phosphodiesterase (PDE)-5 and 3 breakdown cGMP and cAMP, respectively, to limit the duration of vasodilation. Two important vasoconstrictor pathways are conversion of PGH2 to thromboxane A2 (TxA2) by thromboxane synthase and synthesis and release of endothelin-1 (ET-1).

endogenous vasodilator is released by endothelial nitric oxide synthase (eNOS)[6] when stimulated by oxygen.[7,8] NO diffuses to SMCs to stimulate soluble guanylyl cyclase (sGC) which produces cyclic guanosine monophosphate (cGMP)[4,9] to induce vascular smooth muscle relaxation[10,11] (see **Fig. 1**). Phosphodiesterase (PDE)-5 degrades cGMP,[4] and is expressed at high levels in lung tissue, increasing as the fetus approaches term gestation.[12] The disruption in the NO-cGMP pathway in PPHN has been studied in animal models, and a decrease in eNOS expression and activity occurs following prenatal ligation of the ductus arteriosus.[13–15] This decreased expression and activity of eNOS is also seen in neonates suffering from PPHN.[16] Prostaglandins, particularly PGI$_2$ and prostaglandin E$_2$ (PGE$_2$), are important pulmonary vasodilators produced by EC. They induce SMC relaxation by increasing cyclic adenosine monophosphate (cAMP) levels in SMC. Tight control of cAMP levels is mediated by PDE-3, which rapidly breaks down cAMP. Downregulation of PG and cAMP signaling contributes to increased PVR in the PPHN model.[17] Endothelin-1 (ET-1) is released by EC and induces SMC constriction and proliferation[18,19] and promotes the release of the vasoconstrictor, thromboxane.[20] ET-1 levels are elevated in PPHN infants.[21] Thus, the altered balance of vasoactive mediators with increased levels of vasoconstrictors and decreased vasodilators contributes to the pathogenesis of PPHN. Current therapies for PPHN aim to overcome these signaling alterations by increasing cAMP and cGMP levels or antagonizing ET-1 receptors, as summarized in **Fig. 2**.

BRONCHOPULMONARY DYSPLASIA (BPD)-RELATED PULMONARY HYPERTENSION

Pulmonary hypertension affects 16% to 25% of infants with BPD and increases the risks of mortality and long-term complications.[22,23] The mechanisms of pulmonary

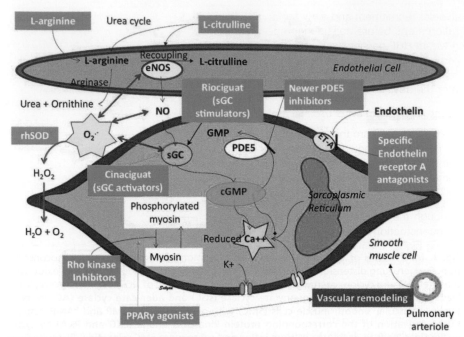

Fig. 2. Emerging targets and therapies for PPHN. L-citrulline-mediated activation of NO and soluble guanylate cyclase (sGC) activators and phosphodiesterase (PDE) 5 inhibitors increase cGMP levels. Rho-kinase inhibitors and specific endothelin receptor – A antagonists (Sitax-sentan and Ambrisentan) reverse vasoconstriction. PPAR γ agonists and antioxidants poten-tially reverse remodeling of pulmonary arteries. These potential new therapies require further evaluation and clinical trials in PPHN. (Reproduced from Lakshminrusimha S, Mathew B, Leach CL. Pharmacologic strategies in neonatal pulmonary hypertension other than nitric oxide. Semin Perinatol. 2016 Apr;40(3):160-73.)

hypertension in BPD-related pulmonary hypertension (BPD-PH) are unclear, and seem to differ from the key alteration of vasoconstrictor-vasodilator imbalance seen in PPHN. The major alteration in BPD-associated pulmonary hypertension is impaired vascular development due to the exposure of the preterm, saccular stage lung to several postnatal injuries like hyperoxia, intermittent hypoxia, barotrauma, inflamma-tion, hemodynamic stress from PDA, and elevated PA pressure.[22] These changes disrupt normal growth factor expression and signaling pathways, resulting in impaired gas diffusion, abnormal vascular remodeling, and simplification of a pulmonary vascular tree from vascular growth arrest.[22,24] Unfortunately, given the unclear path-ogenesis of BPD-associated pulmonary hypertension and paucity of randomized clin-ical trials, there is a lack of evidence-based management strategies for BPD-PH.

APPROACH TO THE MANAGEMENT OF PERSISTENT PULMONARY HYPERTENSION OF THE NEWBORN
General approach

As the clinical manifestation of PPHN is hypoxemic respiratory failure (HRF), the goal of overall management is to maintain adequate oxygen delivery to vital organs and tis-sues. The initial steps should focus on providing adequate oxygen to maintain appro-priate saturations, adequate ventilation and lung recruitment, appropriate fluid resuscitation, and hemodynamic support. Intubation and mechanical ventilation for alveolar recruitment and early surfactant administration are essential to initial stabilization steps before considering specific pulmonary vasodilator therapies. Neonates in whom HRF persists with an OI of greater than 15 (except congenital diaphragmatic hernia (CDH) for reasons addressed in that section) despite establishing adequate ventilation and circulatory resuscitation are candidates for a trial of pulmonary vasodilator therapy.

Pulmonary vasodilators used in the newborn intensive care unit

Oxygen and iNO are the widely used and selective pulmonary vasodilators for infants with PPHN and should be used as first-line therapies. There are several other adjunctive therapies at various stages of investigation that will be summarized in detail in the sections later in discussion.

Oxygen

Although the use of oxygen to correct hypoxemia and minimize hypoxic pulmonary vasoconstriction are important clinical goals in managing neonates with PPHN, maintaining higher than normal blood oxygen tension/content does not lead to additional pulmonary vasodilation and may be potentially harmful.[25] Excess oxygen administration can worsen vasoconstriction by the generation of reactive oxygen species in the PAs which can render other vasodilators like iNO ineffective.[25] We recommend avoiding hyperoxia and targeting goal oxygen saturations of 92% to 97% and/or Pao_2 60 to 90. Hypoxemia in neonates is often secondary to VQ mismatch from parenchymal lung disease; lung recruitment strategies should be adopted in place of reliance primarily on supplemental oxygen.

Inhaled nitric oxide

Inhaled iNO is the only FDA-approved pulmonary vasodilator widely accepted as a standard of care in the management of PPHN in developed countries.[26] Several large randomized clinical trials have demonstrated that iNO therapy decreases the need for ECMO/risk of mortality in full-term and late-preterm ($\geq$34 weeks' gestation) infants with severe hypoxic respiratory failure and pulmonary hypertension.[27–29] Inhaled NO gas reaches alveolar space rapidly and diffuses to the vascular smooth muscle of the adjacent PA causing relaxation by increasing the intracellular cGMP levels. Key facts and considerations are summarized later in discussion.

What makes nitric oxide a selective and ideal pulmonary vasodilator?. Once iNO diffuses from alveolar space into the lumen of PA, it is rapidly bound and inactivated by Hb, limiting its effect on the pulmonary circulation. As iNO gas enters and dilates pulmonary vessels selectively in the ventilated segments of the lungs, it promotes ventilation/perfusion match and thereby improves oxygenation in neonates with parenchymal lung disease. The effect of iNO on pulmonary circulation is also not limited by the presence of extrapulmonary right–left shunts, which often lead to hypotension with intravenous vasodilators.

What is the optimal timing for starting nitric oxide?. We recommend the initiation of iNO therapy when hypoxic respiratory failure progresses and OI reaches 15 to 20 on at least 2 blood gases, based on a clinical trial of iNO for infants in a moderate degree of HRF.[30] Initiation at this OI decreases the progression of HRF, reduces the need for ECMO/incidence of death and decreases length of stay as compared to initiation at OI > 20.

What are the right doses and weaning strategy for nitric oxide?. Previous RCTs have shown that the ideal starting dose for iNO is 20 ppm; higher starting doses do not increase the response to iNO, while potentially increasing the incidence of methemo-globinemia and NO2 exposure.[29] It is important to wean high Fio_2 levels before wean-ing iNO dose. Weaning of iNO as oxygenation improves is well tolerated with reductions in doses from 20 to 10 to 5 and then by 1 ppm decrements , as shown in a previous study that demonstrated the safety of this approach.[31]

Considerations before starting nitric oxide. Before starting any pulmonary vasodi-lator, it is essential to ensure optimum lung recruitment via CPAP or mechanical venti-lation and surfactant administration if there is evidence of parenchymal lung disease.[30] Adequate ventilation is necessary because inhaled NO gets preferentially distributed to the ventilated segments of the lung, resulting in increased perfusion of the ventilated segments, thereby optimizing the ventilation-perfusion matching. As several cyanotic heart diseases can mimic PPHN, an echocardiogram should be performed to confirm the diagnosis and rule out cyanotic heart disease. Inhaled NO is contraindicated in congenital heart diseases with ductal-dependent systemic blood flow and in Total Anomalous Pulmonary Venous Return (TAPVR) whereby the dilation of pulmonary ves-sels in the presence of venous obstruction can worsen pulmonary hypertension.

What is the role of nitric oxide in congenital diaphragmatic hernia?. Despite the widespread use of iNO in neonates with CDH during initial stabilization, randomized controlled trial data and large retrospective studies do not show evidence of improved survival and decreased need for ECMO.[32,33] The questionable benefit and high cost of iNO therapy should prompt clinicians to use this therapy cautiously, ensuring careful patient selection with echocardiographic measures of pulmonary hypertension and normal left ventricular function.[34] In the presence of systolic dysfunction of left ventricle, the rapid rise in pulmonary venous return can overburden a dysfunctional left heart and worsen cardiopulmonary status. iNO treatment did not improve oxygen-ation in patients with LV systolic dysfunction and in this specific subgroup was asso-ciated with greater ECMO rate in a single-center study.[34] We recommend that in instances whereby iNO is initiated based on echo parameters of PH or in acute hyp-oxemic crisis to stabilize for transport and/or ECMO, there should be ongoing evalu-ation of the response and need for continued iNO treatment.

Other pulmonary vasodilators

Pulmonary vasodilators acting via the cyclic guanosine monophosphate pathway
Sildenafil (PDE-5 inhibitor). iNO exerts its vasodilator effect primarily through soluble guanylate cyclase (sGC) and the second messenger, cGMP. Oxidative stress in PPHN oxidizes sGC and decreases cGMP production, and stimulates PDE5 to enhance the breakdown of cGMP, thus rendering iNO ineffective.[35,36] Alternate agents have been investigated for neonates unresponsive to iNO. Among them, PDE-5 inhibitors such as sildenafil have been studied in a few RCTs. Sildenafil increases cGMP levels by pre-venting its breakdown by endogenous PDE-5, resulting in pulmonary vasodilation. Small, randomized trials of sildenafil performed in resource-constrained settings whereby iNO and ECMO were unavailable, reported improved oxygenation and decreased mortality with enteric administration of sildenafil.[37–39] A pilot randomized controlled trial of enteric sildenafil (1–2 mg/kg every 6 hours) in Colombia in a setting whereby ECMO was unavailable showed that it improves oxygenation in neonates with severe PPHN compared with placebo-treated infants. Reported as a proof-of-concept study, this RCT was halted early after 5/6 infants in the placebo group died compared with 1/7 infants in the sildenafil group.[37] Improvement in oxygenation occurred in the sildenafil-treated infants 6 to 12 hours after the first dose. Systemic

hypotension was not observed with enteric sildenafil. Similar results were noted with an RCT in Mexico.[38] This study reported that sildenafil decreased the mortality risk significantly from 40% in the placebo group to 6% in the sildenafil-treated neonates. These RCTs show that sildenafil, used as the primary therapy for PPHN, is effective and safe in resource-limited settings lacking access to iNO.

A small pilot RCT comparing enteric sildenafil + iNO to placebo + iNO did not see improvement in oxygenation in the sildenafil + iNO group.[39] An open-label dose-escalation trial of IV sildenafil in 36 neonates (29 receiving iNO) showed decreased OI starting 4 hours after the administration of the drug. A loading dose of sildenafil 0.4 mg/kg over 3h (0.14 mg/kg/h), followed by 0.07 mg/kg/h (or approximately 1.6 mg/kg/d) continuous infusion provided the intended therapeutic levels as well as clinical benefit.[40] A phase-3 randomized, placebo-controlled trial of IV sildenafil in PPHN investigating short- and long-term outcomes at 12 to 24 months in a group of PPHN neonates already receiving iNO therapy has completed the initial phase. The study found that IV sildenafil (0.1 mg/kg over 30 mins followed by 0.03 mg/kg/h ie, lower doses than the above open-label trial) as an additive therapy to iNO did not reduce the treatment failure rate of need for additional vasodilator/ECMO/death or duration of iNO therapy, compared with placebo.[41] Infants treated with IV sildenafil were more likely to experience hypotension. The results of phase B of this trial, the neurodevelopmental outcomes at 12 to 24 months of age are awaited at this time (NCT01720524). Based on the data available, sildenafil seems to be an effective alternative to iNO in resource-constrained areas as the primary therapy when iNO is not available. The benefit of the addition of sildenafil to infants already on iNO therapy remains unclear. Based on current evidence and our experience, hypotension is more likely with IV than enteric sildenafil, though the latter may have unpredictable absorption.

Pulmonary vasodilators acting via the cyclic adenosine monophosphate pathway
Prostaglandins. Prostacyclin (PGI2) is an arachidonic acid metabolite that stimulates adenyl cyclase in vascular SMCs causing an increase in intracellular cAMP and vasodilation in systemic and pulmonary circulations. There are 3 commercially available prostacyclin or its analog formulations.

(1) Epoprostenol (Flolan) Epoprostenol (Flolan): is a prostacyclin available in IV or aerosolized formulations. There are no RCTs to demonstrate its efficacy and safety profile in neonates with PPHN, and evidence is limited to retrospective reports. Because of its very short half-life ($\sim$6 minutes), it must be administered in a continuous IV or inhaled form. The available evidence is briefly described later in the discussion.

Epoprostenol (FLOLAN) (Intravenous): A prospective case series of 8 consecutive infants showed that IV prostacyclin (epoprostenol) improved ECHO parameters of PAP and oxygenation within a median of 87 hours of administration.[42] Hypotension, resulting from nonselective vasodilation from IV prostacyclins, can be managed with volume expanders and vasopressor medications. A retrospective review of prostacyclin use in critically ill infants with pulmonary hypertension showed acceptable safety and tolerability though the authors did not investigate its ability to modulate pulmonary hypertension severity.[43] There are 3 major limitations to IV prostacyclin: (1) hypoxemia remains a concern in infants with parenchymal lung disease with intravenous administration of epoprostenol, due to continued or increased VQ mismatch from global rather than selective pulmonary vasodilation. However, based on available evidence in the neonatal population, this complication risk remains low. Additionally, given the short half-life of epoprostenol, if appropriate dosing and monitoring are followed, adverse effects can resolve quickly after the discontinuation of the medication. (2) Parenteral administration can lead to systemic hypotension in the presence of right to left shunts across PFO or PDA. (3) The alkaline pH leads to drug compatibility issues, requiring a dedicated line (peripheral or preferably central), which can be challenging for an acutely ill neonate on multiple IV drips and limited access. To overcome these limitations of IV epoprostenol, administration via inhaled route is a preferred alternative.

Epoprostenol (Flolan) (Inhaled): Aerosol administration is given through a nebulizer connected to the breathing circuit of both conventional and high-frequency ventilators. The intravenous formulation of Flolan is dissolved in 20 mL of the manufacturer's diluent (a glycine buffer, pH 10). The effect of such alkaline pH on the neonatal respiratory tract is unknown. Using continuous nebulization at a dose of 50 ng/kg/min, diluted to a volume of 8 mL/h, Kelly and colleagues reported improved oxygenation in 4 infants with PPHN unresponsive to iNO, although one neonate with alveolar capillary dysplasia subsequently deteriorated.[44] Several other case reports and pilot studies reported improved oxygenation status in neonates with aerosolized epoprostenol.[45–47] In a recent retrospective review of 43 critically ill neonates with refractory PPHN, the use of inhaled epoprostenol administered via Aerogen nebulizer was associated with improvement in OI and Fio_2 after 12-h of treatment.[48] Infants with CDH and meconium aspiration were the best responders. None of the infants experienced hypotension with inhaled PGI2 though most were on concomitant inotropes. However, a rebound effect was observed at the end of the continuous nebulization with an increase in OI which was not sustained at 4 hours after the end of treatment.[48] The limitation of these studies is that PPHN infants show labile oxygenation, and it is unclear whether the changes in Pao_2 or OI occurred in response to treatment or as a natural course of their underlying illness. Appropriate monitoring of systemic blood pressure and oxygen saturation should be in place to monitor the rebound effects of interrupted drug delivery.

(2) Iloprost Iloprost, a synthetic analog of prostacyclins, is similar to epoprostenol, but can be given as intermittent nebulizations 6 to 9 times a day due to longer half-life (20–30 minutes) and greater duration of pulmonary vasodilator effect (1–2 hrs). A vibrating mesh nebulizer can be integrated into the inspiratory limb of ventilator circuit as proximal as possible to the endotracheal tube. Nine prospectively enrolled term neonates with PPHN received inhaled iloprost at 1–2 µg/kg every 3 to 4 hours in a center lacking iNO availability.[49] Decreased Fio_2 and improved oxygen saturation were noted in 8/9 patients with no adverse effects reported. A retrospective comparative study of 47 neonates with PPHN in a center without access to iNO, HFV, and ECMO showed that iloprost (1–2.5 µg/kg every 2–4 h) was more effective than oral sildenafil in the time to improvement in OI, duration of drug therapy, mechanical ventilation and inotropic support.[50] However, as with any nebulizer device, some uncertainty will exist regarding the amount of prostacyclin effectively delivered into the alveolar space. DiBlasi and colleagues performed an in vitro study using neonatal test lung model to measure the amount of drug delivered via modern vibrating mesh nebulizers.[51] They found satisfactory iloprost delivery both in conventional and high-frequency ventilation with greater drug delivery when the nebulizer was placed in a proximal position (between patient and circuit) than the distal position, and better delivery with HFOV than conventional ventilation. Evidence of iloprost use in critically ill preterm infants is limited to case reports[52–54] with hypotension noted with IV iloprost but not with inhaled administration.

Based on the available evidence and our experience, aerosolized iloprost or epoprostenol are preferred over IV forms to avoid systemic hypotension and to leverage the pulmonary vasodilator effects in the ventilated segments of the lung. Inhaled prostacyclins overcome the limitation of right to left extrapulmonary shunts (PFO, PDA) which interfere with the delivery of agents to pulmonary circulation. Inhaled route also avoids the need for a dedicated central line required for any IV prostacyclin due to alkaline pH.

(3) **Treprostinil** Treprostinil is a stable tricyclic analog of prostacyclin, which compared with epoprostenol, has a longer half-life, and fewer side effects. It provides an option of a pump for continuous subcutaneous infusion, avoiding the need for central line, as well as means of transitioning to home therapy. Evidence in neonates is limited to small case series or retrospective reviews,[55] though a pilot Phase 2 RCT (NCT02261883) is currently underway. A recent case series provides guidance into transitioning from epoprostenol to Treprostinil.[56] Turbenson and colleagues described 5 patients (three CDH, one 24-week GA preemie with late pulmonary hypertension, one PPHN treated with iNO and sildenafil) that were initiated on IV epoprostenol, escalated to the target dose of epoprostenol and transitioned to IV Treprostinil, followed by switch to subcutaneous Treprostinil.[56] All patients survived to hospital discharge and were sent home on SC Treprostinil with minimal adverse effects. SC Treprostinil has also been used in CDH patients with chronic pulmonary hypertension, resulting in decreased severity of PPHN by ECHO and BNP measurements.[57,58]

(4) **Beraprost** Beraprost sodium is an oral prostacyclin formulation shown to improve pulmonary hypertension in adults[59,60] and children with congenital heart disease.[61,62] The only evidence in neonates is a case series of 7 infants with PPHN; beraprost improved the OI but also decreased systemic blood pressure.[63] Further studies to evaluate the appropriate dose to minimize the risk of systemic hypotension are warranted.

(5) **Prostaglandin E1 (Alprostadil)** PGE1 is typically used in infants with ductal-dependent congenital heart disease. In a small phase I/II open-label clinical trial of 21 infants with PPHN, an inhaled formulation of prostaglandin / (alprostadil) improved the oxygenation without any adverse events.[64] An RCT has attempted to investigate this further but was terminated due to low enrollment.[65] PGE1 can improve right ventricular function by maintaining the patency or reopening a closed ductus arteriosus to provide an outlet to decompress the strained right ventricle and assist systemic blood flow in the presence of LV dysfunction seen in CDH. However, these effects can be inconsistent and potentially increase right-to-left shunt with worsening hypoxemia. In the short term, it may help RV adaptation to high PVR while other agents work to lower pulmonary pressures.

PDE-3 inhibitors
Milrinone. Milrinone inhibits PDE3 in vascular SMCs and cardiac myocytes, leading to increased cAMP levels . Increased cAMP in vascular smooth muscle causes vasorelaxation by improving calcium uptake into the sarcoplasmic reticulum while in the cardiac myocytes, improved calcium uptake leads to increased contractility. Milrinone uniquely induces pulmonary vasodilation, enhances systolic myocardial contractility (inotropy) without increasing myocardial oxygen demand, and promotes diastolic myocardial relaxation (lusitropy). The use of milrinone in refractory PPHN has been supported by several small studies, mostly case series[66-70]; however, evidence from RCTs is lacking. An open-label study in 11 term infants using a bolus of 50 mcg/kg followed by an infusion of 0.33 to 0.99 mcg/kg per min has reported decreases in OI, lactate levels, and base deficit.[67] A small RCT performed in a single-center,

resource-limited setting reported that oral sildenafil plus intravenous milrinone infusion led to a quicker and longer lasting effect on improving PA systolic pressure than either of the agents used alone.[71] Milrinone use may be considered in iNO nonresponders before considering ECMO, with close monitoring of cardiovascular response using clinical parameters and if available, functional echocardiography. The inotropic and lusitropic effects of milrinone may be particularly beneficial in neonates with CDH and left ventricular dysfunction. An RCT evaluating the role of Milrinone in improving oxygenation in CDH infants is ongoing (NCT02951130).

Pulmonary vasodilators acting via the endothelin pathway

Endothelin antagonists

Bosentan. Bosentan is an endothelin-1 antagonist of both endothelin A and B receptors. A small, single-center, randomized study by Mohamed and colleagues in a center lacking iNO and ECMO showed improved oxygenation in the bosentan, compared with the placebo group (80% vs 20%).[72] These data and some other reports suggest that it may have a role in the management of PPHN in resource-constrained settings without access to iNO.[73–76] A multicenter, randomized, double-blind, placebo-controlled trial (FUTURE-4 study) assessed the effects of bosentan (2 mg/kg twice daily via nasogastric tube) as adjuvant therapy in 21 neonates with respiratory failure already receiving iNO.[77] Owing to slow recruitment, the trial was terminated early. In contrast to the observations by Mohamed and colleagues, FUTURE-4 trial showed no additional benefit when given as an adjuvant therapy in terms of time to weaning off iNO, oxygenation status, or need for ECMO. Enteral absorption was slow and unpredictable and took 5 days to reach a steady state. Though no safety concerns were reported in the above trials, the elevation of transaminases has been reported with bosentan use in adult patients with pulmonary hypertension. Anemia and peripheral edema were reported in the FUTURE-4 study. Given the limited evidence of clinical benefit and unreliable pharmacokinetic profile with oral administration, we recommend the cGMP and cAMP targeted therapies as first or second-line options for PPHN.

Steroids

Glucocorticoids are frequently used in critically ill PPHN neonates due to their potent anti-inflammatory and vasopressor effects, reducing right to left shunting. Glucocorticoids increase cGMP levels by normalizing sGC and PDE5 activity and decrease oxidant stress in lambs with PPHN.[78–81] A small randomized 3-arm trial evaluating short courses of IV methylprednisolone, inhaled budesonide, and placebo in meconium-aspiration suggested improvements in the duration of oxygen therapy, radiological clearance of lungs and length of stay in the 2 steroid treated groups.[82] The risk-benefit profile should always be considered due to previously reported concerns for neurodevelopment in premature infants when steroids are used early in life.

A physiology-based approach to pulmonary vasodilators. Some key factors, based on our experience, that may optimize outcomes in PPHN are shown in **Fig. 3**. We recommend a proactive approach to HRF in any late preterm or term infant needing greater than 40% Fio_2 with radiographic findings of parenchymal lung disease. This involves early surfactant and lung recruitment maneuvers like conventional mechanical or high-frequency ventilation. Early initiation of iNO is important to optimize the oxygenation response and to avoid the need for high ventilator settings or Fio_2 or other vasodilator therapies. If there is partial or no response to iNO, we initiate iloprost as it can be given as intermittent nebulizations, while carefully monitoring for hypotension and recognizing its short-half life. If there is a response to iloprost nebulizations, we transition to IV or subcutaneous Treprostinil. All IV prostacyclins require a dedicated

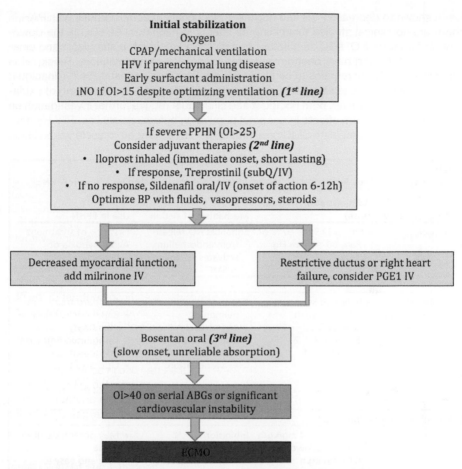

Fig. 3. Suggested approach and timing of interventions for the management of HRF/PPHN. It is important to consider the cardiopulmonary system to be one fully integrated unit and optimize lung recruitment, pulmonary vasodilation, and cardiac function to facilitate a successful transition. The algorithm focuses on vasodilator agents and is not meant to be inclusive of all therapies used in the management of PPHN.

venous line which is often challenging, hence our preference for subcutaneous Treprostinil. If there is evidence of left ventricular dysfunction, milrinone is recommended. IV fluids, pressors, and steroids are administered to optimize blood pressure especially when multiple adjuvant therapies are needed. We prefer enteral over IV sildenafil due to lower risk of hypotension. Weaning process involves weaning oxygen first, before iNO and is based on preductal pulse oximetry and not solely based on Pa_{O_2} from postductal umbilical artery blood gas monitoring. The Goldilocks' principle of 'just the right amount of" oxygen to minimize hypoxic pulmonary vasoconstriction and avoiding hyperoxia lung injury should be adopted by all members of the medical team. Recommendations for vasodilators used in PPHN are summarized in **Table 1**.

Potential future therapeutic approaches. Some newer investigational drugs that target a range of cellular mechanisms are worth mentioning, although their potential application to neonatal care remains unexplored. L-citrulline is converted to L-arginine which is a key substrate for enzyme eNOS that produces NO. Although L-citrulline has been shown to decrease PVR and augment functional capacity in adults with PAH,[83] there are no clinical studies examining its effects in neonates. As sGC is the downstream target for NO, sGC stimulators or activators (riociguat, a stimulator and cinaciguat, an activator) have been investigated as pulmonary vasodilators. Riociguat is used in adult PH but remains to be studied in pediatric and neonatal PH.[84] Cinaciguat induces pulmonary vasodilation in newborn lambs with PPHN in the setting of oxidative stress.[35,85] However, both riociguat and cinaciguat require further investigation on efficacy and long-term effects in neonatal population before clinical use. PPARγ agonists (rosiglitazone) regulate SMC proliferation as well as smooth muscle vasodilation

Table 1
Summary of dosages & practical considerations for pulmonary vasodilator use in PPHN

Drug Category	Administration (Route/Dose)	Mechanism of Action	Use in PPHN
Oxygen	Goal SpO2 92%–97% or Pao$_2$ 60–90 mm Hg	Enhances NO release from endothelium, activates K$^+$ channels in SMC	First line of treatment Avoid hypoxia or hyperoxia
(NO)			
Inhaled nitric oxide (iNO)	Inhalation: Start at 20 ppm, wean gradually 20→ 10→ 5→ 4→ 3→ 2→ 1→0.5→off	Generated within pulmonary endothelial cells, diffuses to smooth muscle cells, ↑cGMP → vasodilation	• Standard treatment • Rapid onset, selective pulmonary vasodilator, improves V/Q match • Optimize lung recruitment/ ventilation before iNO
Phosphodiesterase Inhibitors			
Sildenafil	IV: loading 0.14 mg/kg/h for 3 h followed by 0.07 mg/kg/h PO/NG: 0.5-2 mg/kg/dose Q6-8 h	Inhibition of phosphodiesterase-5 enzyme (responsible for cGMP degradation), ↑cGMP → vasodilation	• May potentiate nitric oxide • Safe and easy to administer enterally • May worsen oxygenation due to the vasodilation of unventilated areas of the lung
Tadalafil	PO/NG: 1 mg/kg/d once daily	Similar to sildenafil	Similar to sildenafil
Milrinone	Term: IV: loading: 50 mcg/kg over more than 60 min; maintenance: 0.25–0.75 mcg/kg/min OR continuous at 0.25–0.75 mcg/kg/min Preterm GA <30 wk: IV: Loading 50mcg/kg/min over more than 3 h; maintenance: 0.2 mcg/kg/min	Inhibition of phosphodiesterase-3 enzyme (responsible for cAMP degradation), ↑cAMP → vasodilation	• May potentiate action of prostaglandins • Should be strongly considered if diminished RV function

(continued on next page)

Table 1
(continued)

Drug Category	Administration (Route/ Dose)	Mechanism of Action	Use in PPHN
Prostaglandins			
PGI 2	Epoprostenol (Flolan) IV: 2–5 ng/kg/min, increments of 2–5 ng/ kg/min Inhalation: 50 ng/kg/ min continuous Iloprost (Inhaled): 0.5–2 mcg/kg/dose Q2-4 h	Produced from arachidonic acid, increases cAMP in pulmonary vascular smooth muscle → vasodilation	• May enhance NO action • Nonspecific pulmonary vasodilator with IV • May cause systemic hypotension (IV > inhalation) • IV formulation needs a dedicated line due to incompatibility with most medications/fluids • Avoid abrupt discontinuation if using continuous Epoprostenol infusion/inhalation • Inhaled route is desirable
PGE1	IV: 0.01–0.1 mcg/kg/min Inhalation: 100–300 ng/ kg/min	Similar to PGI2	Similar to PGI2
Endothelin Receptor Inhibitor			
Bosentan	Oral: 1–2 mg/kg twice daily	Nonspecific antagonist of endothelin A and B receptors	• Limited proven efficacy • LFTs should be monitored

through the inhibition of Rho-kinase. In a rat PH model, activation of PPARγ has decreased RV pressures and vascular remodeling, suggesting its potential role in the management of neonatal PH.[86] Activation of AMP Kinase with metformin ameliorated pulmonary hypertension and improved angiogenesis in the fetal lamb model of PPHN.[87]

Pharmacotherapy in Bronchopulmonary dysplasia-related pulmonary hypertension Current guidelines for BPD-PH recommend the initiation of targeted therapy with pulmonary vasodilators in infants with sustained PH after the optimization of underlying respiratory and cardiac disease.[88] Although these medications are widely used in this population, there is a paucity of data on their safety and efficacy, and effects on long-term outcomes for infants treated with these medications. In the absence of RCT data, the use of PH-targeted medications in infants with BPD is based on expert opinion and clinical experience, emphasizing the need for their comprehensive evaluation in PH centers. A brief review of Pharmacotherapy in BPD-PH is summarized later in discussion along with **Table 2**.

Inhaled nitric oxide: iNO may be beneficial in improving oxygenation during acute deterioration of oxygenation in the setting of worsening BPD-PH, in addition to other cardiorespiratory support. A dose of 10 to 20 PPM may be used for acute PH crises

Table 2
Pharmacotherapy of pulmonary hypertension in BPD

Names	Dose/Titration	Side Effects	Comments
Sildenafil phosphodiesterase-5 inhibitor	PO: 1 mg/kg q 6–8 h; start with low dose (0.3–0.5 mg/kg/dose) and increase gradually to 1 mg/kg/dose as tolerated; slower as outpatient. Maximal dose of 10 mg q 8 h per EMA guidelines for infants. Intravenous:0.25–0.5 mg/kg/dose q 6–8 h (titrate slowly and administer more than 60 min.	Hypotension, GER, irritability (headache), bronchospasm, nasal stuffiness, fever, rarely priapism	Monitor for adverse effects, lower the dose or switch to alternate therapy if not tolerated
Bosentan (Endothelin receptor antagonist)	1 mg/kg PO q 12 h as starting dose; may increase to 2 mg/kg BID in 2–4 wk, if tolerated and liver enzymes stable.	Liver dysfunction especially during viral infections, VQ mismatch, hypotension, anemia (edema and airway issues rare in infants)	Monitor LFTs monthly (earlier with respiratory infections); monitor CBC quarterly. Teratogenicity precautions for caregivers
Inhaled Iloprost	2.5–5 mcg every 2–4 h. Can be given as continuous inhalation during mechanical ventilation. Can titrate dose from 1-5 mcg and frequency from every 4 h to continuous.	Bronchospasm, hypotension, ventilator tube crystallization and clogging, pulmonary hemorrhage, prostanoid side effects (GI disturbances), may be teratogenic to caregivers	Need close monitoring for clogged tubing, may need further dilution. May need bronchodilators or inhaled steroid pretreatment with bronchospasm.
Intravenous Epoprostenol (Flolan)	Start at 1–2 ng/kg/min, titrate up slowly every 4–6 h to 20 ng/kg/min; need to increase the dose at regular intervals because of tachyphylaxis. Further increases as guided by clinical targets and avoiding adverse effects.	Hypotension, VQ mismatch, GI disturbances. Needs dedicated line, very short half-life with high risk for rebound PH with brief interruption of therapy; line-related complications include infection, clogging, breaks in line, thrombosis, arrhythmia	Monitor closely if added to other vasodilator therapies, such as milrinone; careful attention to line care is essential.

(continued on next page)

Names	Dose/Titration	Side Effects	Comments
Treprostinil (Remodulin) IV or Subcutaneous	Start at 2 ng/kg/min and titrate every 4–6 h up to 20 ng/kg/min, then slowly increase dose as tolerated (dose often 1.5–2 times greater than equivalent epoprostenol dose, if switching medications)	SQ: local site pain; IV: similar risks as with epoprostenol, but treprostinil has a longer half-life, which reduces the risk for severe PH with interruption of infusion	Site pain managed with local and systemic measures
Milrinone (IV) (phosphodiesterase-3 inhibitor)	0.15–0.5 mcg/kg/min –lower dosage range when used with other vasodilators	Arrhythmogenic; systemic hypotension and high risk for decreased myocardial perfusion; caution with renal dysfunction	May need to add a pressor, such as vasopressin, to mitigate effects of decrease in systemic pressures.

Table 2 (continued)

Abbreviations: BID, twice a day; CBC, complete blood count; EMA, European Medicines Agency; GER, gastroesophageal reflux; GI, gastrointestinal; IV, intravenous; kg, kilogram; LFT, liver function tests; mcg, microgram; ng, nanogram; PO, oral; SC, subcutaneous; SR, sustained release; VQ, ventilation-perfusion.

Reproduced from Krishnan U, Feinstein JA, Adatia I, Austin ED, Mullen MP, Hopper RK, Hanna B, Romer L, Keller RL, Fineman J, Steinhorn R, Kinsella JP, Ivy DD, Rosenzweig EB, Raj U, Humpl T, Abman SH; Pediatric Pulmonary Hypertension Network (PPHNet). Evaluation and Management of Pulmonary Hypertension in Children with Bronchopulmonary Dysplasia. J Pediatr. 2017 Sep;188:24-34.e1

and weaned after stabilization as tolerated. There is no evidence supporting longer term use of iNO in infants with BPD-PH.

Sildenafil: Sildenafil is widely used in infants with BPD-PH when it persists despite optimizing ventilation and addressing the potential contributing factors (infection, aspiration, airway pathology, and intermittent hypoxia). A study of 25 infants with BPD-PH showed hemodynamic improvement in 88% of patients receiving long-term sildenafil with no safety concerns reported.[89] Several other retrospective reviews have demonstrated an improvement in echocardiographic measurements of PH after sildenafil initiation.[90–93] Whether these improvements were due to sildenafil treatment or evolution of PH over time is difficult to discern in these observational studies with no controls. A recent meta-analysis of chronic sildenafil use in preterm infants with BPD-PH reported an overall mortality of 29.7% per year and demonstrated improvements in estimated pulmonary arterial pressure and respiratory severity scores in patients on sildenafil.[94] The 2012 US FDA warning has been discussed in reviews of BPD-PH and in expert panel recommendations and highlight the importance of optimizing the management of contributing factors and evaluation of vasoreactivity by cardiac catheterization if long-term therapy with sildenafil is being considered.[88]

Prostacyclins *Iloprost:* There are no large studies of iloprost use in BPD-PH patients. In a single-center retrospective study of BPD-PH, its use was discontinued in 17% of patients, most commonly due to increased oxygen requirement.[95] There was higher mortality in the group that received iloprost. However, this was attributed to the underlying severity of illness and its use in acutely deteriorating patients, and not to the medication itself.[95] Given its rapid onset of action, the ease of administration and discontinuation, it may be useful in a select group of patients in acute pulmonary hypertensive crisis. If there is a response, infants can be transitioned to parenteral prostacyclins.[95]

Epoprostenol: There is limited evidence on continuous prostacyclin use in BPD-PH. A case report demonstrated improvement in PA pressures, quality of life, and eventual discontinuation of home ventilation in a child with BPD-PH treated with IV epoprostenol[96] and another case report demonstrated improvement in RV systolic pressures.[97] However, intravenous access can be a significant challenge in premature infants. Hence, subcutaneous treprostinil has been used at some experienced PH centers.

Treprostinil: Subcutaneous treprostinil via a continuous infusion pump was successfully used in 5 patients with BPD-PH as a long term therapy to safely deliver prostacyclin while avoiding the need for central venous access.[98] There was an improvement in echocardiographic measures of PH, decreased need for respiratory support and minimal pump-site specific reactions (pain, redness, swelling).[98] However, this therapy needs a dedicated PH team, committed outpatient follow-up program for dose titration and home nursing support along with extensive education, counseling, and support of caregivers.

Bosentan: Bosentan has been used as an add-on therapy in BPD-PH. A case series of 6 patients with BPD-PH demonstrated improvement in respiratory and hemodynamic status over the course of 2.1 to 2.9 years, 4 of whom were also on sildenafil.[99] Liver function should be monitored cautiously, as 2 of 6 infants had elevated liver enzymes. The long-term efficacy and safety of bosentan from these limited case series remain unknown.

Complexities of persistent pulmonary hypertension of the newborn clinical research Despite decades of work to elucidate molecular pathways and to understand mechanisms using excellent animal models of PPHN, there is a paucity of level 1A evidence in human neonates for various treatment modalities commonly used in bedside management of PPHN. iNO and ECMO are the only clinically proven, effective, life-saving treatment options in severe cases of PPHN. More recent RCT data provide convincing level 1A evidence that early surfactant administration not only in RDS but also for all late preterm and term infants with parenchymal lung disease and hypoxic respiratory failure significantly decreases the need for ECMO.[2,30,100,101] Evidence also suggests that high-frequency ventilation is superior to conventional ventilation for alveolar recruitment in parenchymal lung disease associated with PPHN.[102]

In 30% to 40% cases of PPHN, iNO is either clinically ineffective or provides only transient improvement. Hence, there is an urgent need to conduct high-quality RCTs evaluating the efficacy of additional pulmonary vasodilator therapies in iNO resistant PPHN. Most of the pulmonary vasodilator adjuvant therapies have either not been tested in large multicenter clinical trials or those RCTs have been conducted in low resource settings lacking iNO and ECMO, limiting their generalizability. Many of these studies included small numbers, heterogenous populations with different etiologies of PPHN and lack long-term follow-up. The reasons for the lack of larger RCTs in PPHN are several: (1) PPHN is a rare disease affecting only 1 in 500 infants. Hence, it is difficult to recruit an adequate number of patients at single centers and requires multicenter trials which present logistical challenges. (2) Presentation of severe PPHN is often unexpected in an otherwise uncomplicated pregnancy and may not be known early enough (antenatal/early postnatal) for informed consent. Within a narrow timeframe, discussing the study and consenting parents who are frequently at a distant delivery hospital is challenging. (3) As iNO is the standard of care and available in developed countries, it is not possible to randomize and compare adjuvant therapies versus iNO. (4) iNO has decreased the mortality and ECMO rates remarkably in severe PPHN. Further reductions in mortality or ECMO use would need substantially higher number of infants to be adequately powered to detect the effect size for traditional outcome of ECMO/mortality. Alternate study endpoints need to be used to test the efficacy of other therapies. (5) Parental reluctance and physician bias to use therapies off label rather than enroll infants into a complex RCT that may randomize the infants into the placebo group. The combination of situational, logistical, financial, and ethical considerations in a rare and critically ill patient population challenges the successful recruitment of study subjects into otherwise much needed trials.

SUMMARY

In the absence of RCT evidence of the efficacy of adjuvant pulmonary vasodilator therapies, clinicians are faced with difficult decisions while managing critically ill PPHN infants. As an alternative to traditional RCTs with equal allocation to placebo and treatment groups, alternative trial designs with adaptive and response adaptive clinical trials have been suggested by expert panels. Such trial designs to conduct pragmatic trials in the rare disease population of infants will improve the quality of evidence and allow for timely conduct of trials in this population. Until such randomized trial data are available, clinicians should adopt a physiology-based approach backed by the knowledge of pathophysiology, drug pharmacology, and regular bedside assessment of response to these adjuvant therapies.

Best practices

What is the current practice?
- Inhaled nitric oxide is the only approved pulmonary vasodilator for PPHN in the US and European Union.
- About 30% to 40% of patients do not respond or have incomplete response to iNO, necessitating invasive and expensive treatment modalities like ECMO.
- Alternate pulmonary vasodilator therapies are used commonly as rescue life-saving measures, though there is a lack of high-quality data supporting their efficacy and safety.
- Such alternate therapies (sildenafil, prostacyclins) may be effective and safe in resource-limited settings lacking access to iNO.

What changes in current practice are likely to improve outcome?
- Early surfactant administration and high-frequency ventilation in conjunction with iNO are beneficial for optimal lung recruitment and V-Q matching in PPHN with parenchymal lung disease.
- Avoidance of hyperoxia and maintaining gentle ventilation are lung-protective strategies that will maximize the benefit from pulmonary vasodilators.
- Echocardiography is essential to rule out cyanotic congenital heart disease in babies suspected of having PPHN, before the consideration of vasodilator therapies.
- Functional echocardiography to assess hemodynamics and impact of therapies at the bedside may support better clinical decision making individualized to the infant's pathophysiology.
- Clinician awareness of mechanism, pharmacokinetics, and side-effect profile of adjuvant vasodilator therapies is crucial before their application at the bedside.

Summary statement
- An integrated approach at the bedside to optimize cardiopulmonary support and to minimize injury to the lungs and systemic organs is needed to optimize outcomes for neonates with PPHN. The evidence-based approach presented in this review has led to dramatic reductions in ECMO use for neonates with PPHN over the last 22 years since the approval of iNO for PPHN. Further refinements are needed to test newer therapies using novel trial designs in this rare disease population.

DISCLOSURE

Supported by grants 1R01 HL136597-01from NHLBI, Multiyear Innovation Research grant and Muma Endowed Chair in Neonatology from Children's Research Institute of Children's Wisconsin (G.G. Konduri)

REFERENCES

1. Steurer MA, Jelliffe-Pawlowski LL, Baer RJ, et al. Persistent pulmonary hypertension of the newborn in late preterm and term infants in California. Pediatrics 2017;139(1):e20161165.
2. Konduri GG, Solimano A, Sokol GM, et al. A randomized trial of early versus standard inhaled nitric oxide therapy in term and near-term newborn infants with hypoxic respiratory failure. Pediatrics 2004;113(3 Pt 1):559–64.
3. Rasanen J, Wood DC, Weiner S, et al. Role of the pulmonary circulation in the distribution of human fetal cardiac output during the second half of pregnancy. Circulation 1996;94(5):1068–73.
4. Gao Y, Raj JU. Regulation of the pulmonary circulation in the fetus and newborn. Physiol Rev 2010;90(4):1291–335.
5. Hislop A. Developmental biology of the pulmonary circulation. Paediatr Respir Rev 2005;6(1):35–43.
6. Abman SH, Chatfield BA, Hall SL, et al. Role of endothelium-derived relaxing factor during transition of pulmonary circulation at birth. Am J Physiol 1990; 259(6 Pt 2):H1921–7.
7. Konduri GG, Mattei J. Role of oxidative phosphorylation and ATP release in mediating birth-related pulmonary vasodilation in fetal lambs. Am J Physiol Heart Circ Physiol 2002;283(4):H1600–8.
8. Konduri GG, Mital S, Gervasio CT, et al. Purine nucleotides contribute to pulmonary vasodilation caused by birth-related stimuli in the ovine fetus. Am J Physiol 1997;272(5 Pt 2):H2377–84.
9. Ballou DP, Zhao Y, Brandish PE, et al. Revisiting the kinetics of nitric oxide (NO) binding to soluble guanylate cyclase: the simple NO-binding model is incorrect. Proc Natl Acad Sci U S A 2002;99(19):12097–101.
10. Bloch KD, Filippov G, Sanchez LS, et al. Pulmonary soluble guanylate cyclase, a nitric oxide receptor, is increased during the perinatal period. Am J Physiol 1997;272(3 Pt 1):L400–6.
11. Tzao C, Nickerson PA, Russell JA, et al. Paracrine role of soluble guanylate cyclase and type III nitric oxide synthase in ovine fetal pulmonary circulation: a double labeling immunohistochemical study. Histochem Cell Biol 2003; 119(2):125–30.
12. Corbin JD, Beasley A, Blount MA, et al. High lung PDE5: a strong basis for treating pulmonary hypertension with PDE5 inhibitors. Biochem Biophys Res Commun 2005;334(3):930–8.
13. Afolayan AJ, Eis A, Alexander M, et al. Decreased endothelial nitric oxide synthase expression and function contribute to impaired mitochondrial biogenesis and oxidative stress in fetal lambs with persistent pulmonary hypertension. Am J Physiol Lung Cell Mol Physiol 2016;310(1):L40–9.
14. Shaul PW, Yuhanna IS, German Z, et al. Pulmonary endothelial NO synthase gene expression is decreased in fetal lambs with pulmonary hypertension. Am J Physiol 1997;272(5 Pt 1):L1005–12.

15. Villamor E, Le Cras TD, Horan MP, et al. Chronic intrauterine pulmonary hypertension impairs endothelial nitric oxide synthase in the ovine fetus. Am J Physiol 1997;272(5 Pt 1):L1013–20.
16. Villanueva ME, Zaher FM, Svinarich DM, et al. Decreased gene expression of endothelial nitric oxide synthase in newborns with persistent pulmonary hypertension. Pediatr Res 1998;44(3):338–43.
17. Mahajan CN, Afolayan AJ, Eis A, et al. Altered prostanoid metabolism contributes to impaired angiogenesis in persistent pulmonary hypertension in a fetal lamb model. Pediatr Res 2015;77(3):455–62.
18. Ivy DD, Lee DS, Rairigh RL, et al. Endothelin B receptor blockade attenuates pulmonary vasodilation in oxygen-ventilated fetal lambs. Biol Neonate 2004; 86(3):155–9.
19. Zamora MR, Stelzner TJ, Webb S, et al. Overexpression of endothelin-1 and enhanced growth of pulmonary artery smooth muscle cells from fawn-hooded rats. Am J Physiol 1996;270(1 Pt 1):L101–9.
20. Taddei S, Vanhoutte PM. Endothelium-dependent contractions to endothelin in the rat aorta are mediated by thromboxane A2. J Cardiovasc Pharmacol 1993;22(Suppl 8):S328–31.
21. Rosenberg AA, Kennaugh J, Koppenhafer SL, et al. Elevated immunoreactive endothelin-1 levels in newborn infants with persistent pulmonary hypertension. J Pediatr 1993;123(1):109–14.
22. Mourani PM, Abman SH. Pulmonary hypertension and vascular abnormalities in bronchopulmonary dysplasia. Clin Perinatol 2015;42(4):839–55.
23. Lagatta JM, Hysinger EB, Zaniletti I, et al. The impact of pulmonary hypertension in preterm infants with severe bronchopulmonary dysplasia through 1 year. J Pediatr 2018;203:218–24.e3.
24. Hansmann G, Sallmon H, Roehr CC, et al. Pulmonary hypertension in bronchopulmonary dysplasia. Pediatr Res 2021;89(3):446–55.
25. Lakshminrusimha S, Swartz DD, Gugino SF, et al. Oxygen concentration and pulmonary hemodynamics in newborn lambs with pulmonary hypertension. Pediatr Res 2009;66(5):539–44.
26. Barrington KJ, Finer N, Pennaforte T, et al. Nitric oxide for respiratory failure in infants born at or near term. Cochrane Database Syst Rev 2000;1(2):CD000399.
27. Roberts JD Jr, Fineman JR, Morin FC, et al. Inhaled nitric oxide and persistent pulmonary hypertension of the newborn. The Inhaled Nitric Oxide Study Group. N Engl J Med 1997;336(9):605–10.
28. Clark RH, Kueser TJ, Walker MW, et al. Low-dose nitric oxide therapy for persistent pulmonary hypertension of the newborn. Clinical Inhaled Nitric Oxide Research Group. N Engl J Med 2000;342(7):469–74.
29. Neonatal Inhaled Nitric Oxide Study Group. Inhaled nitric oxide in full-term and nearly full-term infants with hypoxic respiratory failure. N Engl J Med 1997; 336(9):597–604.
30. Konduri GG, Sokol GM, Van Meurs KP, et al. Impact of early surfactant and inhaled nitric oxide therapies on outcomes in term/late preterm neonates with moderate hypoxic respiratory failure. J Perinatol 2013;33(12):944–9.
31. Sokol GM, Fineberg NS, Wright LL, et al. Changes in arterial oxygen tension when weaning neonates from inhaled nitric oxide. Pediatr Pulmonol 2001; 32(1):14–9.
32. Inhaled nitric oxide and hypoxic respiratory failure in infants with congenital diaphragmatic hernia. The Neonatal Inhaled Nitric Oxide Study Group (NINOS). Pediatrics 1997;99(6):838–45.

33. Putnam LR, Tsao K, Morini F, et al. Evaluation of variability in inhaled nitric oxide use and pulmonary hypertension in patients with congenital diaphragmatic hernia. JAMA Pediatr 2016;170(12):1188–94.

34. Lawrence KM, Monos S, Adams S, et al. Inhaled nitric oxide is associated with improved oxygenation in a subpopulation of infants with congenital diaphragmatic hernia and pulmonary hypertension. J Pediatr 2020;219:167–72.

35. Chester M, Seedorf G, Tourneux P, et al. Cinaciguat, a soluble guanylate cyclase activator, augments cGMP after oxidative stress and causes pulmonary vasodilation in neonatal pulmonary hypertension. Am J Physiol Lung Cell Mol Physiol 2011;301(5):L755–64.

36. Farrow KN, Wedgwood S, Lee KJ, et al. Mitochondrial oxidant stress increases PDE5 activity in persistent pulmonary hypertension of the newborn. Respir Physiol Neurobiol 2010;174(3):272–81.

37. Baquero H, Soliz A, Neira F, et al. Oral sildenafil in infants with persistent pulmonary hypertension of the newborn: a pilot randomized blinded study. Pediatrics 2006;117(4):1077–83.

38. Vargas-Origel A, Gómez-Rodríguez G, Aldana-Valenzuela C, et al. The use of sildenafil in persistent pulmonary hypertension of the newborn. Am J Perinatol 2010;27(3):225–30.

39. Al Omar S, Salama H, Al Hail M, et al. Effect of early adjunctive use of oral sildenafil and inhaled nitric oxide on the outcome of pulmonary hypertension in newborn infants. A feasibility study. J Neonatal Perinatal Med 2016;9(3):251–9.

40. Steinhorn RH, Kinsella JP, Pierce C, et al. Intravenous sildenafil in the treatment of neonates with persistent pulmonary hypertension. J Pediatr 2009;155(6):841,e1.

41. Pierce CM, Zhang MH, Jonsson B, et al. Efficacy and safety of IV sildenafil in the treatment of newborn infants with, or at risk of, persistent pulmonary hypertension of the newborn (PPHN): a multicenter, randomized, placebo-controlled trial. J Pediatr 2021;237:154–61.e3.

42. Eronen M, Pohjavuori M, Andersson S, et al. Prostacyclin treatment for persistent pulmonary hypertension of the newborn. Pediatr Cardiol 1997;18(1):3–7.

43. McIntyre CM, Hanna BD, Rintoul N, et al. Safety of epoprostenol and treprostinil in children less than 12 months of age. Pulm Circ 2013;3(4):862–9.

44. Kelly LK, Porta NF, Goodman DM, et al. Inhaled prostacyclin for term infants with persistent pulmonary hypertension refractory to inhaled nitric oxide. J Pediatr 2002;141(6):830–2.

45. Brown AT, Gillespie JV, Miquel-Verges F, et al. Inhaled epoprostenol therapy for pulmonary hypertension: improves oxygenation index more consistently in neonates than in older children. Pulm Circ 2012;2(1):61–6.

46. Soditt V, Aring C, Groneck P. Improvement of oxygenation induced by aerosolized prostacyclin in a preterm infant with persistent pulmonary hypertension of the newborn. Intensive Care Med 1997;23(12):1275–8.

47. Bindl L, Fahnenstich H, Peukert U. Aerosolised prostacyclin for pulmonary hypertension in neonates. Arch Dis Child Fetal Neonatal Ed 1994;71(3):F214–6.

48. Berger-Caron F, Piedboeuf B, Morissette G, et al. Inhaled epoprostenol for pulmonary hypertension treatment in neonates: a 12-year experience. Am J Perinatol 2019;36(11):1142–9.

49. Kim SH, Lee HJ, Kim NS, et al. Inhaled iloprost as a first-line therapy for persistent pulmonary hypertension of the newborn. Neonatal Med 2019;26(4):191–7.

50. Kahveci H, Yilmaz O, Avsar UZ, et al. Oral sildenafil and inhaled iloprost in the treatment of pulmonary hypertension of the newborn. Pediatr Pulmonol 2014; 49(12):1205–13.

51. DiBlasi RM, Crotwell DN, Shen S, et al. Iloprost drug delivery during infant conventional and high-frequency oscillatory ventilation. Pulm Circ 2016;6(1):63–9.
52. Eifinger F, Sreeram N, Mehler K, et al. Aerosolized iloprost in the treatment of pulmonary hypertension in extremely preterm infants: a pilot study. Klin Padiatr 2008;220(2):66–9.
53. Yilmaz O, Kahveci H, Zeybek C, et al. Inhaled iloprost in preterm infants with severe respiratory distress syndrome and pulmonary hypertension. Am J Perinatol 2014;31(4):321–6.
54. Janjindamai W, Thatrimontrichai A, Maneenil G, et al. Effectiveness and safety of intravenous iloprost for severe persistent pulmonary hypertension of the newborn. Indian Pediatr 2013;50(10):934–8.
55. Park BY, Chung SH. Treprostinil for persistent pulmonary hypertension of the newborn, with early onset sepsis in preterm infant: 2 Case reports. Medicine (Baltimore) 2017;96(26):e7303.
56. Turbenson MN, Radosevich JJ, Manuel V, et al. Transitioning from intravenous to subcutaneous prostacyclin therapy in neonates with severe pulmonary hypertension. J Pediatr Pharmacol Ther 2020;25(7):647–53.
57. Olson E, Lusk LA, Fineman JR, et al. Short-term treprostinil use in infants with congenital diaphragmatic hernia following repair. J Pediatr 2015;167(3):762–4.
58. Lawrence KM, Hedrick HL, Monk HM, et al. Treprostinil improves persistent pulmonary hypertension associated with congenital diaphragmatic hernia. J Pediatr 2018;200:44–9.
59. Kunieda T, Nakanishi N, Matsubara H, et al. Effects of long-acting beraprost sodium (TRK-100STP) in Japanese patients with pulmonary arterial hypertension. Int Heart J 2009;50(4):513–29.
60. Ikeda D, Tsujino I, Sakaue S, et al. Pilot study of short-term effects of a novel long-acting oral beraprost in patients with pulmonary arterial hypertension. Circ J 2007;71(11):1829–31.
61. Suzuki H, Sato S, Tanabe S, et al. Beraprost sodium for pulmonary hypertension with congenital heart disease. Pediatr Int 2002;44(5):528–9.
62. Limsuwan A, Pienvichit P, Khowsathit P. Beraprost therapy in children with pulmonary hypertension secondary to congenital heart disease. Pediatr Cardiol 2005;26(6):787–91.
63. Nakwan N, Nakwan N, Wannaro J. Persistent pulmonary hypertension of the newborn successfully treated with beraprost sodium: a retrospective chart review. Neonatology 2011;99(1):32–7.
64. Sood BG, Delaney-Black V, Aranda JV, et al. Aerosolized PGE1: a selective pulmonary vasodilator in neonatal hypoxemic respiratory failure results of a Phase I/II open label clinical trial. Pediatr Res 2004;56(4):579–85.
65. Sood BG, Keszler M, Garg M, et al. Inhaled PGE1 in neonates with hypoxemic respiratory failure: two pilot feasibility randomized clinical trials. Trials 2014; 15:486.
66. Bassler D, Kreutzer K, McNamara P, et al. Milrinone for persistent pulmonary hypertension of the newborn. Cochrane Database Syst Rev 2010;(11):CD007802.
67. McNamara PJ, Shivananda SP, Sahni M, et al. Pharmacology of milrinone in neonates with persistent pulmonary hypertension of the newborn and suboptimal response to inhaled nitric oxide. Pediatr Crit Care Med 2013;14(1):74–84.
68. McNamara PJ, Laique F, Muang-In S, et al. Milrinone improves oxygenation in neonates with severe persistent pulmonary hypertension of the newborn. J Crit Care 2006;21(2):217–22.

69. Patel N. Use of milrinone to treat cardiac dysfunction in infants with pulmonary hypertension secondary to congenital diaphragmatic hernia: a review of six patients. Neonatology 2012;102(2):130–6.

70. James AT, Corcoran JD, McNamara PJ, et al. The effect of milrinone on right and left ventricular function when used as a rescue therapy for term infants with pulmonary hypertension. Cardiol Young 2016;26(1):90–9.

71. El-Ghandour M, Hammad B, Ghanem M, et al. Efficacy of milrinone plus sildenafil in the treatment of neonates with persistent pulmonary hypertension in resource-limited settings: results of a randomized, double-blind trial. Paediatr Drugs 2020;22(6):685–93.

72. Mohamed WA, Ismail M. A randomized, double-blind, placebo-controlled, prospective study of bosentan for the treatment of persistent pulmonary hypertension of the newborn. J Perinatol 2012;32(8):608–13.

73. Nakwan N, Choksuchat D, Saksawad R, et al. Successful treatment of persistent pulmonary hypertension of the newborn with bosentan. Acta Paediatr 2009; 98(10):1683–5.

74. Fatima N, Arshad S, Quddusi AI, et al. Comparison of the efficacy of sildenafil alone versus sildenafil plus bosentan in newborns with persistent pulmonary hypertension. J Ayub Med Coll Abbottabad 2018;30(3):333–6.

75. Goissen C, Ghyselen L, Tourneux P, et al. Persistent pulmonary hypertension of the newborn with transposition of the great arteries: successful treatment with bosentan. Eur J Pediatr 2008;167(4):437–40.

76. Maneenil G, Thatrimontrichai A, Janjindamai W, et al. Effect of bosentan therapy in persistent pulmonary hypertension of the newborn. Pediatr Neonatol 2018; 59(1):58–64.

77. Steinhorn RH, Fineman J, Kusic-Pajic A, et al. Bosentan as adjunctive therapy for persistent pulmonary hypertension of the newborn: results of the randomized multicenter placebo-controlled exploratory trial. J Pediatr 2016;177:90.e3.

78. Chandrasekar I, Eis A, Konduri GG. Betamethasone attenuates oxidant stress in endothelial cells from fetal lambs with persistent pulmonary hypertension. Pediatr Res 2008;63(1):67–72.

79. Konduri GG, Bakhutashvili I, Eis A, et al. Antenatal betamethasone improves postnatal transition in late preterm lambs with persistent pulmonary hypertension of the newborn. Pediatr Res 2013;73(5):621–9.

80. Perez M, Wedgwood S, Lakshminrusimha S, et al. Hydrocortisone normalizes phosphodiesterase-5 activity in pulmonary artery smooth muscle cells from lambs with persistent pulmonary hypertension of the newborn. Pulm Circ 2014;4(1):71–81.

81. Perez M, Lakshminrusimha S, Wedgwood S, et al. Hydrocortisone normalizes oxygenation and cGMP regulation in lambs with persistent pulmonary hypertension of the newborn. Am J Physiol Lung Cell Mol Physiol 2012;302(6):L595–603.

82. Tripathi S, Saili A. The effect of steroids on the clinical course and outcome of neonates with meconium aspiration syndrome. J Trop Pediatr 2007;53(1):8–12.

83. Sharif Kashani B, Tahmaseb Pour P, Malekmohammad M, et al. Oral l-citrulline malate in patients with idiopathic pulmonary arterial hypertension and Eisenmenger Syndrome: a clinical trial. J Cardiol 2014;64(3):231–5.

84. Ghofrani HA, Galiè N, Grimminger F, et al. Riociguat for the treatment of pulmonary arterial hypertension. N Engl J Med 2013;369(4):330–40.

85. Chester M, Tourneux P, Seedorf G, et al. Cinaciguat, a soluble guanylate cyclase activator, causes potent and sustained pulmonary vasodilation in the ovine fetus. Am J Physiol Lung Cell Mol Physiol 2009;297(2):L318–25.

86. Zhang D, Wang G, Han D, et al. Activation of PPAR-γ ameliorates pulmonary arterial hypertension via inducing heme oxygenase-1 and p21(WAF1): an in vivo study in rats. Life Sci 2014;98(1):39–43.

87. Rana U, Callan E, Entringer B, et al. AMP-kinase dysfunction alters notch ligands to impair angiogenesis in neonatal pulmonary hypertension. Am J Respir Cell Mol Biol 2020;62(6):719–31.

88. Krishnan U, Feinstein JA, Adatia I, et al. Evaluation and management of pulmonary hypertension in children with bronchopulmonary dysplasia. J Pediatr 2017; 188:24.e1.

89. Mourani PM, Sontag MK, Ivy DD, et al. Effects of long-term sildenafil treatment for pulmonary hypertension in infants with chronic lung disease. J Pediatr 2009; 154(3):379–84, 384.e1-4.

90. Trottier-Boucher MN, Lapointe A, Malo J, et al. Sildenafil for the treatment of pulmonary arterial hypertension in infants with bronchopulmonary dysplasia. Pediatr Cardiol 2015;36(6):1255–60.

91. Nyp M, Sandritter T, Poppinga N, et al. Sildenafil citrate, bronchopulmonary dysplasia and disordered pulmonary gas exchange: any benefits? J Perinatol 2012;32(1):64–9.

92. Kadmon G, Schiller O, Dagan T, et al. Pulmonary hypertension specific treatment in infants with bronchopulmonary dysplasia. Pediatr Pulmonol 2017;52(1):77–83.

93. Tan K, Krishnamurthy MB, O'Heney JL, et al. Sildenafil therapy in bronchopulmonary dysplasia-associated pulmonary hypertension: a retrospective study of efficacy and safety. Eur J Pediatr 2015;174(8):1109–15.

94. van der Graaf M, Rojer LA, Helbing W, et al. EXPRESS: sildenafil for bronchopulmonary dysplasia and pulmonary hypertension: a meta-analysis. Pulm Circ 2019;(9). 2045894019837875.

95. Nees SN, Rosenzweig EB, Cohen JL, et al. Targeted therapy for pulmonary hypertension in premature infants. Children (Basel) 2020;7(8):97.

96. Zaidi AN, Dettorre MD, Ceneviva GD, et al. Epoprostenol and home mechanical ventilation for pulmonary hypertension associated with chronic lung disease. Pediatr Pulmonol 2005;40(3):265–9.

97. Rugolotto S, Errico G, Beghini R, et al. Weaning of epoprostenol in a small infant receiving concomitant bosentan for severe pulmonary arterial hypertension secondary to bronchopulmonary dysplasia. Minerva Pediatr 2006;58(5):491–4.

98. Ferdman DJ, Rosenzweig EB, Zuckerman WA, et al. Subcutaneous treprostinil for pulmonary hypertension in chronic lung disease of infancy. Pediatrics 2014;134(1):e274–8.

99. Krishnan U, Krishnan S, Gewitz M. Treatment of pulmonary hypertension in children with chronic lung disease with newer oral therapies. Pediatr Cardiol 2008; 29(6):1082–6.

100. Lotze A, Mitchell BR, Bulas DI, et al. Multicenter study of surfactant (beractant) use in the treatment of term infants with severe respiratory failure. Survanta in Term Infants Study Group. J Pediatr 1998;132(1):40–7.

101. Gonzalez A, Bancalari A, Osorio W, et al. Early use of combined exogenous surfactant and inhaled nitric oxide reduces treatment failure in persistent pulmonary hypertension of the newborn: a randomized controlled trial. J Perinatol 2021;41(1):32–8.

102. Kinsella JP, Truog WE, Walsh WF, et al. Randomized, multicenter trial of inhaled nitric oxide and high-frequency oscillatory ventilation in severe, persistent pulmonary hypertension of the newborn. J Pediatr 1997;131(1 Pt 1):55–62.

Withdrawing and Withholding Life-Sustaining Medical Therapies in the Neonatal Intensive Care Unit

Case-Based Approaches to Clinical Controversies

Erin L. Rholl, MD, MA[a], Katie R. Baughman, MD[b],
Steven R. Leuthner, MD, MA[c],*

KEYWORDS

- Withdrawing • Withholding • Life-sustaining medical therapy • End-of-life, nutrition
- Hydration • Ethics • Palliative care

KEY POINTS

- There are situations whereby withholding/withdrawing life-sustaining medical therapy is ethically and morally permissible.
- Withholding/withdrawing artificial nutrition hydration is not morally different from withholding or withdrawing other medical therapies.
- What and when to withdraw should occur through a model of shared decision-making driven by the infant's best interest, the parents' values, and with physician recommendations.

INTRODUCTION

Care of the critically ill neonate focuses on providing care that is in the best interest of the infant, which typically means implementing therapies that prolong life. There are circumstances whereby continuing life-sustaining medical therapies (LSMT) are not considered to be in an infant's best interest and can be withheld or withdrawn. While withholding/withdrawing LSMT (WWLSMT) constitutes most of the pediatric in-hospital deaths in the United States, there remain areas of controversy.[1–4] In this article, we will briefly review the ethical considerations for WWLSMT and discuss

^a Division of Hospital Medicine, PANDA Palliative Care Team, Children's National Medical Center, 111 Michigan Avenue, Washington, DC 20010, USA; ^b Department of Pediatrics, Children's Wisconsin, Medical College of Wisconsin, 8915 W. Connell Court, Milwaukee, WI 53226, USA; ^c Department of Pediatrics, Children's Wisconsin, Medical College of Wisconsin, 999 North 92nd Street, Suite C410, Wauwatosa, WI 53226, USA
* Corresponding author.
E-mail address: sleuthne@mcw.edu

Clin Perinatol 49 (2022) 127–135
https://doi.org/10.1016/j.clp.2021.11.006
0095-5108/22/© 2021 Elsevier Inc. All rights reserved.
perinatology.theclinics.com

the following controversies: what and when to withdraw, withholding/withdrawing artificial nutrition and hydration, and when the infant does not follow the anticipated dying "script." We write under the premise that the infant's best interest is at the center of all recommended care. Definitions associated with WWLSMT can be seen in **Table 1**.

ETHICAL CONSIDERATIONS FOR WITHHOLDING/WITHDRAWING LIFE-SUSTAINING MEDICAL THERAPIES

Medical interventions for pediatric patients are ethically optional if they do not meet typical goals of growth and development, follow parent-specific goals of care, cause significant pain with little pleasure, or lengthen the dying process.[5] Infants are unable to express preferences, so the best interest standard (BIS) guides the medical team and parents in shared decision-making when considering WWLSMT.[5,6] Benefits of treatment are weighed against burdens. Significant burdens are those likely to remain even with maximal therapies such as pain, pharmacologic and nonpharmacologic activity restriction, and seclusion.[6–8] The American Academy of Pediatrics (AAP) and other authorities have issued policy statements supporting WWLSMT.[5] While neonatal providers and families often have personal beliefs about withholding versus withdrawing, there is no moral or ethical distinction between the 2 practices.[9–11]

CASE OF BABY A

The parents of Baby A learned about his diagnoses (congenital heart disease, duodenal atresia (DA), and a limb abnormality) prenatally and were followed at a fetal center. The prenatal counseling focused on the immediate need for cardiac evaluation with suspected single ventricle physiology and the need for surgical interventions for his heart lesion and DA. Baby A was born at 34 weeks due to the premature rupture of membranes and fetal bradycardia and was admitted to the NICU requiring continuous positive airway pressure (CPAP). Immediate postnatal evaluation included a CXR and echocardiogram, which revealed a complex single ventricle and a hypoplastic lung. Baby A was intubated for a CT angiogram to better delineate anatomy, which revealed a cardiac lesion with no immediate surgical need, yet no option for later surgical repair including transplant; the CT also revealed a hypoplastic right lung. The parents were informed about the change in diagnosis and prognosis noting that Baby A's life would certainly be significantly shortened, but life expectancy in an infant with these anomalies was uncertain. The parents initially thought that no need for cardiac surgery was

Table 1 Definitions associated with life-sustaining medical therapies	
Word/Phrase	**Definition**
Live Sustaining Medical Therapy	Treatment that prolongs or extends life without reversing the primary condition.[11] These include mechanical ventilation, renal replacement therapy, inotropic support, extracorporeal membrane oxygenation, and artificial nutrition and hydration.[6,11]
Withholding	Not providing a medical therapy that was considered.[6]
Withdrawing	Starting and stopping a medical therapy.[6]
Artificial Nutrition and Hydration	Nutrition or hydration provided via a physician order and by an artificial means such as a nasogastric, orogastric or gastric tube, or via intravenous access.[15]
Informed Nondissent	Physician does not ask for parent consent but informs them of the plan to WWLSMT and that they will proceed unless they disagree.[13]

good news but started to understand their infant's prognosis with more education on the new expected outcome. The palliative care team was consulted after the change in diagnosis to assist with advanced care planning. The parents identified that their goal was to get Baby A home while doing what was medically appropriate. They did not want their infant to suffer and expressed that they did not want the medical team to do anything that they would not do for their own child.

The team and parents reviewed potential steps forward as Baby A was still intubated and doing poorly on the ventilator, leading the NICU team to think he would not survive without some form of positive pressure support. Without repairing his DA, Baby A could not receive enteral feeds. Given his complex cardiopulmonary anatomy and escalating respiratory needs, the surgeons feared he would not be a good operative candidate. In support of parental goals, the team recommended withdrawing/withholding the ventilator and an altered code. Because the infant was 34 weeks and had appeared to do better on CPAP alone before intubation, the team chose to extubate to CPAP. If he did well, the team could reassess DA surgical potential. The parents agreed to this plan and made Baby A an altered code. The parents also prepared for and expected Baby A to die the day of withdrawal, despite the team preparing them that he may not die immediately.

After extubating to CPAP, Baby A continued to have increased work of breathing and increased CPAP requirements over the next few weeks. While Baby A was still requiring more support than could be provided at home, the parents became more hopeful and used the fact Baby A did not immediately need to be reintubated as a positive prognostic sign. They asked about DA repair and reversed the altered code. Cardiac anesthesia was consulted and recommended against surgery given the significant surgical risks based on Baby A's anatomy and increasing respiratory requirements. The infant's parents initially agreed that if Baby A required intubation, they would consider making Baby A an altered code again. As more time passed, the parents reaffirmed their decision for full code status requesting that the medical team intubate and resuscitate Baby A if the infant's clinical status deteriorated. The parents again sometimes saw the fact that Baby A could not get cardiac repair as a positive that he "did not need" surgery and were hopeful that he could survive to DA repair. The medical team continued to discuss advanced care planning as Baby A's cardiopulmonary status deteriorated. Baby A was reintubated, and despite a significant escalation in ventilator support and initiation of neurosedative drips, he became progressively acidotic. Parents agreed to an altered code, and Baby A died shortly after a while on the ventilator.

What aspects of Baby A's presentation made consideration of WWLSMT appropriate? With the parental goal of wanting to go home, should the trial of extubation be directly to home respiratory support that a baby could go home on rather than provide potential false hope of being OK on CPAP?

CASE OF BABY B

Baby B was born at 31 weeks gestation via an urgent Caesarian section for nonreassuring fetal heart tones. The infant underwent routine care for prematurity, including support with CPAP, and she was described as an active baby. On day of life 5, she developed profound metabolic acidosis and rapid clinical decline. Baby B was intubated for acute respiratory failure and underwent extensive work-up. Her presentation was atypical and initial radiologic studies did not reveal the ultimate diagnosis of atretic bowel and segmental volvulus. Baby B experienced a bowel perforation resulting in emergent surgery, and over the following days, she underwent 3 exploratory laparotomies with small bowel resections. During surgical interventions, she experienced hypotension and after her second operation, she experienced an intraabdominal hemorrhage. Following Baby B's third surgery, there was minimal small bowel remaining; the remaining small bowel and a portion of the large bowel were unhealthy appearing with areas of necrosis.

Baby B's parents were counseled extensively on the surgical findings, the anticipated short gut syndrome, and associated poor prognosis. The findings were also not in isolation. Baby B also experienced prolonged metabolic acidosis, hypotension, shock liver, and electrolyte derangements. Baby B's parents did not want their baby to suffer or to be reliant on prolonged invasive medical support; their values and expectations for quality of life did not align with additional surgical interventions, and the parents chose to redirect goals of care toward comfort care.

Baby B's parents knew that their baby would not be able to survive without additional surgeries, but they were not immediately ready to withdrawal life-sustaining medical therapies. The parents chose to have close family members meet Baby B before extubating or withdrawing medical therapies. During the time of family visits, Baby B's parents consented to a do not attempt resuscitation order and agreed to not escalate support. After spending 3 days of cherished time with Baby B, the parents chose to move forward with extubation. The family was counseled that their infant's condition would ultimately result in her death, but that death following extubation can take minutes, hours, or days. During the days of visitation, the acidosis and electrolyte abnormalities secondary to the ischemic bowel likely began to correct as the tissue completely died, leading to more stability. After extubation, Baby B was able to breathe without mechanical support. During this period, she was also maintained on continuous infusions of neurosedatives for comfort. In the following days, Baby B experienced intermittent periods of profound desaturations and bradycardic episodes but was able to recover. After several days, the family was offered home hospice, including transitioning to sublingual sedatives and withholding of ANH. Baby B went home on room air with sublingual medications for comfort. She died 12 days later.

Though the family and physicians knew Baby B's condition would ultimately result in death, her dying process was slower than anticipated. When an infant does not die as expected, families and medical care teams are left in a state of limbo and faced with multiple questions: Did we make the right decision? Should withholding of ANH occur with extubation? How do we support the baby, the family, and the medical team? Should life-sustaining medical therapies be reinitiated?

WHAT AND WHEN TO WITHDRAW: WHEN TRYING TO HELP PARENTS DECIDE

The approach for WWLSMT should be discussed with clear and open communication with the family and medical team members. There is no uniform plan for what or when WWLSMT is appropriate for all infants. As parents act as surrogate decision-makers for their children, the medical team should explore parents' values before an infant's end-of-life.[12] Once the medical team determines the parents' goals, hopes, and values, they can guide the parents in end-of-life scenarios through shared decision-making.

Regarding what to withhold or withdraw, often families find it easiest to make the decision to WWLSMT in a stepwise fashion. It is common for the family to first agree to an altered code if something should happen, followed by withholding any further escalation of treatments, such as starting or increasing inotropic medications or changing ventilation strategies, as they do not think of settings these limits as being an active decision leading to death as they may in the setting of withdrawal. Withdrawal of a ventilator is often the next step as it is viewed as a high level of technological support and often with death anticipated soon after extubation. In some scenarios, withdrawal of mechanical ventilation alone is followed by an infant's demise. Other infants, like Baby B, are able to breathe without mechanical ventilation and die as a result of their underlying illness over time and often only once artificial nutrition and hydration are discontinued. When WWLSMT is indicated because the prolongation of life is no longer considered in the infant's best interest, medical recommendations should be to withdrawal all life-prolonging medical treatments. A stepwise approach should probably only be done as a way to help families if, through shared conversations, they express that they are more comfortable with this approach. Education and counseling can help many families understand why the stepwise approach can often just lead to a prolongation of the dying process and perhaps prolonged suffering during this process.

Withdrawing in a stepwise fashion can also be driven by provider comfort or standard practices. In the case of Baby A, parents' goals were to try interventions that were appropriate to get their baby home and not cause undo suffering. While the medical team in the case of Baby A talked about uncertainty because they had never seen a case with this specific anatomy, the only detail they were uncertain about was the timing of death from the cardiopulmonary perspective. They were certain that his physiology was not stable enough for surgical repair of his DA, and that his cardiopulmonary physiology would not be maintained on home therapy. None of the providers would have put their own child through any further intervention.

Perhaps a better ethical/medical recommendation, considering the medical facts and directly expressed parental values, would have been to extubate to room air or a low flow nasal cannula to demonstrate that Baby A could not sustain himself at home. Extubating to CPAP put both the family and medical team in a middle ground. The family was willing and prepared to accept their baby's death, but the medical team followed a common practice of deescalating to CPAP, claiming that prematurity may impact the infant's respiratory status and that he had initially looked better on CPAP, was not considering the failing cardiopulmonary status during this time. While some infants born at 34 weeks need CPAP until they have transitioned, the baby was now several weeks old, and no respiratory issues would be related to transition. Using a stepwise medical recommendation did not support the long-term bigger picture of outcomes for this baby. It is important to consider whether provider directed the stepwise withdrawal of LSMT is helpful to parents or could lead to prolongation of the inevitable. What to withdraw, and what to withdraw to, is really a medical not parental decision. This medical decision should be based on the long-term goals of care. Recommending full withdrawal of LSMT, including CPAP, would have prevented weeks of false hopes, prolonged suffering, and moral distress for the family and medical team.

In some scenarios, parents' goals align with WWLSMT but they just cannot make the decision to WWLSMT. If the medical team recognizes this situation based on conversations with the parents, we recommend the practice of informed nondissent. In informed nondissent, the physician does not ask for parent consent but informs the parents of a recommended plan consistent with shared goals, stating that the medical team will proceed with this plan unless the parents disagree.[13] The physician's recommendations are based on the infant's physiology, clinical status, and parent goals. Most inpatient pediatric care follows the practice of informed nondissent. The medical team informs parents of their plan and proceeds unless the parents protest. While the medical team often wants parents to explicitly state they would like to proceed with WWLSMT, parents might not want the burden of requesting WWLSMT. Informed nondissent would have been an appropriate method for Baby A's parents, who recognized they did not want the team to "do anything they would not do for their own child" and did not want him to suffer. Instead of presenting parents with a panel of choices, the team might have recommended a full withdrawal and a focus on comfort care based on the parents' goals. While this approach might seem paternalistic, parents often do not want to state that they would like WWLSMT for their child, especially if they feel guilt or feel like they are giving up on their child.

The timing of withdrawing interventions can have some flexibility, yet sometimes a concern comes up that there is a "window of opportunity" in which withdrawal will lead to a quicker and perhaps more certain death. For example, in the setting of clinical worsening, perhaps in an acute inflammatory state, the withdrawal will lead to a quick death. When an infant has passed this acute inflammatory state before withdrawal, the infant may live longer following WWLSMT. As the case of Baby B demonstrates, the delay in withdrawal to support the family needs led to some level of physiologic recovery that did not change the longer-term life course but allowed the baby to survive longer. While this can lead to caregiver distress and second guessing, appropriate counseling and good palliative care can help reassure everyone that the decision is still ethically appropriate based on long-term concerns, and the length of surviving is more of a psychological issue than an ethical issue.

Personal biases of the medical providers should be recognized and addressed before counseling a family. Medical providers may have differences in opinions about recommendations for families. If there are ethically reasonable options and physicians disagree with each other about what is appropriate, parents should be provided the options and decide based on their values. At the same time, messages portrayed to families should be as consistent as possible. Physicians who are uncomfortable or decline to participate in withdrawal should transfer care to another provider if the withdrawal is ethically reasonable.[6] When there is disagreement among the patient's family and members of the medical team, it is reasonable to obtain a second opinion by consulting the ethics or palliative care teams to assist in shared decision making.[6]

WITHHOLDING/WITHDRAWING ARTIFICIAL NUTRITION AND HYDRATION

There is little controversy regarding the withdrawal of mechanical ventilation and vasopressors in the NICU, but the withdrawal of artificial nutrition and hydration (ANH) still seems to raise controversy.[14] ANH refers to any nutrition or hydration provided by nasogastric tube, gastric tube, or intravenous access and provided as a medical therapy.[5,15] When clinically appropriate, withdrawing/withholding artificial nutrition hydration (WWANH) can be considered and is supported by the AAP and other national organizations.[16] WWANH is not morally or ethically different from other therapies but can cause more moral distress, often due to the emotional connection our society places on feeding an infant. Death after WWANH often takes longer than withdrawing other therapies, which can be wrongly viewed as a prolonged period of suffering.[5] After a period of fasting, the body transitions to ketosis which suppresses appetite and is associated with euphoria.[17] Fasting also decreases burdensome symptoms in chronically ill infants (secretions, coughing, nausea, vomiting, and diarrhea).[17] These positive effects are lost when intermittent nutrition is provided, supporting complete WWANH.[17] If infant cues for feeds, they can be provided oral feedings for comfort but not growth, and parents should be aware if there is a possible safety issue in aspiration, and that even comfort feeds may prolong the dying process.[17] Sometimes these are reasons to only allow nonnutritive support for cues. In the case of Baby B, mechanical ventilation was withdrawn and the infant was maintained on IV fluids to allow for the continuation of IV neurosedatives until the medications were converted to enteral solutions to ensure Baby B's comfort. While this likely prolonged the dying process, it also allowed the parents time to bond with their infant and come to terms with Baby B's prognosis.

WHEN AN INFANT DOES NOT FOLLOW THE SCRIPT

Most WWLSMT occurs with an anticipated time frame and clinical symptoms. Good palliative care includes anticipatory counseling about these expectations. In these cases, the parents and medical team face their grief in an expected timeline. Controversy or moral distress can arise when this script is not followed. This occurred for the parents of both Babies A and B. For Baby A, the family expectation was death shortly after extubation to CPAP, and with each hour to the day he lived, they developed false hope. For the family of Baby B, they were grateful for each day they were able to have; however, each additional day caused them to question their decisions because Baby B's dying process was longer than anticipated.

Withdrawal of life-sustaining therapies in the NICU often occurs when the infant is either experiencing an acute clinical worsening (ie, Baby B) or when an infant is clinically stable but has a chronic disease with an expected poor prognosis (ie, Baby A). In both scenarios, the infant may die quickly, have a prolonged death process, or not die. When an infant does not die as expected, it is important for the medical team and parents to understand that the underlying pathophysiology that led to the decision for WWLSMT has not changed.

Sometimes we as medical providers can set ourselves up for prognostic failure by being too certain of ourselves. Other times we set ourselves up for this "failure" by the timing and/or what we withdraw, as demonstrated by our cases. What this can naturally cause is staff or family to second guess their decision or develop some false hope. When families are counseled on the option of WWLSMT for their infant, they should also be counseled on what to expect following the discontinuation of life-sustaining therapies and on the possibility of a lingering death.[19] Good anticipatory guidance can be helpful to alleviate these concerns and keeping the big/long term reasons for withdrawal in mind can help in accepting that the decisions are still correct. Palliative care services provide excellent support in these times, and can also help in planning the next steps, as the baby is still in a dying process.

SUMMARY

WWLSMT is ethically and morally appropriate for certain neonatal presentations. WWANH is no different from any other medical therapy. Withdrawal of LSMT should be directed by shared decision-making with the infant's best interest and parents' goals and values in mind. Informed nondissent should be considered when intensive medical therapy is not appropriate, but a family has not verbalized the decision to WWLSMT. Physician discomfort should not be the primary reason for stepwise rather than complete WWLSMT. When an infant does not follow the anticipated course after WWLSMT, it is important to remember the physiology that drove the decision to WWLSMT.

BEST PRACTICES BOX

- Recognize that there are clinical situation in which the withholding and/or withdrawing of life sustaining medical treatment is ethically reasonable.

- Decisions should be directed by the infant's best interest as determined throguh shared decision-making.
- Use of Ethics consultation and Palliative Care Services may provide value in situations of discomfort.

DISCLOSURE

The authors have nothing to disclose.

REFERENCES

1. Barton L, Hodgman JE. The contribution of withholding or withdrawing care to newborn mortality. Pediatrics 2005;116(6):1487–91. https://doi.org/10.1542/peds.2005-0392.
2. Dworetz AR, Natarajan G, Langer J, et al. Withholding or withdrawing life-sustaining treatment in extremely low gestational age neonates. Arch Dis Child Fetal Neonatal Ed 2021;106(3):238–43. https://doi.org/10.1136/archdischild-2020-318855.
3. Weiner J, Sharma J, Lantos J, et al. How infants die in the neonatal intensive care unit: trends from 1999 through 2008. Arch Pediatr Adolesc Med 2011;165(7):630–4. https://doi.org/10.1001/archpediatrics.2011.102.
4. de Leeuw R, de Beaufort AJ, de Kleine MJ, et al. Foregoing intensive care treatment in newborn infants with extremely poor prognoses. A study in four neonatal intensive care units in The Netherlands. J Pediatr 1996;129(5):661–6. https://doi.org/10.1016/s0022-3476(96)70146-4.
5. Carter BS, Leuthner SR. The ethics of withholding/withdrawing nutrition in the newborn. Semin Perinatol 2003;27(6):480–7. https://doi.org/10.1053/j.semperi.2003.10.007.
6. Weise KL, Okun AL, Carter BS, et al. Guidance on forgoing life-sustaining medical treatment. Pediatrics 2017;140(3):e20171905. https://doi.org/10.1542/peds.2017-1905.
7. Bester JC. The best interest standard and children: clarifying a concept and responding to its critics. J Med Ethics 2019;45(2):117–24. https://doi.org/10.1136/medethics-2018-105036.
8. Beauchamp TL, Childress JF. Principles of Biomedical ethics. 7th edition. Oxford University Press; 2012.
9. American Academy of Pediatrics Committee on Fetus and Newborn, Bell EF. Noninitiation or withdrawal of intensive care for high-risk newborns. Pediatrics 2007;119(2):401–3. https://doi.org/10.1542/peds.2006-3180.
10. Duff RS, Campbell AG. Moral and ethical dilemmas in the special-care nursery. N Engl J Med 1973;289(17):890–4. https://doi.org/10.1056/NEJM197310252891705.
11. AMA Council on Ethical and Judicial. AMA code of medical ethics' opinions on care at the end of life. AMA J Ethics 2013;13(12):1038–40. https://doi.org/10.1001/virtualmentor.2013.15.12.coet1-1312.
12. Blumenthal-Barby JS, Loftis L, Cummings CL, et al. Should neonatologists give opinions withdrawing life-sustaining treatment? Pediatrics 2016;138(6):e20162585. https://doi.org/10.1542/peds.2016-2585.
13. Kon AA. Informed Nondissent rather than informed assent - CHEST. Chest 2008;133(1):320–1. https://doi.org/10.1378/chest.07-2392.

14. Feltman DM, Du H, Leuthner SR. Survey of neonatologists' attitudes toward limiting life-sustaining treatments in the neonatal intensive. J Perinatol 2012; 32(11):886–92.
15. Porta N, Frader J. Withholding hydration and nutrition in newborns. Theor Med Bioeth 2007;28:443–51. https://doi.org/10.1007/s11017-007-9049-6.
16. Diekema DS, Botkin JR, Committee on Bioethics. Clinical report–Forgoing medically provided nutrition and hydration in children. Pediatrics 2009;124(2):813–22. https://doi.org/10.1542/peds.2009-1299.
17. Winter SM. Terminal nutrition: framing the debate for the withdrawal of nutritional support in terminally ill patients. Am J Med 2000;109(9):723–6. https://doi.org/10.1016/s0002-9343(00)00609-4.

Beyond the Clinical Trials
Off-Protocol Therapeutic Hypothermia

Naomi T. Laventhal, MD, MA*, John D.E. Barks, MD

KEYWORDS

- Therapeutic hypothermia • Hypoxic ischemic encephalopathy • Research ethics
- Neuroprotection • Targeted temperature management

KEY POINTS

- Mild therapeutic hypothermia has been extensively studied and validated as an effective and safe treatment for term and near-term infants with moderate and severe hypoxic encephalopathy meeting narrow inclusion criteria.
- Unanswered questions remain about whether cooling treatment can be optimized to improve outcomes even further, and whether it is reasonable to offer treatment to infants excluded from the foundational studies.
- Consideration of "off-protocol" cooling practices requires methodical review of available evidence and analysis using both a clinical and research ethical framework.

INTRODUCTION

Few advancements in contemporary neonatal medicine have been as paradigm-changing as therapeutic hypothermia (TH) for infants with hypoxic ischemic encephalopathy (HIE). This deceptively simple intervention, both high-tech and counterintuitive - cold, after all, is the enemy in neonatal resuscitation - changed treatment for a sudden and potentially devastating illness from supportive care with watchful waiting to life-saving and life-changing neuroprotection. TH for moderate and severe HIE was systematically evaluated by high-quality randomized control trials. In a meta-analysis, TH was shown to significantly increase survival with normal neurologic function (risk ratio, 1.53; 95% confidence interval [CI], 1.22–1.93, $P<.001$) with a number needed

Attestations: Dr N.T. Laventhal contributed substantially to the conception or design of the work and drafted the work and approved the final version to be published. Dr J.D.E. Barks contributed substantially to the conception or design of the work and revised it critically for important intellectual content and approved the final version to be published.

COI statement: The authors have no conflicts of interest to disclose.

Department of Pediatrics, Division of Neonatal-Perinatal Medicine, Michigan Medicine–University of Michigan Medical School, 8-621 C.S. Mott Children's Hospital, SPC 4254, 1540 East Hospital Drive, Ann Arbor, MI 48105-4254, USA
* Corresponding author.
E-mail address: naomilav@med.umich.edu

to treat of 8 (95% CI, 5–17)[1]; few therapies in the newborn intensive care unit (NICU) offer this magnitude of treatment effect.

Given the complexity and heterogeneity of the condition and the clinical context in which it occurs, trial eligibility criteria were specific and exclusive. For example, the whole-body TH study conducted within the Neonatal Research Network (NRN) of the National Institutes of Health Eunice Kennedy Shriver National Institute of Child Health and Human Development (NICHD) included strict and specific clinical criteria and excluded infants born before 36 completed weeks of gestation, those weighing less than 1800 g, and those with major congenital anomalies.[2] The foundational clinical trials also included detailed protocols for depth and duration of treatment and ancillary clinical monitoring. Although this approach likely contributed to the decisive conclusion that TH initiated within 6 hours of birth offered significant reductions in morbidity and mortality, the narrow inclusion criteria imparted some difficulties for translation of this intervention from the highly regimented confines of a clinical trial to less tidy real-life situations. The promise of improved outcomes for infants with HIE has also led some to consider potentially high-stakes alterations to the originally described cooling procedures.[3,4]

In this article, the authors review some of these challenges by framing them around *clinical* decisions to initiate or carry out this treatment in ways not described in the original research protocols. In broad categories these include the following:

- *Decisions to initiate TH for infants who were specifically excluded by the original research protocol*, including infants born before 35 or 36 weeks, infants with major congenital anomalies and genetic disorders, infants with mild HIE, and infants who would be greater than 6 hours of age at the time of initiation of treatment. Of note, treatment of infants with mild HIE is the topic of a separate article in this issue of *Clinics in Perinatology* and is therefore not explored in depth in this one.
- *Decisions to deviate from published treatment protocols*, including a longer initial period of treatment, early discontinuation of treatment, use of a lower target temperature for treatment. Although adjuvant treatments to potentiate the beneficial effects of TH are a current area of research interest, these are out of the scope of this review. Technical considerations for TH on extracorporeal membrane oxygenation support are also the topic of a growing body of literature but are excluded from this article.
- *Decisions to offer TH for neonatal hypoxic-ischemic brain injury that does not occur in the context of an acute perinatal event.*

"Off-protocol" interventions such as these require careful scientific and ethical analysis, considering available evidence and important principles of clinical and research ethics. For each of these scenarios, the authors undertake this analysis, reviewing both the current state of science and the ethical implications of these decisions. A summary of this work is provided in **Table 1**.

Although expansion of clinical protocols to include a more diverse group of patients or optimize patient outcomes is generally both well intended and based on plausible rationale, doing so requires careful considerations of the risks and benefits, both to individual patients and to future patients using both a clinical and a research ethics framework (**Fig. 1**).

For individual patients, the primary concern is with potential risks versus benefits. Frequently, decisions to include populations not studied in the foundational clinical trials rest on the determination that such patients have something to lose by foregoing the treatment, and that potential risks, known or unknown, are outweighed by the possibility of direct benefit. In general, this argument is easiest to support when the

Table 1
Review of potential off-protocol uses of therapeutic hypothermia

Clinical Decision	Published Empirical Evaluation (Y/N)	Studied by RCT (Y/N)	Evidence Supports Use (Y/N)
Treatment of infants <35 wk' gestational age	Y	Not yet published	N
Treatment of infants <1800 g	N	N	N
Treatment of infants with major congenital anomalies	N	N	N
Initiation of therapeutic hypothermia after 6 h of age	Y	Y	N
Treatment <72 h	Y	Y	1 RCT Eicher*
Treatment >72 h	Y	Y	N
Treatment with lower target temperature	Y	Y	N
Treatment of neonates in NICUs who sustain HIE after nonperinatal sentinel events	N	N	N

Abbreviations: N, no; RCT, randomized clinical trial; Y, yes.

previous strict inclusion criteria had more to do with creating a "clean" data set than in plausible biologic arguments against treatment of certain groups; this distinction will be explored in examples in later discussion. Ethical justification for "what is there to lose?" interventions rests largely on informed consent on the part of the patient (autonomy), or, for infants, the parents (authority). Typically, treatment with unproven interventions of unknown risk is not compelled over parental objection. Critics of such an approach might argue, however, that it is not possible for consent to be truly "informed" when neither the benefits nor risks are known, and that the best parents can do is acknowledge the uncertainty associated with the proposed treatment.[5,6]

Justice arguments may also be applied for and against use of existing therapies in unproven contexts. In the case of interventions that are expensive or use a limited resource, one might make a utilitarian argument that use of the resource off-protocol without sufficient evidence to anticipate cost-effectiveness and maximized collective benefit cannot be morally justified. In the case of long-odds treatments in the face of poor prognosis, such an argument might have some overlap with futility arguments; in patients with an extremely poor prognosis, use of therapies not known or likely to work might both waste precious resources with little hope of return and prolong pain, suffering, or indignity for the patient.

For some interventions, problems arise when clinicians "jump the gun" by expanding therapies to previously excluded patients or altered protocols that have not been studied *yet.* Bringing such practices to prime time without systematically studying them first has the potential to undermine collective clinical equipoise to the point that future (or ongoing) empirical investigation is no longer possible. The result of this is that knowledge of an off-protocol use of a treatment is limited to retrospective study or low-quality evidence, challenging the ideal state that all patient care is based on soundly obtained scientific knowledge. Balancing duty to collective groups of future patients and the needs of a specific patient in real time remains a challenge as use of TH for neonates evolves. Finally, even when informed consent for clinical care is consistently sought from parents and documented, poor outcomes associated with "experimental" treatment can undermine public trust in biomedical research.

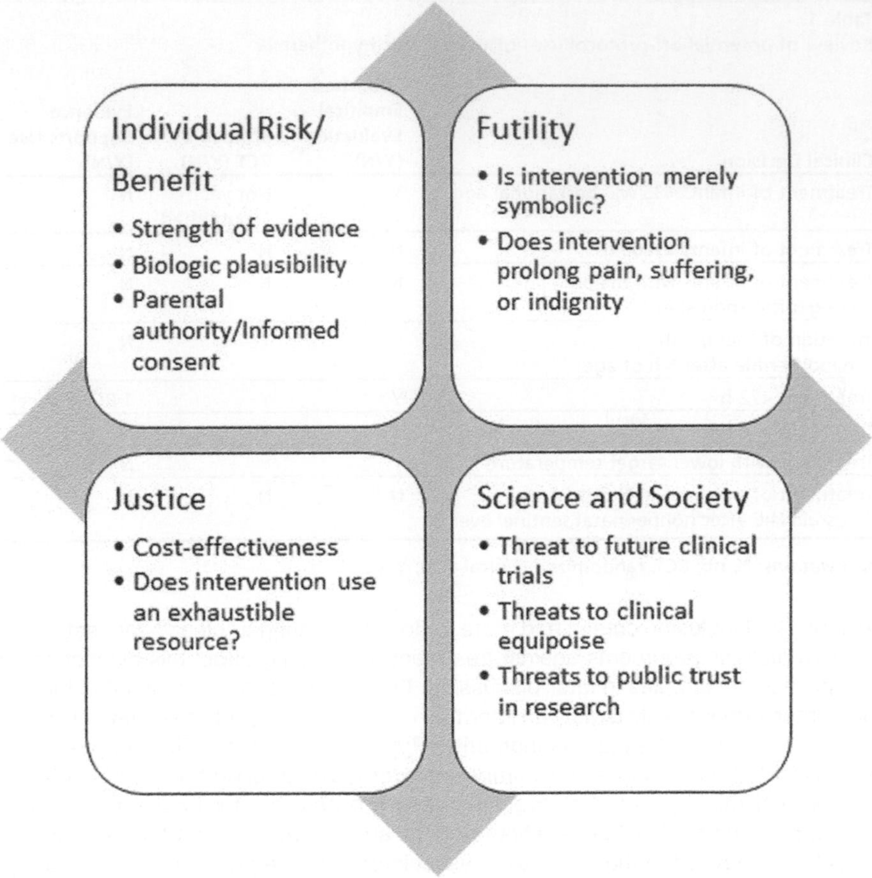

Individual Risk/Benefit

- Strength of evidence
- Biologic plausibility
- Parental authority/Informed consent

Futility

- Is intervention merely symbolic?
- Does intervention prolong pain, suffering, or indignity

Justice

- Cost-effectiveness
- Does intervention use an exhaustible resource?

Science and Society

- Threat to future clinical trials
- Threats to clinical equipoise
- Threats to public trust in research

Fig. 1. The moral landscape of off-protocol usage of clinical trial-proven interventions for an infant.

DECISIONS TO INITIATE THERAPEUTIC HYPOTHERMIA FOR INFANTS WHO WERE SPECIFICALLY EXCLUDED BY THE ORIGINAL RESEARCH PROTOCOL

The foundational clinical trials of TH excluded infants born before 35 or 36 completed gestational weeks and those weighing less than 1800 g and infants with a "major congenital abnormality." Given the need to discern clinically meaningful differences in neurodevelopmental outcome, it was rational to exclude infants with other, easily identifiable risk factors for neurodevelopmental impairment. Diagnostic precision for HIE in preterm infants imparts additional challenges.[7] Furthermore, given the paucity of data about potential risks of TH, including concern about coagulopathy, exclusion of infants at higher-than-baseline risk of intraventricular hemorrhage (IVH) was similarly rational. However, continued exclusion of these patient groups has raised clinical and ethical concern.

Therapeutic Hypothermia for Infants Born Before 36 weeks' Gestation and/or Weighing less than 1800 g

Given what is now known about the risks of TH for both term and late preterm infants, offering this intervention to premature infants, particularly those with a low absolute risk of IVH (3% and 1% in 34- and 35-week infants, respectively,[8,9] 16% in a cohort of 37 infants 32–36 weeks, none of whom developed grade 3 or 4 IVH[10]), is a matter of practice variation and debate.[11] Similarly, the weight threshold of 1800 g is subject to interpretation: historically, weight thresholds have been used for research in populations with limited access to prenatal care, as a proxy for gestational age. Furthermore, for infants with reasonably accurate gestational dating, severe intrauterine growth restriction (IUGR) can be accompanied by thrombocytopenia, evidence of systemic malperfusion, and a wide array of other comorbidities given the diverse potential causes of IUGR, all of which impart uncertainty regarding the safety, feasibility, and tolerability of TH. Despite these concerns, prohibition against a generally well-tolerated intervention that reduces the incidence of death and disability for infants who *already* have risk factors for poor outcomes raises the questions of whether the unknowns about the safety and efficacy of TH in this population justify continuing to withhold it.

Although some early studies did include some preterm infants, subgroup analyses stratified by gestational age were not reported.[12] A small pilot study (4 patients) of premature infants (as young as 32 weeks' gestation at birth) identified important safety, feasibility, and clinical trial design concerns for this population.[13] A 2021 study by Shipley and colleagues[14] reported that among 635 late preterm infants (34- and 35-weeks' gestation) diagnosed with any grade of HIE, 259 (~41%) were treated with TH, with an increase in use of TH over time (2011–2013 vs 2014–2016) but without a change in mortality in this population. Herrera and colleagues[12] reported outcomes of 30 infants born before 36 weeks that underwent TH, with treatment procedures aligned with the previously published NICHD NRN trial[2]; although all the infants in the cohort completed a full course of treatment, three-quarters experienced a complication. Results of the "Preemie Hypothermia for Neonatal Encephalopathy," a randomized controlled trial to assess safety and effectiveness of whole-body hypothermia for 72 hours in preterm infants 33 to 35 weeks' gestational age, have not yet been published.[15] The American Academy of Pediatrics Clinical Report "Hypothermia and Neonatal Encephalopathy," published in 2014 concludes that "[c]ooling infants who are born at less than 35 weeks' gestation... should only be performed in a research setting and with informed parental consent."[16]

No studies target small-for-gestational-age patients weighing less than 1800 g. Although technical problems may arise in trying to achieve and maintain target temperatures in extremely growth-restricted infants, no data support or prohibit attempts to provide TH for infants born at or after 35 and 0/7 weeks who weigh less than 1800 g for that reason alone.

More than one approach to ethical decision making for more premature and smaller infants exist. Those placing a high value on parental authority might argue that given the risks of mortality and morbidity that accompany HIE, and the low incidence of critical adverse events, TH for smaller and younger infants should be offered and initiated when parents provide informed consent. However, those who prioritize more restraint around insufficiently studied interventions might emphasize a nonmaleficence-based argument against use of unproven, potentially risky treatments, and point out the difference between providing informed consent with *known* risks versus consent with *unknown* risks. Research ethicists might emphasize protection over access, and the importance of maintaining clinical equipoise until appropriately designed studies are completed.

Therapeutic Hypothermia for Infants with Major Congenital Anomalies

Exclusion of infants with major congenital anomalies raises additional moral concerns. The term "major congenital anomalies" includes numerous conditions with a favorable prognosis for survival and neurodevelopment,[17] including Trisomy 21/Down syndrome. Intellectual and physical disabilities generally do not justify withholding of medical treatment, and doing so may represent discrimination and be unlawful.[18] Unless the identified anomaly specifically imparts a *medical contraindication* to TH, the infant is moribund, or TH does not align with the broader goals of care for the infant, as determined before birth, categorical exclusion of infants from TH solely based on the presence of one or more major congenital anomalies is not ethically justifiable. More practical reasons not to withhold TH for infants with congenital anomalies also exist, particularly if these were not identified before birth. Given the narrow window for initiation of therapy, thoughtful discussion with families about prognosis and goals of care might not be possible, and preservation of neurodevelopmental potential while continuing to collect information and engage families and specialists in medical decision making prospectively may be preferable. Infants with some underlying conditions might be at higher risk for intrapartum brain injury, which may be very difficult to distinguish from underlying neurologic dysfunction immediately after birth. Treatment of *potentially reversible* brain injury is appropriate, even if the possibility of *irreversible* structural brain abnormalities is identified.

DECISIONS TO PROVIDE THERAPEUTIC HYPOTHERMIA WITH CHANGES TO THE TREATMENT PROTOCOL THAT WAS STUDIED IN CLINICAL TRIALS

As use of TH for term and near-term infants with moderate or severe HIE moved from experimental to routine, both the challenges and the potential of this treatment emerged as hot topics of debate and exploration among neonatologists.

Initiation of Therapeutic Hypothermia after 6 hours of Age

The use of the 6-hour initiation deadline in the foundational trials and subsequent routine clinical practice is derived from early animal model research.[19] The regionalization of neonatal intensive care coupled with the technical requirements for providing TH brought to light the considerable constraints imparted by the 6-hour threshold for initiating TH after birth. Clinical manifestations of HIE might not be apparent (or appreciated) immediately after birth, and travel times and transport team constraints could result in failure to evaluate and initiate cooling for infants "in time," with the suboptimal result of infants not receiving state-of-the-art neuroprotective care. Although the development of cooling systems that can be used during transport, and gradual institution of clinical cooling procedures in more community hospital NICUs have reduced the likelihood of missed opportunities to initiate TH,[20] late presentation and recognition of HIE and continued logistic obstacles to timely initiation of treatment perpetuate the desire to understand whether late initiation of treatment is appropriate.

In a 2012 report from the Vermont Oxford Network Neonatal Encephalopathy registry, Pfister and colleagues[21] reported that more than one-third of infants were not admitted to a NICU until after 6 hours of age. Early attempts at in-transit TH via passive cooling raised concerns for excessive cooling,[22,23] causing some to question whether late initiation of treatment was a safer alternative to uncontrolled hypothermia in transit. In a study comparing infants with HIE who were initiated with TH before 6 hours of age, with those initiated between 6 and 12 hours of age, Jia and colleagues[24] reported comparable benefit of cooling for infants initiated late who had moderate HIE but no benefit of cooling when initiated after 6 hours in infants with severe HIE, using the surrogate outcomes of amplitude integrated electroencephalography findings and neuron-specific enolase levels. An NICHD randomized control trial in 168 infants with HIE presenting late (6–24 hours of age), of TH initiated at 6 to 24 hours of age versus routine supportive care, reported a modest and "nonconclusive" effect: "76% probability of any reduction in death or disability, and a 64% probability of at least 2% less death or disability at 18 to 22 months."[25] Importantly, this study extended the duration of hypothermia from 72 hours to 96 hours based on preclinical data, suggesting that a longer period of treatment was needed at later initiation times.

Delay in initiation of TH because of geographic isolation, lack of access to a hospital that can offer routine TH for infants with moderate or severe HIE, or lack of a regional center capable of cooling infants during transport raise important concerns about distributive justice, and the need to address access at an organizational or regional and policy level, particularly given the potential for racial, cultural, and socioeconomic inequities, which may impact families who reside in rural, remote, or underresourced areas. Although complex issues about equitable access to high-quality obstetric and newborn care have been explored and warrant attention, an extensive review of this is outside of the scope of this review.

Treatment for Less Than 72 Hours

Routine TH for infants with HIE is generally done for a period of 72 hours, with gradual rewarming to follow. For some infants, particularly those who did not develop respiratory failure and/or multisystem organ dysfunction and rapidly normalized from a neurologic perspective, continuing this treatment for 3 days can be difficult for providers and families. Infants being cooled cannot be held, cannot be fed by mouth, and may experience discomfort caused by low body temperature and lack of consoling measures, such as swaddling and rocking. One might rationally ask the question whether any infants can derive the potential benefits of TH while being treated for a shorter period. This justification for early termination of TH should be distinguished for cessation of treatment that no longer serves the goals of care, that is, when the infant is transitioned to comfort care, and adverse events that can be decisively attributed to the treatment (rather than the underlying condition) and cannot be remedied by other supportive interventions (collective experience with TH suggests that the latter occurs quite rarely).

All but one of the foundational trials of TH used a 72-hour cooling duration; in one trial, infants randomized to TH were cooled to 33°C for 48 hours.[26,27] The combined outcome of death or severe motor abnormalities at 12 months age was reduced with cooling, and there were no safety concerns. However, no clinical trial has directly compared 48 versus 72 hours' cooling duration. Despite this, evidence exists that some infants' treatment is electively discontinued before 72 hours of treatment.[28,29] This practice is not supported by in-human trials or preclinical data, leading HIE experts to conclude: "Given the low risk of side effects from therapeutic hypothermia, its cost-effectiveness, the preclinical evidence of worse, outcomes associated with stopping early and lack of evidence from controlled trials of shorter duration of hypothermia, we strongly recommend that at present, except for palliation, once hypothermia has been started, it should be continued for 72 hours in infants with HIE."[30] Whether a shorter period of treatment might be appropriate for infants with mild HIE is a question worthy of exploration, but treatment of mild HIE is not addressed in this review.

From an ethical point of view, it is worth considering the dilemma that might arise if parents of a well-appearing or clinically improving infant insist that rewarming be undertaken early. Ideally, this situation is avoided by methodical anticipatory guidance at the time of treatment initiation, including explanation of rewarming procedures. However, in a scenario in which parents are not able to be persuaded that early rewarming is not advisable, the decision about whether to respect the parents' authority as surrogate decision-makers and conclude treatment prematurely, or invoke legal mechanisms to treat over parental objection, must be individualized, balancing the potential risks and benefits of early discontinuation of TH. Abrupt rewarming without following appropriate procedures is not ethically justifiable by either the principle of best interest or the "harm principle" as originally described by Diekema.[31]

"Optimizing" Cooling: Treatment greater than 72 hours and/or Treatment with Lower Target Temperature

The possibility that a longer duration of cooling might offer incremental improvement in outcome over the "standard" 72-hour duration was evaluated in the NICHD NRN "Optimizing Cooling" trial, which was halted by its data safety monitoring board for safety and efficacy concerns at approximately 50% enrollment. Cooling for 120 hours did not reduce death or disability.[32] Results of preclinical studies in a fetal lamb HIE model were consistent with the lack of benefit of prolongation beyond 72 hours in the Optimizing Cooling trial.[33] Thus, cooling for HIE of longer duration than 72 hours is not supported by evidence and not clinically justifiable.

At least one uncontrolled case series suggested that cooling to a lower temperature might offer incremental benefit.[34] The possibility that cooling to a lower core temperature (32 C) versus a "standard" core temperature (33.5 C) was also evaluated in the NICHD NRN "Optimizing Cooling" randomized controlled trial[32]; cooling to the lower temperature offered no benefit versus standard temperature.

For both described practices, withholding these treatments, even if the individual clinician wishes to improve the outcome for a specific patient (or group of patients), and even if parents' wish to treat more aggressively to prevent an undesirable outcome, rests on the principle of nonmaleficence. Parental acknowledgment of known and potential risks is an insufficient process by which to justify exploration of these treatment possibilities outside of a controlled clinical trial.

DECISIONS TO OFFER THERAPEUTIC HYPOTHERMIA FOR HYPOXIC-ISCHEMIC BRAIN INJURY THAT DOES NOT OCCUR IN THE CONTEXT OF AN ACUTE PERINATAL EVENT

The use of TH to improve outcomes for other groups of patients, including older children and adults who arrest in out-of-hospital settings has been systematically evaluated.[35,36] Although the results of clinical studies of "targeted temperature management" (TTM) in children do not decisively support this treatment,[37] the 2019 International Consensus on Cardiopulmonary Resuscitation and Emergency Cardiovascular Care Science with Treatment Recommendations from the International Liaison Committee on Resuscitation advises that it is reasonable to consider TTM (32 C to 34 C or 36 C to 37.5 C) in infants as young as 24 hours of age who remain comatose after out-of-hospital or in-hospital cardiac arrest. This raises the question of whether neonates cared for in a NICU are candidates for TH following a nonperinatal sentinel event.[38] One case report describes this being done in the NICU setting.[39] Presently, clinical research on TTM in infants is done in the pediatric intensive care unit setting and has little applicability to NICUs. The foundational and subsequent studies relevant to newborn populations continue to focus on intrapartum brain injury and do not offer clinical support for treating infants who sustain their brain injury after birth. If TTM is considered for such infants, it is advisable to do so in consultation with a *pediatric* critical care team that can provide this care in a protocolized fashion in a pediatric intensive care unit.

SUMMARY

In this review, we have explored potential uses of TH for infants with HIE beyond those that were studied in the foundational clinical trials. Decisions about initiating TH in this context require careful examination of available evidence, and viewing the clinical decision through an ethical lens, considering the principles of parental authority, infant best interest, beneficence, nonmaleficence, and justice. Application of principles of research ethics, including clinical equipoise, informed consent, and trust in the scientific enterprise, imparts additional complexity. Regarding infants excluded from initial trials owing to gestational age, birth weight, underlying genetic conditions, chronologic age, and cause of brain injury, we find that presently empirical evidence and ethical analysis support treating infants as young as 35 completed weeks' gestational age, infants less than 1800 g provided that small size does not impart specifically identified technical obstacles, and infants with congenital anomalies. We conclude that initiation of treatment of infants younger than 35 weeks, after 6 hours of age, treatment for less than or more than 72 hours, and to a lower target temperature is not advisable, nor is treatment of infants who did not sustain brain injury during an intrapartum event. It is our hope that current and future clinical research will provide more insight into these scenarios and offer guidance to clinicians in improved and enhanced outcomes for neonates with brain injury, and that current practice will support these scientific endeavors by way of rigorously developed and implemented clinical trials.

Best Practices

- Mild hypothermia to a core temperature of 33.5 degrees Celsius for 72 hours following a clearly defined hospital protocol should be initiated within six hours of birth for infants born at or above 36 weeks' gestational age who weigh at least 1800 grams unless contraindications are identified, and should be considered for infants born at or after 35 weeks' gestation and for infants who weigh less than 1800 grams; further deviation from empirically evaluated treatment protocols should only be done in the context of a clinical trial.

- Categorical exclusion of infants from TH solely based on the presence of one or more major congenital anomalies is not ethically justifiable.

- The Newborn Intensive Care Unit is generally not an appropriate setting for therapeutic hypothermia for indications other than perinatal hypoxic-ischemic encephalopathy, which should only be undertaken in a clinical setting with expertise, experience, and clinical protocols to support this practice.

REFERENCES

1. Edwards AD, Brocklehurst P, Gunn AJ, et al. Neurological outcomes at 18 months of age after moderate hypothermia for perinatal hypoxic ischaemic encephalopathy: synthesis and meta-analysis of trial data. BMJ 2010;340:c363.
2. Shankaran S, Laptook AR, Ehrenkranz RA, et al. Whole-body hypothermia for neonates with hypoxic-ischemic encephalopathy. N Engl J Med 2005;353(15):1574–84.
3. Parga-Belinkie J, Foglia EE, Flibotte J. Caveats of cooling: available evidence and ongoing investigations of therapeutic hypothermia. NeoReviews 2019; 20(9):e513–9.
4. Burnsed J, Zanelli SA. Neonatal therapeutic hypothermia outside of standard guidelines: a survey of U.S. neonatologists. Acta Paediatr 2017;106(11):1772–9.
5. Laventhal N, Tarini BA, Lantos J. Ethical issues in neonatal and pediatric clinical trials. Pediatr Clin North Am 2012;59(5):1205–20.
6. Laventhal NT, Barks JD, Kim SY. Off-protocol use of therapeutic hypothermia for infants with hypoxic-ischemic encephalopathy. Virtual Mentor 2012;14(10): 784–91.

7. Amiel-Tison C. Neurological evaluation of the maturity of newborn infants. Arch Dis Child 1968;43(227):89–93.

8. Nakasone R, Fujioka K, Kyono Y, et al. Neurodevelopmental outcomes at 18 months of corrected age for late preterm infants born at 34 and 35 gestational weeks. Int J Environ Res Public Health 2021;18(2):640.

9. Mitha A, Chen R, Altman M, et al. Neonatal morbidities in infants born late preterm at 35-36 weeks of gestation: a Swedish Nationwide Population-based Study. J Pediatr 2021;233:43–50.e45.

10. Jin JH, Yoon SW, Song J, et al. Long-term cognitive, executive, and behavioral outcomes of moderate and late preterm at school age. Clin Exp Pediatr 2020; 63(6):219–25.

11. Gunn AJ, Bennet L. Brain cooling for preterm infants. Clin perinatology 2008; 35(4):735–48, vi-vii.

12. Herrera TI, Edwards L, Malcolm WF, et al. Outcomes of preterm infants treated with hypothermia for hypoxic-ischemic encephalopathy. Early Hum Dev 2018; 125:1–7.

13. Walsh W. Report of a pilot study of cooling four preterm infants 32-35 weeks gestation with HIE. J Neonatal-Perinatal Med 2015. https://doi.org/10.3233/NPM-15814078.

14. Shipley L, Gale C, Sharkey D. Trends in the incidence and management of hypoxic-ischaemic encephalopathy in the therapeutic hypothermia era: a national population study. Arch Dis Child Fetal Neonatal Ed 2021;106(5):529–34.

15. ClinicalTrials.gov Preemie hypothermia for neonatal encephalopathy NCT01793129. 2021. 2021. Available at: https://clinicaltrials.gov/ct2/show/results/NCT01793129?term=preterm&cond=Hypoxic-Ischemic+Encephalopathy&draw=2&rank=7. Accessed July 15, 2021.

16. Papile LA, Baley JE, Benitz W, et al. Hypothermia and neonatal encephalopathy. Pediatrics 2014;133(6):1146–50.

17. Birth Defects Surveillance Toolkit 1.4 congenital anomalies—definitions. 2020. 2021. Available at: https://www.cdc.gov/ncbddd/birthdefects/surveillancemanual/chapters/chapter-1/chapter1-4.html. Accessed July 15, 2021.

18. Discrimination on the basis of disability. 2021. 2021. Available at: https://www.hhs.gov/civil-rights/for-individuals/disability/index.html. Accessed July 16, 2021.

19. Gunn AJ, Gunn TR. The 'pharmacology' of neuronal rescue with cerebral hypothermia. Early Hum Dev 1998;53(1):19–35.

20. Akula VP, Joe P, Thusu K, et al. A randomized clinical trial of therapeutic hypothermia mode during transport for neonatal encephalopathy. J Pediatr 2015;166(4):856–61.e1-2.

21. Pfister RH, Bingham P, Edwards EM, et al. The Vermont Oxford Neonatal Encephalopathy Registry: rationale, methods, and initial results. BMC Pediatr 2012; 12:84.

22. Fairchild K, Sokora D, Scott J, et al. Therapeutic hypothermia on neonatal transport: 4-year experience in a single NICU. J Perinatol 2010;30(5):324–9.

23. Hallberg B, Olson L, Bartocci M, et al. Passive induction of hypothermia during transport of asphyxiated infants: a risk of excessive cooling. Acta Paediatr 2009;98(6):942–6.

24. Jia W, Lei X, Dong W, et al. Benefits of starting hypothermia treatment within 6 h vs. 6-12 h in newborns with moderate neonatal hypoxic-ischemic encephalopathy. BMC Pediatr 2018;18(1):50.

25. Laptook AR, Shankaran S, Tyson JE, et al. Effect of therapeutic hypothermia initiated after 6 hours of age on death or disability among newborns with hypoxic-

ischemic encephalopathy: a randomized clinical trial. JAMA 2017;318(16): 1550–60.

26. Eicher DJ, Wagner CL, Katikaneni LP, et al. Moderate hypothermia in neonatal encephalopathy: safety outcomes. Pediatr Neurol 2005;32(1):18–24.

27. Eicher DJ, Wagner CL, Katikaneni LP, et al. Moderate hypothermia in neonatal encephalopathy: efficacy outcomes. Pediatr Neurol 2005;32(1):11–7.

28. Mehta S, Joshi A, Bajuk B, et al. Eligibility criteria for therapeutic hypothermia: from trials to clinical practice. J Paediatr Child Health 2017;53(3):295–300.

29. Oliveira V, Singhvi DP, Montaldo P, et al. Therapeutic hypothermia in mild neonatal encephalopathy: a national survey of practice in the UK. Arch Dis Child Fetal Neonatal Ed 2018;103(4):F388–90.

30. Davidson JO, Battin M, Gunn AJ. Evidence that therapeutic hypothermia should be continued for 72 hours. Arch Dis Child Fetal Neonatal Ed 2019;104(2):F225.

31. Diekema DS. Parental refusals of medical treatment: the harm principle as threshold for state intervention. Theor Med Bioeth 2004;25(4):243–64.

32. Shankaran S, Laptook AR, Pappas A, et al. Effect of depth and duration of cooling on death or disability at age 18 months among neonates with hypoxic-ischemic encephalopathy: a randomized clinical trial. JAMA 2017;318(1):57–67.

33. Davidson JO, Yuill CA, Zhang FG, et al. Extending the duration of hypothermia does not further improve white matter protection after ischemia in term-equivalent fetal sheep. Sci Rep 2016;6:25178.

34. Compagnoni G, Bottura C, Cavallaro G, et al. Safety of deep hypothermia in treating neonatal asphyxia. Neonatology 2008;93(4):230–5.

35. Rasmussen TP, Bullis TC, Girotra S. Targeted temperature management for treatment of cardiac arrest. Curr Treat Options Cardiovasc Med 2020;22(11):39.

36. Moler FW, Silverstein FS, Holubkov R, et al. Therapeutic hypothermia after out-of-hospital cardiac arrest in children. N Engl J Med 2015;372(20):1898–908.

37. Mick NW, Williams RJ. Pediatric cardiac arrest resuscitation. Emerg Med Clin North Am 2020;38(4):819–39.

38. Duff JP, Topjian AA, Berg MD, et al. 2019 American Heart Association focused update on pediatric advanced life support: an update to the American Heart Association guidelines for cardiopulmonary resuscitation and emergency cardiovascular care. Pediatrics 2020;145(1):e904–14.

39. Roychoudhury S, Mohammad K, Yusuf K, et al. Successful Outcome of Therapeutic Hypothermia in A Case of Sudden Postnatal Cardiac Arrest and Asphyxia: A Case Report and Literature Review. J Pediatr Care 2017;3(2). https://doi.org/10.21767/2471-805X.100030. Available at: https://pediatrics.imedpub.com/successful-outcome-of-therapeutic-hypothermia-in-a-case-of-sudden-postnatal-cardiac-arrest-and-asphyxia-a-case-report-and-literatu.php?aid=19170.

Percutaneous Closure of Patent Ductus Arteriosus

Megan Barcroft, DO[a], Christopher McKee, DO[a,b,c], Darren P. Berman, MD[a,c], Rachel A. Taylor, MD[a,c], Brian K. Rivera, MS[d], Charles V. Smith, PhD[e], Jonathan L. Slaughter, MD, MPH[a,d,f], Afif El-Khuffash, MD[g,h], Carl H. Backes, MD[a,c,d],*

KEYWORDS

- Patent ductus arteriosus • Very low birth weight infant • Preterm infant
- Percutaneous closure • Catheter-based closure

KEY POINTS

- Percutaneous-based patent ductus arteriosus (PDA) closure is technically feasible among infants ≤1.5 kg, but inconsistent reporting of adverse events, including anesthesia-related complications, obscures contemporary assessments of safety profiles.
- Limitations of existing data underscore the critical need for clinical studies with well-delineated inclusion and exclusion criteria that target populations of infants with hemodynamically significant PDA.
- Primary end point for RCTs comparing percutaneous closure versus alternative treatment strategies should include longer-term outcomes of importance to health care providers and patient families.

INTRODUCTION

The ductus arteriosus is a vital component of fetal circulation, providing a conduit for blood to bypass the high-resistance pulmonary vascular bed.[1,2] Among term infants, the ductus typically closes within 72 hours of birth. In contrast, the ductus remains open (patent) in approximately 70% of extremely preterm infants (<28 weeks of gestation) at 1-month postnatal.[1,2] Patent ductus arteriosus (PDA) is the most

Funding Source: The authors (C.H. Backes and J.L. Slaughter) are funded by the National Heart, Lung, and Blood Institute of the National Institutes of Health (R01HL145032).
^a Department of Pediatrics, The Ohio State University Wexner Medical Center, Columbus, OH, USA; ^b Department of Anesthesiology, Nationwide Children's Hospital, Columbus, OH, USA; ^c The Heart Center, Nationwide Children's Hospital, Columbus, OH, USA; ^d Center for Perinatal Research, The Abigail Wexner Research Institute at Nationwide Children's Hospital, Columbus, OH, USA; ^e Center for Integrated Brain Research, Seattle Children's Research Institute, Seattle, WA, USA; ^f Division of Epidemiology, College of Public Health, The Ohio State University, Columbus, OH, USA; ^g Department of Neonatology, The Rotunda Hospital, Dublin, Ireland; ^h Department of Paediatrics, The Royal College of Surgeons in Ireland, Dublin, Ireland
* Corresponding author. Center for Perinatal Research, Nationwide Children's Hospital, 700 Children's Drive, Columbus, OH 43205.
E-mail address: Carl.Backes@nationwidechildrens.org

common cardiovascular condition among preterm infants, and is associated with adverse short- and longer-term outcomes, including mortality.[3–5]

Uncertainty on the optimal approach to treat PDA has led to marked variation across US children's hospitals.[6] Pharmacologic therapy is often used in the first month postnatal to induce ductal closure.[7,8] Despite pharmacologic treatment, PDA fails to close in 30% to 50% of extremely preterm infants.[9,10] In this subgroup of infants, procedural closure is the only remaining option for definitive closure. Surgical ductal ligation via thoracotomy was the traditional method of procedural closure following failed pharmacologic management.[11,12] Over the last decade, associations between surgical PDA ligation and vocal cord paralysis, chylothorax, postligation syndrome, and neurodevelopmental delays have been reported.[11–14] These observations have led to growing interest among health care providers in alternative therapies for definitive ductal closure among extremely preterm infants following failed pharmacologic therapy.[15–17]

Percutaneous PDA closure is the procedure of choice for definitive ductal closure in adults, children, and infants greater than 6 kg.[18,19] Over the past decade, evidence on the safety and feasibility of percutaneous ductal closure among smaller and more premature infants has been emerging.[15,17] In 2019, the Food and Drug Administration approved a novel percutaneous PDA closure device among infants greater than 3 postnatal days and greater than 700 g.[20] Despite Food and Drug Administration approval, the strength of the available evidence in among smaller, more premature infants ($\leq$1.5 kg) remains uncertain.[21] Focused on this subgroup of infants, the goals of the present review are to: (1) assess the technical success (feasibility) and short-term safety profile of the intervention, with particular attention to the risks of post–device closure syndrome (PDCS); (2) provide a general overview of the procedure, including recent modifications to optimize risk/benefit profiles; (3) characterize strategies to minimize anesthesia-related complications; and (4) address fundamental gaps in knowledge and summarize the necessary components in the design of a clinical trial of percutaneous closure.

PROCEDURAL FEASIBILITY, RISKS, AND POST–DEVICE CLOSURE SYNDROME

Feasibility (technical success) of percutaneous PDA closure is defined as successful placement of the device in the PDA.[22] In contrast, technical failure is commonly defined as cases where the device is placed, but requires surgical or catheter-based removal.[19,22] In a recent meta-analysis that included 28 studies of 373 infants less than or equal to 1.5 kgs, technical success with percutaneous PDA closure was 96% (95% confidence interval, 93%–98%).[21] Among the cases (10/373; 3%) with technical failure, reasons included: cardiac perforation or tamponade (n = 4), device protrusion into the left pulmonary artery or descending aorta (n = 4), dissection of the inferior vena cava following sheath advancement (n = 1), and device embolization requiring surgical ligation (n = 1). Importantly, even following adjustment for weight, type of device, or year of publication, the likelihood of technical failure was inversely related to postnatal age in days at the time of procedure (odds ratio, 0.9; 95% confidence interval, 0.83–0.97; P = .009).[21]

Evidence that the risk of an adverse event (AE) following percutaneous ductal closure is inversely related to postnatal age is mixed.[19,21] Compared with 773 infants with procedural weights of 1.5 to 6 kg, 373 infants with weights less than or equal to 1.5 kg undergoing percutaneous closure had similar risk of major AEs (8.4% vs 6.9%; P = .40) and lower risk of minor AEs (13.4% vs 9.1%; P = .034).[21] However, marked heterogeneity across studies in definitions for AEs, timing (intraprocedural, post-procedural) of AE reporting, and adjudication of procedural-related complications limits the interpretation of available data on the risks of AEs following percutaneous PDA closure. To secure more accurate estimates of the risks of complications following percutaneous closure, health care providers need to achieve consensus on the optimal strategies to independently adjudicate procedure-related AEs in the context of procedural (eg, type of device), center (eg, hospital procedural volume), and patient (postnatal age) specific factors that may influence the likelihood of AE rates.

Despite the lack of consensus nomenclature, most investigators use the term "post-ligation cardiac syndrome" to describe decreased cardiorespiratory performance following surgical ligation of the ductus.[12,17,23–27] Evidence suggests that, compared with presurgery status, 40% to 50% of infants undergoing surgical ligation require increased respiratory or inotropic support to address decreases in cardiac performance (shortening fraction, ejection fraction) and maintain cardiorespiratory stability.[23,25,26,28–30] Abrupt decreases in preload and increases in systemic vascular resistance are likely contributing mechanisms to the observed findings.[26,31,32]

Given the risks of surgical ligation, we performed a comprehensive review of existing literature on cardiorespiratory consequences following percutaneous PDA closure among infants less than or equal to 1.5 kg, termed PDCS. For consistency, we applied a standardized definition across studies.[33] The results of our comprehensive search of existing literature are shown in **Table 1**.[15–17,27,34–47] Contemporary evidence suggests that the risk of cardiorespiratory compromise is less following percutaneous device closure than following surgical ligation.[21,23,26,30,43] However, marked inconsistency in the timing (postnatal age) of postnatal closure, illness severity at procedure, and definitions used may contribute to observed differences in rates of cardiorespiratory complications following percutaneous closure versus surgical ligation.

PROCEDURAL STEPS AND RECENT MODIFICATIONS

Over the past decade, the pediatric interventional cardiology community has collaborated with industry partners and neonatal colleagues to increase feasibility and decrease AEs for lower-weight infants undergoing percutaneous PDA closure.[15,18,48] Herein, we provide a general overview of the procedure, with an emphasis on recent procedural modifications to optimize risk/benefit profiles (**Fig. 1**).

Preprocedural Assessment

Adoption of a standardized approach to identifying candidates for percutaneous closure is essential. Transthoracic echocardiography (TTE) remains the gold standard for evaluating the PDA (**Fig. 2**). To that end, TTE is used to determine candidacy for device closure and also during the procedure (**Table 2**). In general, the PDA in extremely low-birthweight infants is long and tubular; however, marked variability in ductal length is acknowledged.[16,17] Increased ductal length facilitates procedural success to position a device (eg, Piccolo Occluder, Abbott Medical, Plymouth, MN) without device protrusion into the descending aorta or left pulmonary artery.

Procedural and Post-procedural Considerations

Once positioned appropriately on the catheterization table, a short fluoroscopic image of the chest confirms endotracheal tube position, lung symmetry, and adequacy of ventilation. The femoral vein is accessed using the modified Seldinger technique, often with ultrasound guidance. Given the risks of arterial injury (eg, thrombosis), femoral arterial access is avoided.[18] Following femoral venous access, a 4F catheter is advanced into the right ventricle via the femoral venous sheath under fluoroscopic guidance. A floppy-tipped wire is advanced through this catheter and across the

Table 1
Post–device closure syndrome[a] among infants ≤1.5 kg

Last Name, Publication Year	Procedural Weight[b]	# Infants	Devices	Evidence of PDCS,[a] Standardized Definition	Evidence (Any) of Cardiorespiratory Compromise
Francis et al,[37] 2010	1.1 ± 0.1	7	Coil	None reported	None
Baspinar et al,[35] 2015[c]	1.4 ± 0.2	7	ADO II-AS	None reported	None
Zahn et al,[17] 2016[d]	1.25 (0.76–2.24)	17	AVP 2	None reported	None
Sathanandam et al,[44] 2017	1.1 ± 0.2	11	MVP	None reported	None
Morville and Akhavi,[38] 2017[e]	1.06 (0.75–1.50)	21	ADO II-AS	None reported	5 infants (23.8%) required dopamine post-closure
Pamukcu et al,[41] 2018[f]	0.97 (0.75–1.45)	13	ADO II-AS	None reported	None
Rodriguez Ogando et al,[43] 2018[g,h]	1.20 (1.00–1.45)	20	ADO II-AS	None reported	Surgical group required greater use of inotropic therapy post-procedure that percutaneous group
Auriau,[34] 2019	1.19 (1.00–1.40)	6	ADO II-AS	None reported	None
Berry et al,[36] 2019	1.5 (1.20–3.30)	9	MVP	None reported	None
Serrano et al,[27] 2020	1.2 ± 0.2	10	MVP	None reported	No cases in the catheterization group required initiation of hemodynamic support; surgical group had higher peak F_{IO2} and a greater absolute increase in peak F_{IO2} post-procedurally
Chien et al,[45] 2020	1.16 (0.59–2.30)	14	ADO II-AS, AVP	None reported	None
Malekzadeh-Milani et al,[47] 2020	0.9 ± 0.1	80	Piccolo, MVP	None reported	None
Sathanandam et al,[15] 2020	1.25 ± 0.60	100	ADO II-AS	None reported	None

Abbreviations: ADO-II AS, Amplatzer Duct Occluder 2 – Additional Sizes; AVP, Amplatzer Vascular Plug; F_{IO2}, fraction of inspired oxygen; MVP, microvascular plug.

[a] PDCS defined as a composite requirement of inotrope and/or pressor support and oxygenation and/or ventilation failure within 24 hours of procedure.[33]

[b] Mean ± standard deviation and/or median (range).

[c] Includes two cases reported in Sungur and coworkers.[46]

[d] Includes four cases reported in Zahn and coworkers.[16]

[e] Includes 16 cases reported in Morville and coworkers.[39]

[f] Includes 10 cases reported in Narin and coworkers.[40]

[g] Cases also reported in Rodriguez Ogando and coworkers.[42]

[h] Includes infants from the ≤1 kg and 1–2 kg subgroups (procedural weight of 1–2 kg subgroup reported as 1.33 ± 0.23 kg).

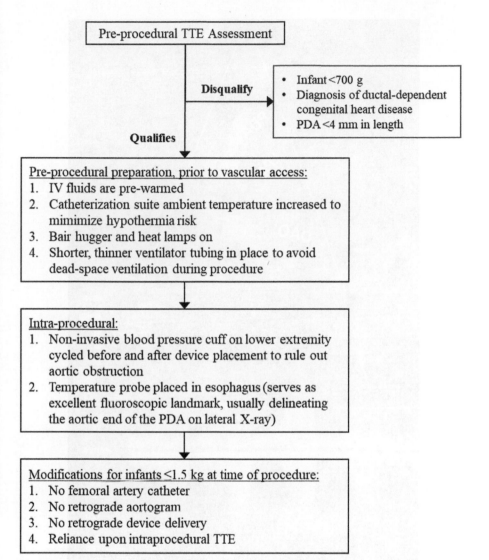

Fig. 1. Preprocedural intraprocedural flowchart. IV, intravenous; TTE, transthoracic echocardiography.

pulmonary valve through the PDA and down the descending aorta. Over this wire, the existing catheter in the right ventricle is removed and the 4F delivery catheter is advanced over the wire through the right heart and across the PDA into the thoracic descending aorta. To minimize the risk of injury to the tricuspid valve, a known complication of this procedure, every effort should be made to avoid "mismatch" between the delivery catheter and the wire as it advances across the tricuspid valve and through the heart. To minimize the risk of this mismatch of the delivery catheter over the coronary wire, a microcatheter is advanced ahead of the delivery catheter to smooth the transition through the tricuspid valve (**Fig. 3**).[15] Once in the aorta via the PDA, diluted contrast is introduced through this catheter to image the aorta, PDA, and pulmonary arteries (**Fig. 4**).

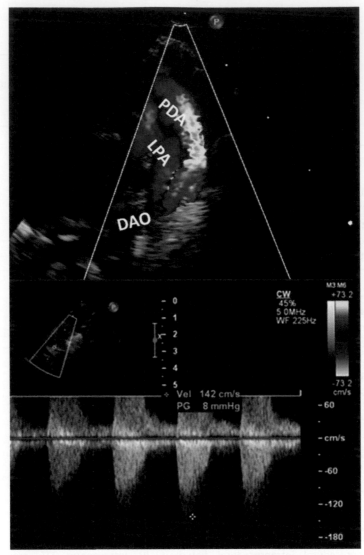

Fig. 2. Transthoracic echocardiography to assess the size of the PDA (*A*), and obtain baseline Doppler velocities of descending aorta (DAO) (*B*) and left pulmonary artery (LPA).

Based on the baseline procedural TTE and angiogram, an appropriately sized device is chosen. The device is advanced through the delivery catheter already in place within the aorta, and the device is deployed entirely intraductally under fluoroscopic and TTE guidance (**Fig. 5**). With the device deployed (but before release from the delivery cable), repeat detailed TTE images are obtained and compared with the baseline procedural images. If no obstruction is present and device position is appropriate, the device is released (**Fig. 6**). Following release of the device, TTE evaluation of all pertinent structures is repeated, assessing device position, residual shunt (if any), aortic and LPA flows by color and spectral Doppler, left ventricular (LV) function, and presence of new tricuspid valve regurgitation. A post-procedural radiograph and TTE are performed within 24 hours of the procedure to confirm device positioning (**Fig. 7**).

Table 2
Considerations in transthoracic echocardiography studies for percutaneous ductal closure

Preprocedure	Intraprocedural
1. Evaluation for presence of other congenital heart disease, especially ductal-dependent forms, including coarctation of the aorta.	1. Ductal length from origin at the aorta to insertion on the pulmonary artery.
2. Evaluation for severe ductal-dependent pulmonary hypertension as evidenced by the PDA shunt Doppler pattern.	2. Ductal diameter at origin, insertion, and at significant caliber changes along the length.
3. Assessment of left atrial and left ventricular size.	3. Baseline Doppler (color and spectral) interrogation of flow across the PDA.
4. Assessment of mitral valve and left ventricular function.	4. Baseline Doppler (color and spectral) interrogation of flow across the proximal descending aorta at the ductal origin.
5. Determination of aortic arch sidedness.	5. Baseline Doppler (color and spectral) interrogation of flow across the left pulmonary artery at insertion of the ductus.

ANESTHETIC CONSIDERATIONS IN PERCUTANEOUS PATENT DUCTUS ARTERIOSUS CLOSURE

In most settings, percutaneous PDA closure necessitates exposure to general anesthesia; thus, thoughtful consideration of optimal anesthesia and sedation practices are necessary. A growing body of evidence suggests that anesthetic and sedative medications alter neuronal architecture in preterm animal models.[49–51] In fact, most widely used anesthetic medications (**Table 3**) for percutaneous PDA closure cases have been shown to be associated with neurotoxicity.[52–54] However, the impact of anesthetic exposure on the neurocognitive development of infants and young children remains a subject of tremendous debate and controversy (**Table 4**).[54–56] Although data are mixed, some investigators have reported that lower-weight infants (<4 kg at the time of procedure) are at the greatest risk for such anesthesia- and sedation-related complications

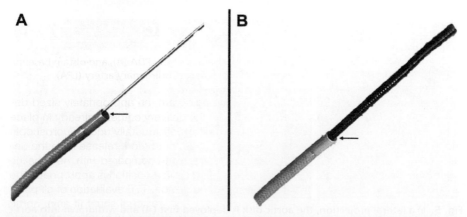

A **B**

Fig. 3. To minimize the mismatch of the delivery catheter over the coronary wire (*A*), a microcatheter is advanced ahead of the TorqVue delivery catheter to smooth the transition through the tricuspid valve (*B*).

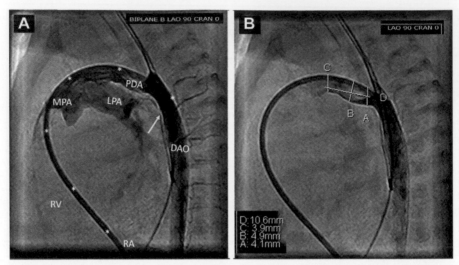

Fig. 4. (*A*) A wire (*asterisks*) courses through the delivery catheter from the inferior vena cava to the right atrium (RA), right ventricle (RV), and main pulmonary artery (MPA), across the PDA, and to the DAO. (*B*) The TorqVue delivery catheter is withdrawn to the aortic ampulla to facilitate angiography and obtain measurements of ductus. An esophageal temperature probe (*arrow*) typically serves as a surrogate marker for the aortic ampulla. This patient also has a feeding tube.

among pediatric populations.[57] A recent study reported 30-day mortality rates for neonates undergoing procedures requiring general anesthesia were 376.4 per 10,000 anesthetics, of which 10 (2.7%) cases were attributed to complications from general anesthesia.[53] However, in contrast to multiple exposures, investigators have not reported evidence of neurotoxicity in infants and younger pediatric patients following single exposures to anesthetic agents.[58–60]

Several anesthesia-related considerations in preterm infants undergoing percutaneous PDA closure warrant careful attention. First, among infants with large,

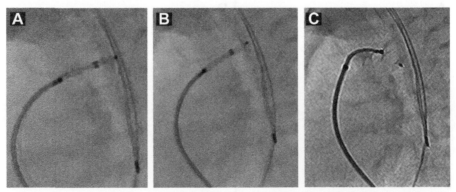

Fig. 5. In a lateral projection, the aortic disk is deployed first (*A*) and withdrawn into aortic ampulla (*B*) before delivery of central body and pulmonary artery disk (*C*). The device may reorient during delivery process with loss of tension on delivery cable. The device remains attached to delivery cable at this stage.

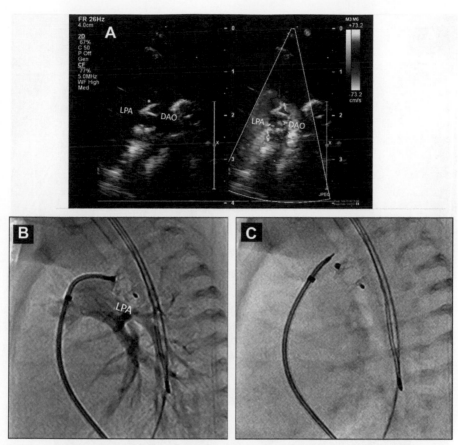

Fig. 6. Before release, echocardiography is performed of the LPA (*A*) and aortic arch, demonstrating no obstruction of flow to the DAO nor LPA. The device (*asterisk*) is positioned within the ductus, and there is trivial residual shunt (*arrow*) through device. Additional considerations may include MPA angiography through the delivery catheter (*B*). When satisfied with TTE, examination, and fluoroscopic/angiographic assessments, the device is released by unscrewing the delivery cable (*C*).

hemodynamically significant PDAs, percutaneous closure of the ductus leads to alterations in oxygen delivery, cardiac contractility, and vasomotor tone, with consequent clinical manifestations that may include coronary ischemia and cerebral and renal hypoperfusion.[33] Thus, consistent with the American Society of Anesthesia, surveillance for infants undergoing percutaneous PDA closure must include electrocardiogram, blood pressure, pulse oximetry, temperature, and inspired gas and end-tidal carbon dioxide monitoring.[61] Second, preterm infants may also benefit from a second pulse oximeter, which allows preductal and postductal monitoring, and cerebral near-infrared spectroscopy to assess oxygen delivery.[62] Third, current understanding of the safety profile of anesthesia exposure among extremely preterm infants is obscured by small procedural volumes at single centers, failure to adjudicate anesthesia-related complications in a consistent and transparent manner, and lack of adjustment for potential confounding factors (procedure and patient complexity). To better understand optimal anesthesia and sedation practices among infants undergoing percutaneous

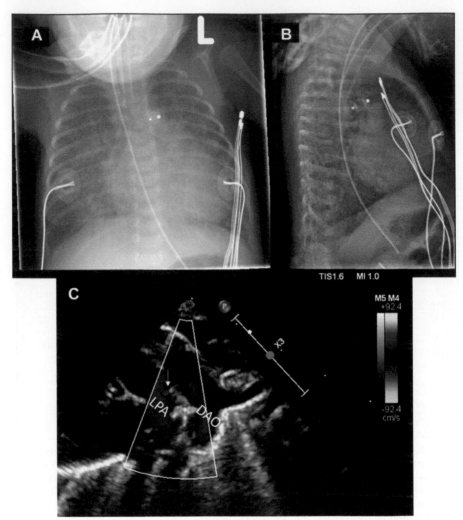

Fig. 7. Anteroposterior (*A*) and cross-table lateral (*B*) chest radiographs are obtained the day following the procedure, demonstrating stable lung findings and the device in stable position. Post-procedural echocardiography (*C*) demonstrates trivial residual shunt (*arrow*), which was no longer visualized on subsequent echocardiograms in this patient.

closure, an emphasis on better reporting practice, including detailed information on the type and nature of anesthesia exposure, is warranted.

CONSIDERATIONS IN THE DESIGN OF A CLINICAL TRIAL OF PERCUTANEOUS CLOSURE
Patient Selection in Clinical Trials

One of the major limitations of PDA trials, to date, is the lack of coherent approaches to patient selection for inclusion. This stems from the failure to accurately characterize hemodynamic significance of the ductus, including the presence of pulmonary over-circulation; systemic hypoperfusion; and physiologic precursors to the development

Table 3
Anesthetic agents associated with neuronal alterations in preclinical studies

Benzodiazepines	Barbiturates	Halogenated Vapor	GABA Agonists	NMDA Antagonists
Midazolam	Thiopental	Isoflurane	Propofol	Ketamine
Lorazepam	Pentobarbital	Sevoflurane	Etomidate	Nitrous oxide

Abbreviations: GABA, γ-aminobutyric acid; NMDA, *N*-methyl-D-aspartate.

of clinically relevant outcomes, such as bronchopulmonary dysplasia and necrotizing enterocolitis. Unfortunately, previous studies have used arbitrary and inconsistent selection criteria of echocardiography and clinical parameters for entry into PDA treatment trials that are not related to important outcomes.[63] For the studies most needed presently, the inclusion process should be geared to selecting infants with

Table 4
Anesthesia exposure and neurodevelopment consequences

First Author, Year Published	Study Design	Primary Finding
Bartels et al,[70] 2009	Retrospective	Among discordant twin pairs, where one received anesthesia and one did not, academic outcomes were similar
Wilder et al,[71] 2009	Retrospective	Patients with >1 exposure to anesthesia before age 4 had nearly twice the risk of a school referral for learning disability than infants without any exposure to anesthesia
Ing et al,[72] 2012	Retrospective	Exposure to 1 anesthetic before age of 3 y had an increased risk of language and cognitive deficits at age 10 y
Graham et al,[73] 2016	Retrospective	Modest increase in risk for developmental disability after a single anesthetic exposure between ages 2 and 4 y
Sun et al,[60] 2016	Retrospective and prospective phases	No meaningful differences in IQ between siblings in which one was exposed to a single anesthetic
Glatz et al,[74] 2017	Retrospective	Modest decrease in IQ with anesthetic exposures before the age of 4 y in military recruits
Hu et al,[75] 2017	Retrospective	Patients with >1 exposure to anesthesia before the age of 3 y were found to be at increased risk for school difficulties
Warner et al,[76] 2018	Retrospective and prospective phases	No significant differences in IQ between children <3 y of age exposed to anesthesia and those not exposed to anesthesia
O'Leary et al,[77] 2019	Retrospective	No increased risk of developmental difficulties in anesthesia-exposed siblings when compared with nonexposed siblings
Zaccariello et al,[78] 2019	Retrospective and prospective phases	Children with multiple exposures to anesthesia were at risk for processing speed and fine motor abilities
Davidson & Vutskits,[79] 2020	Prospective	No differences in IQ between infants exposed to general anesthesia vs regional anesthesia at <60 wk postmenstrual age

large PDAs that are associated with high rates of the outcomes of interest (eg, chronic lung disease or death before discharge) and unlikely to close spontaneously. This focus facilitates the selection of infants most likely to benefit from treatment and shunt elimination.

Defining Hemodynamic Significance

Hemodynamic significance remains a difficult entity to characterize and quantify. It is likely a complex interaction between echocardiography markers (measured at the optimal time) and clinical characteristics that serve as effect modifiers. A comprehensive appraisal of hemodynamic significance of the ductus is likely to be most helpful if it incorporates the following components: (1) an assessment of shunt volume and the degree of associated pulmonary overcirculation and systemic hypoperfusion, (2) measurement of LV diastolic function to quantify the ability of the heart to handle the increased pulmonary return, and (3) consideration of clinical features that are likely to contribute to the detrimental effect of shunting across the PDA.[64]

Accurate estimation of shunt volume using echocardiography remains a challenge, because of the dynamic nature of the ductal diameter, the tortuosity of the vessel, the varying viscosity of the blood, and the changing pressure gradients between the systemic and pulmonary circulations. Therefore, effort should be directed to the measurements of surrogate markers of increased pulmonary blood flow and decreasing systemic blood flow. Those markers have been described in detail elsewhere.[65] In addition, the degree of LV diastolic dysfunction should be quantified and incorporated in the hemodynamic assessments of PDAs.

Premature birth is associated with significant diastolic dysfunction secondary to poor LV compliance. Recent evidence suggests that this may contribute to pulmonary venous congestion and respiratory morbidity in the setting of increased pulmonary venous return.[66] The increase in left atrial pressure leads to pulmonary venous hypertension and this may increase right ventricular afterload resulting in a fall in contractility.[67] Finally, the consideration of important clinical factors, such as gestational age, growth restriction, lack of antenatal steroid administration, and other important AEs that are likely to contribute to the evolution of the morbidities of interest in the setting of PDA shunting, should be incorporated into the assessment.

Timing of Patent Ductus Arteriosus Evaluation

The timing of PDA assessment also warrants careful consideration. A balance needs to be struck between an assessment carried out too early following birth, where a high pulmonary vascular resistance prevents significant shunting from taking place, or carried out too late, when the effects of the pathophysiologic shunting may be too late to arrest or mitigate.[68]

Patent Ductus Arteriosus Scoring System

Incorporation of all of the markers mentioned into a scoring system that can identify infants with PDAs that are unlikely to close spontaneously and are associated with high rates of chronic lung disease and/or death before discharge has been attempted. The PDA severity score recently developed by El-Khuffash and colleagues,[68] to incorporate markers of pulmonary overcirculation, LV diastolic function, and clinical characteristics, can predict chronic lung disease or death before discharge. In their observational study, the group demonstrated that the PDA severity score was able to distinguish between infants less than 29 weeks gestation that developed a persistent PDA with associated morbidities and those with a PDA that underwent spontaneous closure and had a low incidence of morbidities. The score was recently tested in a pilot randomized controlled trial that demonstrated the ability to identify infants with large PDAs that were not likely to close spontaneously. In their studies, most infants who were deemed low risk (and were not randomized but were followed to discharge) closed their PDAs spontaneously and had low rates of morbidity.[69]

SUMMARY

The data reviewed herein demonstrate that percutaneous-based PDA closure is technically feasible among infants less than or equal to 1.5 kg. However, marked heterogeneity in the type and nature of AEs and anesthesia exposures among infants undergoing percutaneous closure obscures current understanding of the safety profile of the procedure. Although data on the risks and benefits of PDCS remain promising, lack of comparative trials and consistent definitions across published studies obscure confidence in estimates provided to date. These observations underscore the critical need for clinical studies with well-delineated inclusion and exclusion criteria that target populations of infants with hemodynamic significance of the ductus. To minimize risk and yield the greatest benefits, clinical studies of PDA treatment should consider incorporating more robust assessments (eg, PDA scores), to ensure that infants at greatest risk for adverse ductal consequences are included. For percutaneous PDA closure among infants less than or equal to 1.5 kg to be considered standard of care, primary end points for future randomized controlled trials comparing percutaneous closure versus alternative treatment strategies should be longer-term outcomes of importance to health care providers and patient families, rather than ductal closure.

Best Practices

- Recent procedural modifications, including the avoidance of femoral arterial access, have improved the safety profile of percutaneous PDA closure among infants <1.5 kgs.

- In the absence of comparative trials, available evidence suggests that the risks of cardiorespiratory compromise following percutaneous device closure is less than those following surgical closure.

- Well-designed, large, randomized clinical studies with strict inclusion criteria (PDA scoring system), consistent adverse event reporting, and longer-term outcomes, are greatly needed.

DISCLOSURE

The authors have no financial relationships relative to this article to disclose. All authors have no conflicts of interest to disclose.

REFERENCES

1. Clyman RI, Couto J, Murphy GM. Patent ductus arteriosus: are current neonatal treatment options better or worse than no treatment at all? Semin Perinatol 2012; 36(2):123–9.
2. Koch J, Hensley G, Roy L, et al. Prevalence of spontaneous closure of the ductus arteriosus in neonates at a birth weight of 1000 grams or less. Pediatrics 2006; 117(4):1113–21.
3. Brown ER. Increased risk of bronchopulmonary dysplasia in infants with patent ductus arteriosus. J Pediatr 1979;95(5 Pt 2):865–6.
4. Mirza H, Garcia J, McKinley G, et al. Duration of significant patent ductus arteriosus and bronchopulmonary dysplasia in extremely preterm infants. J Perinatol 2019;39(12):1648–55.

5. Noori S, McCoy M, Friedlich P, et al. Failure of ductus arteriosus closure is associated with increased mortality in preterm infants. Pediatrics 2009;123(1): e138–44.

6. Bixler GM, Powers GC, Clark RH, et al. Changes in the diagnosis and management of patent ductus arteriosus from 2006 to 2015 in United States neonatal intensive care units. J Pediatr 2017;189:105–12.

7. Slaughter JL, Reagan PB, Bapat RV, et al. Nonsteroidal anti-inflammatory administration and patent ductus arteriosus ligation, a survey of practice preferences at US children's hospitals. Eur J Pediatr 2016;175(6):775–83.

8. Slaughter JL, Reagan PB, Newman TB, et al. Comparative effectiveness of nonsteroidal anti-inflammatory drug treatment vs no treatment for patent ductus arteriosus in preterm infants. JAMA Pediatr 2017;171(3):e164354.

9. Hagadorn JI, Brownell EA, Trzaski JM, et al. Trends and variation in management and outcomes of very low-birth-weight infants with patent ductus arteriosus. Pediatr Res 2016;80(6):785–92.

10. Ohlsson A, Shah PS. Paracetamol (acetaminophen) for patent ductus arteriosus in preterm or low birth weight infants. Cochrane Database Syst Rev 2020;1: CD010061.

11. Benitz WE. Patent ductus arteriosus: to treat or not to treat? Arch Dis Child Fetal Neonatal Ed 2012;97(2):F80–2.

12. Ulrich TJB, Hansen TP, Reid KJ, et al. Post-ligation cardiac syndrome is associated with increased morbidity in preterm infants. J Perinatol 2018;38(5):537–42.

13. Benjamin JR, Smith PB, Cotten CM, et al. Long-term morbidities associated with vocal cord paralysis after surgical closure of a patent ductus arteriosus in extremely low birth weight infants. J Perinatol 2010;30(6):408–13.

14. Hamrick SEG, Sallmon H, Rose AT, et al. Patent ductus arteriosus of the preterm infant. Pediatrics 2020;146(5).

15. Sathanandam SK, Gutfinger D, O'Brien L, et al. Amplatzer Piccolo Occluder clinical trial for percutaneous closure of the patent ductus arteriosus in patients >/ =700 grams. Catheter Cardiovasc Interv 2020;96(6):1266–76.

16. Zahn EM, Nevin P, Simmons C, et al. A novel technique for transcatheter patent ductus arteriosus closure in extremely preterm infants using commercially available technology. Catheter Cardiovasc Interv 2015;85(2):240–8.

17. Zahn EM, Peck D, Phillips A, et al. Transcatheter closure of patent ductus arteriosus in extremely premature newborns: early results and midterm follow-up. JACC Cardiovasc Interv 2016;9(23):2429–37.

18. Backes CH, Cheatham SL, Deyo GM, et al. Percutaneous patent ductus arteriosus (PDA) closure in very preterm infants: feasibility and complications. J Am Heart Assoc 2016;5(2).

19. Backes CH, Rivera BK, Bridge JA, et al. Percutaneous patent ductus arteriosus (PDA) closure during infancy: a meta-analysis. Pediatrics 2017;139(2): e20162927.

20. Backes CH, Giesinger RE, Rivera BK, et al. Percutaneous closure of the patent ductus arteriosus in very low weight infants: considerations following US Food and Drug Administration approval of a novel device. J Pediatr-us 2019;213: 218–21.

21. Bischoff AR, Jasani B, Sathanandam SK, et al. Percutaneous closure of patent ductus arteriosus in infants 1.5 kg or less: a meta-analysis. J Pediatr 2021;230: 84–92 e14.

22. El-Said HG, Bratincsak A, Foerster SR, et al. Safety of percutaneous patent ductus arteriosus closure: an unselected multicenter population experience. J Am Heart Assoc 2013;2(6):e000424.
23. Harting MT, Blakely ML, Cox CS Jr, et al. Acute hemodynamic decompensation following patent ductus arteriosus ligation in premature infants. J Invest Surg 2008;21(3):133–8.
24. Jain A, Sahni M, El-Khuffash A, et al. Use of targeted neonatal echocardiography to prevent postoperative cardiorespiratory instability after patent ductus arteriosus ligation. J Pediatr 2012;160(4):584–9.e1.
25. Teixeira LS, Shivananda SP, Stephens D, et al. Postoperative cardiorespiratory instability following ligation of the preterm ductus arteriosus is related to early need for intervention. J Perinatol 2008;28(12):803–10.
26. El-Khuffash AF, Jain A, Weisz D, et al. Assessment and treatment of post patent ductus arteriosus ligation syndrome. J Pediatr 2014;165(1):46–52 e41.
27. Serrano RM, Madison M, Lorant D, et al. Comparison of 'post-patent ductus arteriosus ligation syndrome' in premature infants after surgical ligation vs. percutaneous closure. J Perinatol 2020;40(2):324–9.
28. Moin F, Kennedy KA, Moya FR. Risk factors predicting vasopressor use after patent ductus arteriosus ligation. Am J Perinatol 2003;20(6):313–20.
29. Noori S, Friedlich P, Seri I, et al. Changes in myocardial function and hemodynamics after ligation of the ductus arteriosus in preterm infants. J Pediatr 2007; 150(6):597–602.
30. McNamara PJ, Stewart L, Shivananda SP, et al. Patent ductus arteriosus ligation is associated with impaired left ventricular systolic performance in premature infants weighing less than 1000 g. J Thorac Cardiovasc Surg 2010;140(1):150–7.
31. El-Khuffash AF, Jain A, Dragulescu A, et al. Acute changes in myocardial systolic function in preterm infants undergoing patent ductus arteriosus ligation: a tissue Doppler and myocardial deformation study. J Am Soc Echocardiogr 2012;25(10): 1058–67.
32. Kimball TR, Ralston MA, Khoury P, et al. Effect of ligation of patent ductus arteriosus on left ventricular performance and its determinants in premature neonates. J Am Coll Cardiol 1996;27(1):193–7.
33. Nealon E, Rivera BK, Cua CL, et al. Follow-up after percutaneous patent ductus arteriosus occlusion in lower weight infants. J Pediatr 2019;212:144–50.e3.
34. Fraisse A, Bautista-Rodriguez C, Burmester M, et al. Transcatheter Closure of Patent Ductus Arteriosus in Infants With Weight Under 1,500 Grams. Front Pediatr 2020;8:558256.
35. Baspinar O, Sahin DA, Sulu A, et al. Transcatheter closure of patent ductus arteriosus in under 6 kg and premature infants. J Interv Cardiol 2015;28(2):180–9.
36. Berry JM, Hiremath G, Heal E, et al. Echocardiographic imaging of the Medtronic Micro Vascular Plug during off label placement in the premature infant with patent ductus arteriosus. Echocardiography 2019;36(5):944–7.
37. Francis E, Singhi AK, Lakshmivenkateshaiah S, et al. Transcatheter occlusion of patent ductus arteriosus in pre-term infants. JACC Cardiovasc Interv 2010;3(5): 550–5.
38. Morville P, Akhavi A. Transcatheter closure of hemodynamic significant patent ductus arteriosus in 32 premature infants by Amplatzer Ductal Occluder additional size-ADOIIAS. Catheter Cardiovasc Interv 2017;90(4):612–7.
39. Morville P, Douchin S, Bouvaist H, et al. Transcatheter occlusion of the patent ductus arteriosus in premature infants weighing less than 1200 g. Arch Dis Child Fetal Neonatal Ed 2018;103(3):F198–201.

40. Narin N, Pamukcu O, Baykan A, et al. Percutaneous PDA closure in extremely low birth weight babies. J Interv Cardiol 2016;29(6):654–60.

41. Pamukcu O, Tuncay A, Narin N, et al. Patent ductus arteriosus closure in preterms less than 2kg: surgery versus transcatheter. Int J Cardiol 2018;250:110–5.

42. Rodriguez Ogando A, Ballasteros Tejerizo F, Blanco Bravo D, et al. Transcatheter occlusion of patent ductus arteriosus in preterm infants weighing less than 2 kg with the Amplatzer Duct Occluder II additional sizes device. Rev Esp Cardiol 2018;71(10):865–6.

43. Rodriguez Ogando A, Planelles Asensio I, de la Blanca ARS, et al. Surgical ligation versus percutaneous closure of patent ductus arteriosus in very low-weight preterm infants: which are the real benefits of the percutaneous approach? Pediatr Cardiol 2018;39(2):398–410.

44. Sathanandam S, Justino H, Waller BR 3rd, et al. Initial clinical experience with the Medtronic Micro Vascular Plug in transcatheter occlusion of PDAs in extremely premature infants. Catheter Cardiovasc Interv 2017;89(6):1051–8.

45. Chien YH, Wang HH, Lin MT, et al. Device deformation and left pulmonary artery obstruction after transcatheter patent ductus arteriosus closure in preterm infants. Int J Cardiol 2020;312:50–5.

46. Sungur M, Karakurt C, Ozbarlas N, et al. Closure of patent ductus arteriosus in children, small infants, and premature babies with Amplatzer Duct Occluder II additional sizes: multicenter study. Catheter Cardiovasc Interv 2013;82(2): 245–52.

47. Malekzadeh-Milani S, Akhavi A, Douchin S, et al. Percutaneous closure of patent ductus arteriosus in premature infants: a French national survey. Catheter Cardiovasc Interv 2020;95(1):71–7.

48. Apalodimas L, Waller BR Iii, Philip R, et al. A comprehensive program for preterm infants with patent ductus arteriosus. Congenit Heart Dis 2019;14(1):90–4.

49. Boscolo A, Starr JA, Sanchez V, et al. The abolishment of anesthesia-induced cognitive impairment by timely protection of mitochondria in the developing rat brain: the importance of free oxygen radicals and mitochondrial integrity. Neurobiol Dis 2012;45(3):1031–41.

50. Brambrink AM, Back SA, Riddle A, et al. Isoflurane-induced apoptosis of oligodendrocytes in the neonatal primate brain. Ann Neurol 2012;72(4):525–35.

51. Brambrink AM, Evers AS, Avidan MS, et al. Ketamine-induced neuroapoptosis in the fetal and neonatal rhesus macaque brain. Anesthesiology 2012;116(2): 372–84.

52. Cabrera OH, O'Connor SD, Swiney BS, et al. Caffeine combined with sedative/anesthetic drugs triggers widespread neuroapoptosis in a mouse model of prematurity. J Matern Fetal Neonatal Med 2017;30(22):2734–41.

53. Houck CS, Vinson AE. Anaesthetic considerations for surgery in newborns. Arch Dis Child Fetal Neonatal Ed 2017;102(4):F359–63.

54. Soriano SG, McCann ME. Is anesthesia bad for the brain? Current knowledge on the impact of anesthetics on the developing brain. Anesthesiol Clin 2020;38(3): 477–92.

55. Grabowski J, Goldin A, Arthur LG, et al. The effects of early anesthesia on neurodevelopment: a systematic review. J Pediatr Surg 2021;56(5):851–61.

56. Ing C, Jackson WM, Zaccariello MJ, et al. Prospectively assessed neurodevelopmental outcomes in studies of anaesthetic neurotoxicity in children: a systematic review and meta-analysis. Br J Anaesth 2021;126(2):433–44.

57. Lin CH, Desai S, Nicolas R, et al. Sedation and anesthesia in pediatric and congenital cardiac catheterization: a prospective multicenter experience. Pediatr Cardiol 2015;36(7):1363–75.
58. Davidson AJ, Disma N, de Graaff JC, et al. Neurodevelopmental outcome at 2 years of age after general anaesthesia and awake-regional anaesthesia in infancy (GAS): an international multicentre, randomised controlled trial. Lancet 2016;387(10015):239–50.
59. Davidson AJ, Sun LS. Clinical evidence for any effect of anesthesia on the developing brain. Anesthesiology 2018;128(4):840–53.
60. Sun LS, Li G, Miller TL, et al. Association between a single general anesthesia exposure before age 36 months and neurocognitive outcomes in later childhood. JAMA 2016;315(21):2312–20.
61. Odegard KC, Vincent R, Baijal R, et al. SCAI/CCAS/SPA expert consensus statement for anesthesia and sedation practice: recommendations for patients undergoing diagnostic and therapeutic procedures in the pediatric and congenital cardiac catheterization laboratory. Catheter Cardiovasc Interv 2016;88(6): 912–22.
62. Zulueta JL, Vida VL, Perisinotto E, et al. Role of intraoperative regional oxygen saturation using near infrared spectroscopy in the prediction of low output syndrome after pediatric heart surgery. J Cardiovasc Surg 2013;28(4):446–52.
63. Zonnenberg I, de WK. The definition of a haemodynamic significant duct in randomized controlled trials: a systematic literature review. Acta Paediatr 2012; 101(3):247–51.
64. Smith A, El-Khuffash AF. Defining "haemodynamic significance" of the patent ductus arteriosus: do we have all the answers? Neonatology 2020;117(2):225–32.
65. van Laere D, van Overmeire B, Gupta S, et al. Application of NPE in the assessment of a patent ductus arteriosus. Pediatr Res 2018;84(Suppl 1):46–56.
66. Bussmann N, Breatnach C, Levy PT, et al. Early diastolic dysfunction and respiratory morbidity in premature infants: an observational study. J Perinatol 2018; 38(9):1205–11.
67. Bussmann N, El-Khuffash A, Breatnach CR, et al. Left ventricular diastolic function influences right ventricular-pulmonary vascular coupling in premature infants. Early Hum Dev 2018;128:35–40.
68. El-Khuffash A, James AT, Corcoran JD, et al. A patent ductus arteriosus severity score predicts chronic lung disease or death before discharge. J Pediatr 2015; 167(6):1354–61.e2.
69. El-Khuffash A, Bussmann N, Breatnach CR, et al. A pilot randomized controlled trial of early targeted patent ductus arteriosus treatment using a risk based severity score (the PDA RCT). J Pediatr 2020;229:127–33.
70. Bartels M, Althoff RR, Boomsma DI. Anesthesia and cognitive performance in children: no evidence for a causal relationship. Twin Res Hum Genet 2009; 12(3):246–53.
71. Wilder RT, Flick RP, Sprung J, et al. Early exposure to anesthesia and learning disabilities in a population-based birth cohort. Anesthesiology 2009;110(4): 796–804.
72. Ing C, DiMaggio C, Whitehouse A, et al. Long-term differences in language and cognitive function after childhood exposure to anesthesia. Pediatrics 2012; 130(3):e476–85.
73. Graham MR, Brownell M, Chateau DG, et al. Neurodevelopmental assessment in kindergarten in children exposed to general anesthesia before the age of 4 Years: a retrospective matched cohort study. Anesthesiology 2016;125(4):667–77.

74. Glatz P, Sandin RH, Pedersen NL, et al. Association of anesthesia and surgery during childhood with long-term academic performance. JAMA Pediatr 2017; 171(1):e163470.

75. Hu D, Flick RP, Zaccariello MJ, et al. Association between exposure of young children to procedures requiring general anesthesia and learning and behavioral outcomes in a population-based birth cohort. Anesthesiology 2017;127(2): 227–40.

76. Warner DO, Zaccariello MJ, Katusic SK, et al. Neuropsychological and behavioral outcomes after exposure of young children to procedures requiring general anesthesia: the Mayo Anesthesia Safety in Kids (MASK) study. Anesthesiology 2018; 129(1):89–105.

77. O'Leary JD, Janus M, Duku E, et al. A population-based study evaluating the association between surgery in early life and child development at primary school entry. Anesthesiology 2016;125(2):272–9.

78. Zaccariello MJ, Frank RD, Lee M, et al. Patterns of neuropsychological changes after general anaesthesia in young children: secondary analysis of the Mayo Anesthesia Safety in Kids study. Br J Anaesth 2019;122(5):671–81.

79. Davidson AJ, Vutskits L. Anesthesia in childhood and neurodevelopmental outcome. Anesthesiology 2020;133(5):967–9.

Exome and Whole Genome Sequencing in the Neonatal Intensive Care Unit

Michael Muriello, MD

KEYWORDS

- Genomic sequencing • Exome sequencing • Whole genome sequencing

KEY POINTS

- Genomic sequencing (GS) should be used in the neonatal intensive care unit to diagnose patients with suspected genetic disorders.
- GS is cost-effective and has high diagnostic and clinical utility.
- The decision to pursue standard- or rapid-turnaround GS depends on the level of concern for a genetic condition, the level of acuity, and the availability of testing.
- GS is not recommended without the support of medical geneticists and genetic counselors.

INTRODUCTION

There has in the past been controversy about the role of genetic testing in the inpatient setting that has led to our current situation with usage of advanced sequencing in the intensive care unit (ICU) limited to a few academic medical centers. Several arguments have been made against inpatient genetic testing: genetic testing is too expensive, the turnaround time (TAT) of the tests are too slow to affect management, as it cannot be made available before discharge, and that genetic testing does not affect management in a timely manner or in enough instances. However, in the last 2 decades there has been a revolution in genetic testing with improvements in both technology and bioinformatic analysis that may have made these concerns obsolete. The cost of genetic testing has plummeted: today the cost of even large gene panels and genomic sequencing are insignificant in comparison to the potential benefit (see **Box 1** for definitions). The TAT of testing has similarly diminished: in the critical care setting results of rapid whole genome sequencing (WGS) can be provided in less than 48 hours (the world record is 19 hours). This chapter reviews the growing body of evidence that as of 2021 clearly supports the use of genomic testing in the critical care setting for appropriate patients.

Division of Genetics, Medical College of Wisconsin, 9000 W Wisconsin Avenue, MS 716, Milwaukee, WI 53226, USA
E-mail address: mmuriello@mcw.edu

Clin Perinatol 49 (2022) 167–179
https://doi.org/10.1016/j.clp.2021.11.018
0095-5108/22/© 2021 Elsevier Inc. All rights reserved.

Box 1	
Definitions	
Exome sequencing (ES)	Genetic testing of the sequence of all exons of all known genes
Whole genome sequencing (WGS)	Genetic testing of the sequence of all regions of the genome including exons, introns, and intergenic regions
Genomic sequencing	Either ES or WGS
Turnaround time (TAT)	Time from drawing the patient's blood to reporting of results
Trio sequencing	GS that tests both the patient and parents, allowing immediate determination of *de novo* and *trans* or *cis* status of variants
Copy number variants (CNVs)	Deletions and/or duplications of any size segment of DNA

Genetic disorders are an important and common cause of morbidity and mortality in the neonatal ICU (NICU), accounting for as many as 20% of all infant deaths[1]; this includes 23% to 28% of deaths[2–4] and 51% of death in those younger than 1 year in the United States.[5] These are likely underestimates, as many patients with suspected genetic disorders go undiagnosed, including those who undergo thorough genetic evaluation. Although the prevalence of genetic disorders detected by newborn screening is 1 in 500 births,[6] other evidence suggests the true prevalence is much higher. One study found 9% of all patients admitted to the NICU ended up with a genetic diagnosis.[7] In a study of European data there was a 2.7% prevalence of congenital malformations, ~15% of which were attributable to a genetic disorder[8]; this is undoubtedly an underestimate as 78% of congenital malformations were "nonsyndromic," a significant portion of which may have an identifiable genetic cause if they were to undergo genetic testing. The prevalence of genetic disorders in a cohort of 154 "healthy" newborns evaluated by exome sequencing identified genetic disorders conferring risk for childhood-onset disease in 9.4.[9] Outside of the neonatal period genetic disorders continue to be a significant source of morbidity in general accounting for 16% of all hospitalizations in one study.[10] This burden of illness has led some to advocate for the collection of blood and skin tissue for a "molecular autopsy" in all unexplained or undiagnosed neonatal and infant deaths.[3]

HISTORY/BACKGROUND
Types of Clinical Genetic Testing

The evolution of genetic testing began with the advent of chromosome visualization and banding (aka karyotype) in 1959, progressing to "Sanger sequencing" in 1977, fluorescence in situ hybridization in 1982, massively parallel sequencing in 1992, and comparative genomic hybridization in 1998. Older technologies continue to find usage in the NICU, especially G-banded karyotype for aneuploidies and sanger sequencing for single gene testing. Chromosomal microarray, which detects copy number variants (CNVs) as small as 50 to 100,000 base pairs, has long been the standard of care for evaluation of neonates with suspected genetic disorders. Microarray for many years has been considered the standard of care for infants with multiple congenital malformations in the NICU.[11] The human genome project launched in 1990 that led to the first publication of the core sequence was completed in 2003, which opened the door to genomic sequencing. Clinical exome sequencing was validated in the research setting for diagnosis of rare or undiagnosed disease in the late 2000s. The first clinical genetic diagnosis was made by exome sequencing in 2009,[12] and the technology entered routine clinical practice after 2010.

Genomic sequencing technology has improved rapidly in the decades since the first sequence of the human genome was completed, which has led to increased utilization and a precipitous drop in the cost of genomic sequencing.[13] The TAT to complete sequencing has fallen alongside overall cost: what once took several months can now be achieved in a few days. Today genomic sequencing is no longer cost prohibitive and is used in routine clinical care in both the inpatient and outpatient setting for the diagnosis of rare genetic disorders.

Exome Versus Whole Genome Sequencing

Understanding the differences between exome sequencing (ES) and WGS is important, as each have their own strengths and limitations. ES targets all known exons that represent approximately 1% of all DNA and harbor greater than 99% of all known disease-causing variants. WGS is untargeted and generates sequence data for the entire genome. ES is readily available in many clinical laboratories and is becoming more widely accepted as a necessary test by insurance in both the inpatient and outpatient settings. GS is more expensive than ES due to the need to generate, store, and bioinformatically process more data and is not covered in most circumstances by insurance (at the time of publication). CNVs can be more readily and directly detected by WGS owing to relatively even read-depth coverage of all genomic regions. CNVs can be extrapolated from ES data but there are still reservations of absolute accuracy comparative to true microarray/comparative genomic hybridization and WGS. As the target-capture step of ES is not needed for sample preparation with WGS, it can be initiated and completed more rapidly than ES. Rapid WGS with an optimized process can achieve a 2- to 4-day TAT from receipt of sample but many laboratories still work on 10- to 14-day TAT. The published "record" for clinical WGS TAT is 19 hours.[14] Some studies have shown that WGS provides better coverage of exons, especially for the first exons of genes.[15] Finally, WGS data can be used to identify some pathogenic repeat expansions with high specificity[16,17] although as of 2021 few laboratories have clinically validated this bioinformatic process.

WGS provides an estimated ~5 and 10% increase in the diagnostic yield of ES, primarily by detection of CNVs and deep intronic.[15] Although intergenic variation is detected, the limited ability to interpret variants has prevented these variants from leading to an appreciable increase in yield. As ES technology has improved the increase in yield from WGS has become smaller over time, and some studies have found no increase in yield.[18]

The best diagnostic yield is achieved by "trio" genomic sequencing (testing samples from both parents) that allows for immediate phasing of variants. Confirming whether variants in dominant genes are de novo (new in the proband) or variants in recessive genes are in trans (affecting both copies of the gene) is crucial evidence to prove pathogenicity. On the other hand, several studies have demonstrated that proband-only ("singleton") ES and WGS have a diagnostic yield either equivalent to or only moderately diminished in comparison to trio sequencing, including rapid testing in the NICU.[18–21] Trio sequencing is more expensive (testing more individuals) and may slow the testing process if parents are not immediately available.

CURRENT EVIDENCE
Impact on Management in the Intensive Care Unit

Arguments made against inpatient genetic testing often focus on the idea that the test will not affect immediate inpatient care. Many, if not most, genetic disorders may inform prognosis and some aspects of long-term management. There are several ways in which genetic testing can have an immediate influence on critical care decision-making:

1. Disease-specific medications, procedures, therapies, or diet

2. Avoiding or discontinuing specific medications, therapies, or procedures
3. Identifying risks to other organ systems that prompts additional diagnostic testing or specialist consultation
4. Ruling out specific disorders of concern, thereby avoiding other diagnostic tests
5. Providing prognostic information that helps direct the goals of care discussion

Examples are plentiful:

• A child with congenital onset spondyloepiphyseal dysplasia is at risk for increased intracranial pressure and c-spine instability.
• An infant with Alagille syndrome might avoid a diagnostic liver biopsy by first receiving a molecular diagnosis.
• A child with Leigh disease due to coenzyme Q10 deficiency receives CoQ10 early in the disease course.
• Children with inborn errors of metabolism are at greater risk for catabolic decompensation when under increased stress of illness, and managing their energy metabolism needs appropriately improves outcomes.
• A neonate with status epilepticus is given high-dose pyrixodine therapy when pyridoxine-dependent epilepsy is molecularly diagnosed.
• Identification of pharmacogenetic variants may guide dosing or medication choice.

There have been a large number of studies that have assessed the diagnostic yield, medical management, and cost of inpatient sequencing (**Table 1**). Study parameters varied in each test (ES or WGS), rapid or standard TAT, age group (neonatal, infantile, pediatric), and location (NICU, multiple ICUs, any inpatient setting). TATs dropped precipitously from the earliest studies, and overall ranged from 24 hours to 40 days. In general inclusion criteria were nonspecific, similar to the indications for genomic testing laid out in **Box 2**. The diagnostic yield was 43% (median, range 21% to 69%), including only definite diagnoses defined as likely pathogenic or pathogenic results. Similarly, a meta-analysis of 18 studies before 2020 (1049 patients) found an overall diagnostic yield of 43% (95% confidence interval 36%–50%) and did not find a significant difference between ES and WGS.[34]

Although easily comparable figures are complicated to discern from studies, it is clear that among diagnosed patients, immediate management change (diet, procedures, surgical planning, medication, goals of care) is common. Across all studies medical management was reported to be changed in 43% (median, range 21%–100%) of diagnosed patients and of 24% (median, range 12%–60%) of all patients tested. In general there was a higher rate of change in management in patients recruited from the NICU. The 3 studies exclusive to NICU patients showed a management change in more than 50% of all patients tested.[14,22,23] Despite variability in study design and in what was considered a change in management, no study reported a change in less than 10% of those tested. This should be taken as a clear demonstration of the utility of genomic sequencing in appropriate patients The impact of a negative test was not included in most of the studies, as it is more difficult to assess. The 2 studies that did report on the impact of a negative test both noted a change in management in ~11% of cases without a diagnosis.[23,38] In general the most commonly reported changes in management were implementing targeted medical therapy, avoiding surgery or altering the choice of surgical approach, implementing curative bone marrow transplant, and transitioning from high intensity intervention to palliative.

The primary endpoints, diagnostic yield and change in management, do not tell the whole story. The first randomized controlled trial of rapid WGS versus "standard care"

Table 1
Studies of exome and whole genome sequencing in pediatric inpatient populations

Publication (First Author, Ref#), Year	Study Population[a]	Study Type	Test[b]	Turnaround Time	Diagnostic Rate	Change in Management[c]
Studies with all patients located in NICU						
Clark et al,[14] 2019	n = 7, neonates; NICU	Prospective	GS (trio)	20 h (median)	43%	100% of diagnosed (43% of tested)
Elliot et al,[22] 2019	n = 25, neonates; NICU	Prospective	ES (trio)	7 d (mean)	60%	83% of diagnosed (60% of tested)
Freed et al,[23] 2020	n = 46, neonates; NICU	Prospective	ES (trio)	9 d (mean)	43%	95% of diagnosed (52% of tested)
Studies with patients in mixed ICU settings						
Willig et al,[24] 2015	n = 35, infants; NICU or PICU	Retrospective	GS	23 d (median)	57%	65% of diagnosed (37% of tested)
van Diemen et al,[25] 2017	n = 23, infants; NICU or PICU	Prospective	GS	12 d (median)	30%	71% of diagnosed (22% of tested)
Meng et al,[26] 2017	n = 63, infants; any ICU	Retrospective	ES	13 d (median)	37%	52% of diagnosed (19% of tested)
Petrikin et al,[27] 2018	n = 32, infants; NICU or PICU	RCT	GS	14 d (median)	31%	48% of diagnosed (15% of tested)
Mestek-Boukhibar et al,[28] 2018	n = 24, infants; PICU	Prospective	GS (trio)	8.5 d (median)	42%	100% of diagnosed (24% of tested)
French et al,[29] 2019	n = 195, pediatric; NICU or PICU	Prospective	GS (trio)	4.5 wk (median)	21%	65% of diagnosed (13% of tested)
Sanford et al,[30] 2019	n = 33, pediatric; PICU	Retrospective	GS	13 d (mean)	45%	24% of diagnosed (12% of tested)
Wu et al,[31] 2019	n = 40, pediatric; PICU	Prospective	ES	6 d (mean)	52%	81% of diagnosed (25% of tested)

(continued on next page)

Table 1
(continued)

Publication (First Author, Ref#), Year	Study Population[a]	Study Type	Test[b]	Turnaround Time	Diagnostic Rate	Change in Management[c]
Wang et al,[32] 2020	n = 33, infants; NICU or PICU	Prospective	ES	24 h (median)	69%	43% of diagnosed (23% of tested)
Wang et al,[33] 2020	n = 130, pediatric; NICU or PICU	Prospective	GS (trio)	3.8 d (median)	48%	48% of diagnosed (23% of tested)
Chung et al,[34] 2020	n = 102, pediatric; NICU or PICU	Prospective	ES	11 d (median)	31%	88% of diagnosed (27% of tested)
Wu et al,[35] 2021	n = 202, pediatric; PICU	Prospective	GS (trio)	7 d (median)	36%	21% of diagnosed ("immediate" changes only; 8% of tested)
Studies with patients in ICU or inpatient setting						
Sweeney et al,[36] 2021	n = 24, infants; NICU or CICU	Retrospective	GS	5–10 d	43%	45% of diagnosed (20% of tested)
Farnaes et al,[37] 2018	n = 42, infants; any ICU or inpatient ward	Retrospective	GS	23 d (median)	43%	72% of diagnosed (31% of tested)
Lunke et al,[38] 2020	n = 108, neonates; NICU, PICU or inpatient ward	Prospective	ES	3 d (range 2–7)	51%	76% with and 11% without diagnosis (44% of all tested)

Abbreviation: PICU, pediatric intensive care unit.

[a] Inclusion criteria and patient populations not uniform across studies. In general, "neonate is less than 2 months of age, "infant" less than 12 months, and "pediatric" less than 10 years. Most patient populations had a wide variety of organ system involvement. Amount of prior genetic workup also variable.

[b] If not noted, sequencing was either proband-only or a mix of proband-only, trio, and other familial approaches.

[c] Excluding cases where only change was genetic counseling, familial risk assessment, outpatient referral, or long-term management change. Not including impact of negative cases or variants of uncertain significance, except where specified.

> **Box 2**
> **Indications for genomic sequencing**
>
> Phenotype and/or family history strongly suggest congenital or neurodevelopmental disorder
>
> - Multiple congenital anomalies concerning for a genetic cause
> - Metabolic abnormalities that suggest an inborn error of metabolism (ie hyperammonemia, lactic acidosis)
> - Neurologic abnormalities (severe hypotonia, seizures) unexplained by hypoxic-ischaemic encephalopathy
> - First-degree relative with sudden unexplained death in infancy or childhood
> - Unexplained dysfunction of multiple organ systems
> - Intellectual disability or developmental regression
>
> AND at least one of the following:
>
> Clinical features not specific to single genetic disorder (eg, trisomies, VACTERL would be excluded)
>
> Atypical disease course (severity, duration, failure of or abnormal response to therapy)
>
> Atypical or complex combinations of signs, symptoms, and laboratory findings not explained by clinical presentation.
>
> More than one genetic test is justifiable based on differential diagnosis.

in the NICU was terminated due to lack of equipoise, when the investigators deemed "standard care" inferior to the study intervention.[25] Both critical care faculty and parents perceived high clinical utility from the NISGHT2 trial, with only a minority of parents endorsing distress as a result of the testing.[39] Parents also place high value on negative results, emphasizing that diagnostic yield is not a predictor of perceived utility.[40] Two recurring observations support the use of genomic over targeted sequencing: the clinical phenotype or differential diagnosis frequently does not align with the molecular diagnosis, and in a some of cases, dual diagnoses lead to a confounding phenotype[23,37,38] It is possible to analyze all genomic content present including nonhuman DNA ("metagenomics"), demonstrated by Wu and colleagues,[34] who were able identify the causative pathogens in 6 critically ill septic infants as part of their WGS analysis.

All studies that have performed cost analysis found a significant reduction in health care costs from inpatient genomic sequencing.[21,34,36,37,39,41] The cost savings were mostly attributable to reduction in length of hospital stay and reduction of invasive interventions. Supporting the utility of rapid testing, Dimmock and colleagues reported that the cost differential was not due to the acquired data but the expediency at which the data could be provided. Their control study arm that followed conventional genetic and molecular workup did not show the same cost savings as the study group that underwent rapid genome sequencing.

DISCUSSION
Practical Aspects of Inpatient Genomic Sequencing

The appropriate time to consider genomic sequencing in the ICU remains a subjective decision. Patients in the ICU setting often have severe illness with rapid decompensation, and time may be a limited resource for the patient and caregivers. In these situations shortening the time to diagnosis may have outsized impact in comparison to an outpatient diagnostic odyssey. In general guide one should consider rapid genome sequencing for any patient in a critical decompensated state who has no clear cause for their circumstance and for whom a genetic disorder is possible. Clinical situations that should raise this concern are listed in **Box 2**. This list is incomplete, and there may be other phenotypic clues or family history that suggest a mendelian disorder.

Genetic counseling by a certified professional should be required before ordering genomic sequencing, and when possible, consultation with a medical geneticist is strongly recommended. The drawbacks of any GS test include the identification of variants of uncertain significance or incorrect interpretation of results leading to false-positive diagnoses, negative impact on family dynamics or communication, negative psychosocial impact, and reduction or loss of privacy.[42] It should be noted that recent studies have shown that provider and parent perception of harm is very limited.[39,40] Given the potential negative impact of genomic testing on families, informed consent is crucial. Genetic counseling aids in setting expectations regarding potentially confusing results, cost and TAT, diagnoses unrelated to the indication for testing (incidental findings), and whether secondary findings are going to be reported. Medical genetics expertise is especially useful when deciding how to interpret and follow-up on variants of uncertain significance.

There are several considerations when selecting the most appropriate test (**Fig. 1**). First, inpatient genetic testing (even karyotype or microarray) is not universally accessible, especially outside of academic health centers or when genetics consultative service is not readily available. The choice to implement genetic testing in such circumstances must be purposeful, ideally through an institutional agreement with

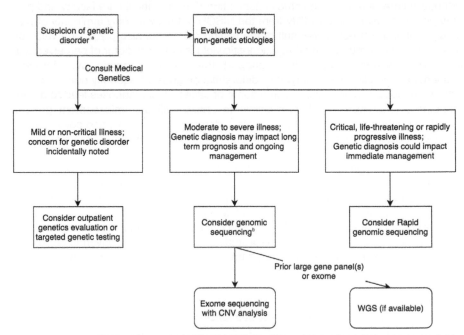

Fig. 1. A proposed algorithm to help the decision-making process for when to pursue inpatient genomic sequencing, rapid testing, and exome versus whole genome sequencing. [a]See **Box 2**. [b]The choice between exome and whole genome sequencing may depend on the specifics of the available tests.

large genomic centers. Clear protocols should be established to guide decision support. Second is the acuity of illness, which directs the decision to pursue rapid testing (3- to 7-day TAT), standard genomic sequencing (usually 1- to 3-month TAT), or outpatient genetics referral. In the setting of subacute or chronic medical concerns with incidentally noted concern for a genetic disorder outpatient genetics referral or targeted testing may be appropriate. When there is moderate to severe illness but little risk of decompensation, death, or imminent morbidity, standard turnaround ES testing would be an appropriate choice to reduce the overall burden to health care expenditure. In critically ill neonates and children, the seeking rapid testing should be considered, as the speed to reaching a diagnosis may have significant consequences and impact on outcome. As of 2021 ES should probably still be considered a first-line test because the difference in diagnostic yield between ES and WGS has narrowed due to improvements in modern exome sequencing technology, and the cost of WGS is still significantly higher. However, this decision will need to be situation specific. For example, if rapid ES is available but does not include CNV calling, for a critically ill child rapid WGS will have a higher yield and is the better test. Third is the disease process (symptoms, differential diagnosis) and prior genetic testing. Some differential diagnoses are better evaluated by nongenomic sequencing (ie spinocerebellar ataxias caused by repeat expansions, imprinting disorders) or other tests (ie, biochemical testing). If both genome wide CNV analysis and genomic testing are indicated, either WGS or ES with CNV analysis (not available at every ES laboratory) is advisable. If there is negative prior testing (especially large gene panels or ES) WGS should be considered. If ES or WGS has been completed in the past (at least 1 year) and the patient remains undiagnosed, reanalysis is always recommended.

SUMMARY

Genetic testing is an important part of the diagnostic evaluation of neonates and infants, as genetic disorders are a common cause of morbidity and mortality in the NICU. The use of inpatient genomic sequencing is currently not widespread due in part to concerns about clinical utility and cost. The rapid evolution of sequencing technology and bioinformatic processes in the last decade has drastically reduced the cost and TAT of ES and WGS. Results of rapid sequencing can now routinely be returned in less than 7 days and in some circumstances much faster. For patients in whom a genetic disorder is possible or suspected the diagnostic yield of genomic sequencing in the ICU is close to 40%. Immediate clinical management (ie medication, diagnostic testing, surgical planning, diet, goals of care) affects ~40% of diagnosed patients and 24% of all patients tested (medians). Cost analyses of studies of GS for infants in the ICU have consistently shown net cost-savings in health care expenditures, primarily through reduction of hospital length of stay. The evidence is sufficient to support GS in all NICU patients with an appropriate indication, as part of standard care. The most important remaining barrier to widespread implementation of genomic sequencing in the NICU is access to medical geneticists and genetic counselors.

CLINICS CARE POINTS

- Genetic disorders are common causes of morbidity and mortality in the NICU, and a high index of suspicion for genetic disorders should be maintained for unexplained symptomatology.
- Genomic sequencing (exome or whole genome) should be considered early in the diagnostic process when a genetic disorder is a reasonable possibility.

- Rapid genomic sequencing should be considered in any patient for whom a genetic disorder is possible and whose acuity is high (critical or imminently life-threatening illness, progressively worsening disease).
- Improvements in technology and bioinformatic processes have reduced the cost and TAT of genomic sequencing, which can now reliably be resulted within 7 days.
- The diagnostic yield of genomic sequencing for infants in pediatric ICU settings is greater than 40% and may be higher in the NICU.
- Immediate impacts on management from an early genetic diagnosis include changes to medications, disease-specific therapies or diets, avoiding diagnostic procedures or unnecessary surgeries, and informing goals of care discussions of disease-specific prognoses.
- Changes in short-term management occur in close to 20% of all critically ill pediatric patients who undergo genomic sequencing in whom a genetic diagnosis is possible or suspected.
- Cost analyses have found significant reductions in health care costs from inpatient genomic sequencing.
- The choice between ES and WGS whole genome sequencing should depend on patient acuity, the specifics of the available tests, and the extent of prior genetic testing.
- Genomic sequencing without the direct involvement of medical geneticists and genetic counselors is not recommended.

BEST PRACTICES

- Improving utilization of genomic sequencing in the NICU for appropriate patients will lead to more diagnoses, reductions in morbidity, and disease-specific therapy and management.
- A clinical algorithm for ordering genomic sequencing in the NICU should include consultation with medical genetics and assessments of the likelihood of a genetic disorder and the acuity of illness, and workukp non-genetic etiologies (clinical algorithm is in text, figure 1)
- Initiating rapid genomic testing early in the disease course has the highest likelihood of impacting clinical care

DISCLOSURE

The author has no commercial or financial conflicts of interests and no external funding sources.

REFERENCES

1. Matthews TJ, MacDorman MF, Thoma ME. Infant mortality statistics from the 2013 period linked birth/infant death data set. Natl Vital Stat Rep 2015;64(9):1–30.
2. Hudome SM, Kirby RS, Senner JW, et al. Contribution of genetic disorders to neonatal mortality in a regional intensive care setting. Am J Perinatol 1994; 11(2):100–3. https://doi.org/10.1055/s-2007-994565.
3. Wojcik MH, Brodsky D, Stewart JE, et al. Peri-mortem evaluation of infants who die without a diagnosis: focus on advances in genomic technology. J Perinatol 2018;38(9):1125–34. https://doi.org/10.1038/s41372-018-0187-7.
4. Wojcik MH, Schwartz TS, Yamin I, et al. Genetic disorders and mortality in infancy and early childhood: delayed diagnoses and missed opportunities. Genet Med 2018;20(11):1396–404. https://doi.org/10.1038/gim.2018.17.

5. Stevenson DA, Carey JC. Contribution of malformations and genetic disorders to mortality in a children's hospital. Am J Med Genet A 2004;126-A(4):393–7. https://doi.org/10.1002/ajmg.a.20409.

6. Feuchtbaum L, Carter J, Dowray S, et al. Birth prevalence of disorders detectable through newborn screening by race/ethnicity. Genet Med 2012;14(11):937–45. https://doi.org/10.1038/gim.2012.76.

7. Swaggart KA, Swarr DT, Tolusso LK, et al. Making a genetic diagnosis in a level IV neonatal intensive care unit population: who, when, how, and at what cost? J Pediatr 2019;213:211–7.e4. https://doi.org/10.1016/j.jpeds.2019.05.054.

8. Moorthie S, Blencowe H, Darlison MW, et al. Estimating the birth prevalence and pregnancy outcomes of congenital malformations worldwide. J Community Genet 2018;9(4):387–96. https://doi.org/10.1007/s12687-018-0384-2.

9. Ceyhan-Birsoy O, Murry JB, Machini K, et al. Interpretation of genomic sequencing results in healthy and ill newborns: results from the BabySeq project. Am J Hum Genet 2019;104(1):76–93. https://doi.org/10.1016/j.ajhg.2018.11.016.

10. Gjorgioski S, Halliday J, Riley M, et al. Genetics and pediatric hospital admissions, 1985 to 2017. Genet Med 2020;22(11):1777–85. https://doi.org/10.1038/s41436-020-0871-9.

11. Miller DT, Adam MP, Aradhya S, et al. Consensus statement: chromosomal microarray is a first-tier clinical diagnostic test for individuals with developmental disabilities or congenital anomalies. Am J Hum Genet 2010;86(5):749–64. https://doi.org/10.1016/j.ajhg.2010.04.006.

12. Choi M, Scholl UI, Ji W, et al. Genetic diagnosis by whole exome capture and massively parallel DNA sequencing. Proc Natl Acad Sci U S A 2009;106(45):19096–101. https://doi.org/10.1073/pnas.0910672106.

13. van Dijk EL, Auger H, Jaszczyszyn Y, et al. Ten years of next-generation sequencing technology. Trends Genet 2014;30(9):418–26. https://doi.org/10.1016/j.tig.2014.07.001.

14. Clark MM, Hildreth A, Batalov S, et al. Diagnosis of genetic diseases in seriously ill children by rapid whole-genome sequencing and automated phenotyping and interpretation. Sci Transl Med 2019;11(489):eaat6177. https://doi.org/10.1126/scitranslmed.aat6177.

15. Bick D, Jones M, Taylor SL, et al. Case for genome sequencing in infants and children with rare, undiagnosed or genetic diseases. J Med Genet 2019;56(12):783–91. https://doi.org/10.1136/jmedgenet-2019-106111.

16. Dolzhenko E, van Vugt JJFA, Shaw RJ, et al. Detection of long repeat expansions from PCR-free whole-genome sequence data. Genome Res 2017;27(11):1895–903. https://doi.org/10.1101/gr.225672.117.

17. Tankard RM, Bennett MF, Degorski P, et al. Detecting expansions of tandem repeats in cohorts sequenced with short-read sequencing data. Am J Hum Genet 2018;103(6):858–73. https://doi.org/10.1016/j.ajhg.2018.10.015.

18. Clark MM, Stark Z, Farnaes L, et al. Meta-analysis of the diagnostic and clinical utility of genome and exome sequencing and chromosomal microarray in children with suspected genetic diseases. NPJ Genom Med 2018;3:16. https://doi.org/10.1038/s41525-018-0053-8.

19. Brockman DG, Austin-Tse CA, Pelletier RC, et al. Randomized prospective evaluation of genome sequencing versus standard-of-care as a first molecular diagnostic test. Genet Med 2021;23(9):1689–96. https://doi.org/10.1038/s41436-021-01193-y.

20. Stark Z, Tan TY, Chong B, et al. A prospective evaluation of whole-exome sequencing as a first-tier molecular test in infants with suspected monogenic disorders. Genet Med 2016;18(11):1090–6. https://doi.org/10.1038/gim.2016.1.

21. Yeung A, Tan NB, Tan TY, et al. A cost-effectiveness analysis of genomic sequencing in a prospective versus historical cohort of complex pediatric patients. Genet Med 2020;22(12):1986–93. https://doi.org/10.1038/s41436-020-0929-8.

22. Elliott AM, du Souich C, Lehman A, et al. RAPIDOMICS: rapid genome-wide sequencing in a neonatal intensive care unit—successes and challenges. Eur J Pediatr 2019;178(8):1207–18. https://doi.org/10.1007/s00431-019-03399-4.

23. Freed AS, Clowes Candadai SV, Sikes MC, et al. The impact of rapid exome sequencing on medical management of critically ill children. J Pediatr 2020; 226:202–12.e1. https://doi.org/10.1016/j.jpeds.2020.06.0201.

24. Willig LK, Petrikin JE, Smith LD, et al. Whole-genome sequencing for identification of Mendelian disorders in critically ill infants: a retrospective analysis of diagnostic and clinical findings. Lancet Respir Med 2015;3(5):377–87. https://doi.org/10.1016/S2213-2600(15)00139-3.

25. van Diemen CC, Kerstjens-Frederikse WS, Bergman KA, et al. Rapid targeted genomics in critically ill newborns. Pediatrics 2017;140(4):e20162854. https://doi.org/10.1542/peds.2016-2854.

26. Meng L, Pammi M, Saronwala A, et al. Use of exome sequencing for infants in intensive care units: ascertainment of severe single-gene disorders and effect on medical management. JAMA Pediatr 2017;171(12):e173438. https://doi.org/10.1001/jamapediatrics.2017.3438.

27. Petrikin JE, Cakici JA, Clark MM, et al. The NSIGHT1-randomized controlled trial: rapid whole-genome sequencing for accelerated etiologic diagnosis in critically ill infants. NPJ Genom Med 2018;3:6. https://doi.org/10.1038/s41525-018-0045-8.

28. Mestek-Boukhibar L, Clement E, Jones WD, et al. Rapid Paediatric Sequencing (RaPS): comprehensive real-life workflow for rapid diagnosis of critically ill children. J Med Genet 2018;55(11):721–8. https://doi.org/10.1136/jmedgenet-2018-105396.

29. French CE, Delon I, Dolling H, et al. Whole genome sequencing reveals that genetic conditions are frequent in intensively ill children. Intensive Care Med 2019; 45(5):627–36. https://doi.org/10.1007/s00134-019-05552-x.

30. Sanford EF, Clark MM, Farnaes L, et al. Rapid whole genome sequencing has clinical utility in children in the PICU. Pediatr Crit Care Med 2019;20(11): 1007–20. https://doi.org/10.1097/PCC.0000000000002056.

31. Wu E-T, Hwu W-L, Chien Y-H, et al. Critical trio exome benefits in-time decision-making for pediatric patients with severe Illnesses. Pediatr Crit Care Med 2019; 20(11):1021–6. https://doi.org/10.1097/PCC.0000000000002068.

32. Wang H, Qian Y, Lu Y, et al. Clinical utility of 24-h rapid trio-exome sequencing for critically ill infants. NPJ Genom Med 2020;5(1):1–6. https://doi.org/10.1038/s41525-020-0129-0.

33. Wang H, Lu Y, Dong X, et al. Optimized trio genome sequencing (OTGS) as a first-tier genetic test in critically ill infants: practice in China. Hum Genet 2020; 139(4):473–82. https://doi.org/10.1007/s00439-019-02103-8.

34. Chung CCY, Leung GKC, Mak CCY, et al. Rapid whole-exome sequencing facilitates precision medicine in paediatric rare disease patients and reduces healthcare costs. Lancet Reg Health West Pac 2020;1:100001. https://doi.org/10.1016/j.lanwpc.2020.100001.

35. Wu B, Kang W, Wang Y, et al. Application of full-spectrum rapid clinical genome sequencing improves diagnostic rate and clinical outcomes in critically ill infants in the China neonatal genomes project. Crit Care Med 2021. https://doi.org/10.1097/CCM.0000000000005052.

36. Sweeney NM, Nahas SA, Chowdhury S, et al. Rapid whole genome sequencing impacts care and resource utilization in infants with congenital heart disease. NPJ Genom Med 2021;6:29. https://doi.org/10.1038/s41525-021-00192-x.
37. Farnaes L, Hildreth A, Sweeney NM, et al. Rapid whole-genome sequencing decreases infant morbidity and cost of hospitalization. NPJ Genom Med 2018;3:10. https://doi.org/10.1038/s41525-018-0049-4.
38. Lunke S, Eggers S, Wilson M, et al. Feasibility of ultra-rapid exome sequencing in critically ill infants and children with suspected monogenic conditions in the Australian public health care system. JAMA 2020;323(24):1–9. https://doi.org/10.1001/jama.2020.7671.
39. Dimmock DP, Clark MM, Gaughran M, et al. An RCT of rapid genomic sequencing among seriously ill infants results in high clinical utility, changes in management, and low perceived harm. Am J Hum Genet 2020;107(5):942–52. https://doi.org/10.1016/j.ajhg.2020.10.003.
40. Cakici JA, Dimmock DP, Caylor SA, et al. A prospective study of parental perceptions of rapid whole-genome and -exome sequencing among seriously ill infants. Am J Hum Genet 2020;107(5):953–62. https://doi.org/10.1016/j.ajhg.2020.10.004.
41. Stark Z, Lunke S, Brett GR, et al. Meeting the challenges of implementing rapid genomic testing in acute pediatric care. Genet Med 2018;20(12):1554–63. https://doi.org/10.1038/gim.2018.37.
42. Manickam K, McClain MR, Demmer LA, et al. Exome and genome sequencing for pediatric patients with congenital anomalies or intellectual disability: an evidence-based clinical guideline of the American College of Medical Genetics and Genomics (ACMG). Genet Med 2021;1–9.

Biomarkers of Necrotizing Enterocolitis: The Search Continues

Aarthi Gunasekaran, MD[a], Christa Devette, MD, PhD[b],
Samuel Levin, MD[a], Hala Chaaban, MD[a],*

KEYWORDS

- Necrotizing enterocolitis • Biomarkers • Proteomics • Transcriptomics
- Metabolomics

KEY POINTS

- Necrotizing enterocolitis (NEC) is a devastating disease that primarily affects preterm infants.
- Despite advances in clinical care, mortality and morbidity from NEC have not improved partly due to lack of accurate biomarkers.
- Significant barriers exist in finding optimal biomarkers including the lack of a robust case-definition that can differentiate NEC from non-NEC entities.
- Single or multi-omics approaches hold promise in identifying biomarkers that will aid in the prediction, early diagnosis, or prognosis of NEC, but will require validation in larger studies.

INTRODUCTION

Necrotizing enterocolitis (NEC) is the most devastating gastrointestinal (GI) pathology in preterm infants.[1,2] NEC results in significant morbidity, and mortality rates range up to 50% in premature infants who undergo surgical intervention.[3–6] This unacceptably high mortality and morbidity are partly due to the complexity of the pathogenesis, and the lack of appropriate biomarkers for early diagnosis and treatment.[7]

The current diagnosis of NEC is made by a combination of nonspecific clinical signs, symptoms, and radiological findings.[7,8] The early signs and symptoms of NEC, such as temperature instability, apnea, feeding intolerance, and abdominal distension, are difficult to distinguish from other common pathologies such as GI dysmotility or sepsis-induced intestinal ileus. Moreover, early radiologic features and pneumatosis

[a] Neonatal-Perinatal Medicine, The University of Oklahoma Health Sciences Center, 1200 N Everett Drive, Oklahoma City, OK 73104, USA; [b] Department of Pediatrics, The University of Oklahoma Health Sciences Center, 1200 N Everett Drive, Oklahoma City, OK 73104, USA
* Corresponding author.
E-mail addresses: Christa-Devette@ouhsc.edu (C.D.); Samuel-Levin@ouhsc.edu (S.L.); Hala-chaaban@ouhsc.edu (H.C.)

Clin Perinatol 49 (2022) 181–194
https://doi.org/10.1016/j.clp.2021.11.011
0095-5108/22/© 2021 Elsevier Inc. All rights reserved.
perinatology.theclinics.com

intestinalis are difficult to interpret and have low sensitivity for diagnosing NEC.[9,10] Thus, a specific biomarker or a panel of biomarkers that can identify infants with NEC early is critical for improving outcomes.[9,11]

CHALLENGES IN IDENTIFYING THE IDEAL NECROTIZING ENTEROCOLITIS BIOMARKER(S)

The biggest obstacle in identifying optimal diagnostic/prognostic biomarkers is that NEC is likely not a single clinical entity.[10,12] Several pathways lead to the "endpoint" of intestinal necrosis or injury. Classical or preterm NEC differs from the NEC-like intestinal injuries seen in term infants with cyanotic heart disease, perinatal asphyxia, gastroschisis, food protein-induced enterocolitis syndrome, or Hirschsprung's.[13,14] Unfortunately, the current diagnostic criteria and definitions used do not differentiate classical NEC from these non-NEC diseases.[15–17] Furthermore, the misconception that the radiological finding of pneumoperitoneum or pneumatosis intestinalis is diagnostic of NEC, irrespective of gestational age, has led to a significant overlap between NEC and the "NEC mimics", limiting the value of the biomarkers studied to date.[10] Therefore, to facilitate biomarkers discovery, researchers and clinicians must establish a consensus "gold standard" definition for NEC that can be used both in clinical practice and for studies.[15] Newer proposed definitions that take into account gestational age, postnatal age, and radiological signs seem to be superior to the conventional Bell staging, but their use in clinical practice is still limited.[12,17]

CHARACTERISTICS OF THE IDEAL BIOMARKER(S) FOR NECROTIZING ENTEROCOLITIS

A biomarker is defined as "A characteristic that is measured as an indicator of normal biological processes, pathogenic processes, or response to an exposure or intervention."[12] The following suggested criteria could aid clinicians at the bedside and help reduce the burden of NEC[18–20]:

- Must have a well-defined "cut-off" value with a rapid increase or decrease (preferably before clinical manifestation).
- High specificity and positive predictive value to enhance its ability to detect NEC from non-NEC entities.
- Alternatively, have a high sensitivity and negative predictive values to "rule out" NEC to reduce unnecessary antibiotics and interventions.
- Prognostic markers should have the ability to predict the severity of NEC, the development of complications, surgical needs, and mortality.
- Ideally noninvasive or requires a small volume of blood.

Other important laboratory aspects include molecular stability, the ability to perform the test in-house, and relatively low cost.

Serum Biomarkers for Necrotizing Enterocolitis

Numerous serum biomarkers, such as white blood cell (WBC) and platelet counts,[21–24] acute-phase proteins,[25–27] cytokines,[28] chemokines,[28,29] have been studied for the diagnosis or prognostication of NEC (**Table 1**). None demonstrated sufficient specificity and sensitivity to be used in clinical practice. Intestinal-specific inflammatory mediators have been studied in a limited capacity and show various specificity and sensitivities. For example, serum intestinal fatty acid-binding protein (I-FABP)[30,31] and intestinal trefoil factors (TFF3)[32] seem to be promising but have not been rigorously assessed in large studies.

Table 1 Serum biomarkers for NEC		
Biomarker	**Description**	**Limitations**
Complete blood count	• High total WBC count, immature/mature ratio associated with increased mortality.[21] • Lower lymphocytes, monocytes, neutrophils, and platelets associated with fulminant NEC.[22] • Fall in Absolute monocyte count >20% (modest sensitivity of 0.70 and specificity of 0.71, and negative predictive value of 88%[23]) • Thrombocytopenia was seen in 50%–90% of NEC within 24–72 h.[33] • Lower platelet counts are associated with worse outcomes.[22,24]	• Low to moderate sensitivity • Not sensitive or specific for NEC.
C- reactive protein (CRP)	• Persistently elevated CRP associated with complications from NEC (strictures) or surgical NEC.[25,26] • A CRP/Albumin ratio of ≥ 3 on day 2 of NEC could be associated with a higher likelihood for surgery and mortality.[34]	• Relatively sensitive (91%) but not specific to NEC (∼65%).
Procalcitonin (PCT)	• Could differentiate NEC from septic ileus (low in NEC compared with septic patients[27]).	• Limited studies • Not sensitive or specific to NEC.
Cytokines	• Low blood TGF-β levels are associated with an increased risk of NEC.[28] • Elevated IL-6, IL-8, IL-10, IL-2 in NEC.[28,29] • Consistently elevated IL-8 is associated with increased severity.[35] • IP-10, IL-1β elevated in NEC and sepsis.[18]	• Will not differentiate NEC from sepsis or other causes of inflammation.
Complement component 5a (C5a)	• Elevated in NEC and potentially superior to IL-6 and CRP in predicting surgical NEC and mortality.[36]	• Not sensitive or specific to NEC.

(continued on next page)

Table 1 (*continued*)		
Biomarker	Description	Limitations
Inter-Alpha Inhibitor Protein (IAIP)	• Significantly lower in NEC than controls.[37] • Potentially superior to CRP in the diagnosis of NEC. • Could differentiate NEC from spontaneous intestinal perforation.[38]	• Not specific to NEC (levels are also low in sepsis).
Intestinal Fatty Acid Binding Protein (I-FABP)	• Released from damaged enterocytes. • Potentially useful for determining the severity of NEC (medical vs surgical, complicated vs uncomplicated.[39] • Plasma I-FABP levels are associated with the length of bowel resection in surgical NEC.[40]	• High specificity to gut injury but low sensitivity and predictive values.[30,31] • Limited value for early diagnosis due to variable concentration in healthy premature infants and the short half-life.[40]
Ischemia-modified Albumin (IMA)	• Significantly increased in NEC than sepsis. • Could predict severity of NEC (medical vs surgical, and mortality).[41]	• Not specific for NEC. • Levels could be elevated from other ischemic diseases from other organs.
Intestinal Trefoil Factors (TFF3)	• Could differentiate NEC from sepsis. Level significantly higher in infants with NEC than those with neonatal sepsis.	• Moderate sensitivity (85%) but nonspecific marker (59%) for NEC
Serum Amyloid-A Protein	• Increased in NEC, could determine severity and response to therapy.[42] • Could differentiate NEC from sepsis.[42] • Levels of SAA decreased earlier than CRP and PCT in NEC in a small study.[26]	• Limited evaluation • Will need validation
Resistin-like molecule β (RELMβ)	• RELMβ levels in the NEC group were significantly higher than the control group with a sensitivity and specificity of 71.4% and 91.7%, respectively.[32] • Combined with low platelet count increases sensitivity and specificity to 82.89% and 93.21%, respectively.	• Small sample size • Will need validation

Urine Biomarkers (Table 2)

Biological proteins and peptides filtered in urine have been used as diagnostic tools for multiple pathologies.[43,44]

Advantages of urine biomarkers are the following:

- Obtaining samples is easy and noninvasive.

Table 2
Urine biomarkers for NEC

Urine Biomarker	Description	Limitations
Intestinal Fatty Acid Binding Protein (I-FABP)	• Peaks 8–24 h after onset of NEC.[46,47] • Distinguish medical from surgical NEC[48] and correlates with extent of intestinal necrosis.[40] • High levels before re-feeding after NEC correlates with poor outcomes.[49]	• Rapidly cleared by the kidneys with short half-life of ~11 min.[50] • Low sensitivity and specificity for NEC (Pooled performance statistics from meta-analysis by Yang and colleagues).[39]
Serum Amyloid A Protein (SAA)	• Can differentiate medical from surgical NEC.[51,52] • Early enteral feeding established when levels of SAA low. • When combined with urinary I-FABP and L-FABP, can predict portal venous gas.[51]	• Limited studies • A cut off value of 42.2 pg/nmol had a low sensitivity of 41% and specificity of 91% for NEC diagnosis.[53]
Trefoil Factor −3 (TFF3)	• Co-secreted along with mucin from goblet cells of small and large intestine at sites of intestinal injury. • Elevated TFF3 levels in stage III B NEC as compared with Stage II A, IIB, and IIIA.[51] • Can predict pneumatosis intestinalis when combined with SAA and I-FABP.[51]	• Not specific for NEC, elevated in sepsis as well. • Limited studies.
Claudins	• In a small pilot study, Claudin-2 was elevated in NEC.[54] • Claudin-3, a sealing tight junction elevated in NEC.[55]	• Low sensitivity of 71% and specificity of 81%.[55]
Prostaglandin E Major Urinary Metabolite (PGE-MUM)	• Levels correlate with NEC disease severity and length of intestine affected.[56] • Sensitivity of 92.3% and specificity of 81.5%.[56]	• Not specific for NEC, metabolites of cyclooxygenase are upregulated in all inflammatory conditions. • Levels measured may be affected in the presence of chronic lung disease.[57–67]

- Availability to collect in a relatively large amount.
- Could be collected continuously, allowing for the detection of biomarkers of early disease, progression, and response to treatment.

Disadvantages of urine biomarkers for infants with NEC:

- Could be limited in oliguric patients, a common complication of NEC.[45]
- Lack of established normative values for gestational age for most of the protein components .

FECAL BIOMARKERS (TABLE 3)

Fecal markers have been used as a diagnostic tool and to monitor disease activity for inflammatory bowel disorders for almost a decade.[68] They offer the advantage of being noninvasive and potentially early detection of local inflammation/injury before systemic involvement. The main disadvantage, however, is the difficulty in obtaining stool samples in infants with ileus secondary to NEC.

The Application of High-Throughput Data and Large-Scale Data to NEC Biomarker Discovery

Advances in the fields of transcriptomics, proteomics, and metabolomics, offer a huge promise for medical research and biomarker discovery.[81] By understanding how each level of gene and protein regulation is involved in NEC, the identification of key disease biomarkers and therapeutic targets will be much more attainable.

Table 3
Fecal biomarkers for potential biomarkers of NEC

Biomarker	Strengths	Limitation
Calprotectin	• Fecal levels elevated in NEC.[55,69–71] • Most recent meta-analysis which included 528 patients showed a pooled sensitivity of 86% and specificity of 79%.[72]	Variability in the levels in normal infants, limiting its value as a screening tool for NEC.[73]
S100A12	• In a prospective study of 145 preterm infants, levels were significantly higher in NEC infants (n = 18) at the time of diagnosis, with a sensitivity of 67% and a specificity of 78%.[74] • Correlated with increase in the total bacterial/E. coli count[75]	Limited studies.
Volatile Organic compounds (VOC)	• VOC profiles can discriminate infants with NEC from controls, days before the onset of disease.[76] • Promising noninvasive tool for early screening and detection of NEC.[77]	Limited studies.
Fecal miRNA	• Fecal miR- 223 and miR-451 significantly higher in NEC than non-NEC.[78–80]	Low specificity and Positive predictive value.

Transcriptomics: identification of necrotizing enterocolitis biomarkers on the RNA level

Much headway has been made in using host transcriptomes as potential biomarkers in NEC. Several studies support miRNA as sentinel markers for NEC progression. miRNA are 18 to 24 nucleotide small noncoding RNAs that bind specific mRNAs to posttranscriptionally inhibit gene expression. A large-scale meta-analysis using the NIH GEO database miRNA chips showed that miRNA-429/200a/b and miRNA-141/200c clusters were poorly expressed in intestinal tissues from 4 newborns with NEC compared with 4 controls.[82] Ng and colleagues,[83] identified elevated plasma miR-1290 as a potential biomarker that can differentiate NEC from neonatal sepsis with high sensitivity, specificity, and predictive values. Finally, miR-431 and the target gene Forkhead Box A1 (FOXA1) in intestinal tissues of NEC infants predicted surgical versus medical management of NEC.[84] The authors later confirmed that the miR-431-FOXA1 axis plays a role in the intensification of the inflammatory response and potentially contributes to the proinflammatory pathophysiology in NEC. These studies highlight the role of transcriptomics in biomarker discovery and advancing our understanding of the pathogenesis of NEC.

Table 4
Proteomic studies evaluating potential markers for the diagnosis of NEC

Proteomic Studies	Description	Results
Murgas Torrazza et al.[86]	• Preterm infants with BW <1250g, GA <32 wks enrolled and followed for radiologic evidence of NEC (n = 10) vs matched controls (n = 10). • Buccal swabs at 2 and 3 weeks, before NEC development.	• IL-1RA is decreased before NEC onset.
Sylvester et al.[87]	• A proteomic cohort study of urine samples from premature infants with NEC or Late-onset sepsis (LOS). • Urine was obtained from premature infants (85 NEC, 17 LOS, 17 control) at the time of initial clinical concern for NEC or sepsis.	• A panel of seven urine biomarkers (alpha-2-macroglobulin-like protein 1, cluster of differentiation protein 14, cystatin 3, fibrinogen alpha chain, pigment epithelium-derived factor, retinol-binding protein 4, and vasolin) was identified for distinguishing NEC vs Sepsis (AUC 0.98) and medical NEC vs surgical NEC (AUC 0.98).
Stewart et al.[88,89]	• Case-control study with proteomic analysis of serum from preterm infants with NEC and LOS • Serum obtained ± 2 wk surrounding and at time of diagnosis from NEC/LOS cases matched with controls • NEC/LOS cases (n = 10) matched with controls (n = 9) serum underwent proteomic (LC-MS/MS) and metabolomic analysis	• Panel of 8 serum NEC-associated proteins was identified (CRP, macrophage migration inhibitory factor, serum amyloid A-2 protein, TGF-β induced protein ig-h3, ant others.) • Panel of 4 serum LOS-associated proteins was identified (Haptoglobin, transthyretin, U5 small nuclear ribonucleoprotein 200 kDa helicase, and Isoform XK of plasma membrane calcium transporting ATPase 4).

Proteomics: the study of protein expression in necrotizing enterocolitis biomarker discovery

Proteomics is the study of the whole proteome or all the proteins from a tissue, cell, or from a biological fluid. Jiang and colleagues[85] conducted a proteomic analysis of tissues from the small intestine and colon of preterm infants with NEC. They showed that heat shock proteins (HSPA5 and HSP27), histamine receptor, cytoskeletal proteins, among other acute phase reactants to be differentially expressed in NEC versus controls. Other compelling studies in the past 15 years have since identified candidate

Table 5
Metabolomics studies evaluating diagnostic markers for NEC

Metabolomic Studies	Description	Results
Morrow et al.[90]	• Cohort study of 32 early preterm (<29 wk) infants and <1200g of which 11 developed NEC (Bell's Stage II, III) and 21 matched controls. • Stool samples underwent bacterial microbiome analysis with 16S rRNA gene sequencing. • Urine metabolomic profiles were assessed by NMR.	• Infants who developed NEC had lower microbiome diversity with 2 distinct phenotypes, one predominately proteobacteria and the other firmicutes. • No metabolites distinguished NEC from controls. • Alanine, pyridoxine, and histidine distinguished suspected NEC (NEC stage I) from II. • A high alanine/histidine ratio was associated with dysbiosis and NEC.
Sylvester et al.[91]	• Retrospective cohort study using 94,110 state newborn screening samples (744 NEC, 93,366 controls) of preterm infants <37 wks for model development over 4 y from 2005 to 2008. • Subsequent validated with preterm infants born (22,992 infants).	• Acylcarnitine profiles in combination with patient characteristics (birth weight and parenteral nutrition) were able to predict NEC with AUC 0.89.
Rusconi et al.[92]	• A case-control study with stool 1–5 days before NEC onset, 9 cases (Bell's Stage ≥ II NEC), and 19 matched controls.	• Differences in certain ceramides and sphingolipids were evident in NEC Bell's Stage I vs II/III, which had 73% accuracy for NEC classification by machine learning and hierarchical clustering. • Limitation includes high false positives and failure to encompass many NEC cases.
Thomaidou et al.[93]	• A case-control study with urine collected on day 1 of suspected NEC from NEC preterm infants. • Samples were analyzed by H1 NMR (nontargeted acquisition) and Hydrophilic interaction chromatography (HILICLC-MS/MS) (targeted acquisition).	• Prical component analysis and clustering of metabolites revealed significant changes in NEC infants, and ultimately a panel of 25 metabolites with 3 in particular (*Tyrosine, Arginine, and Riboflavin*) holding most potential as NEC biomarkers.

biomarkers in NEC using numerous source samples and tissues from preterm. Four of those pilot studies are described in **Table 4**.

Metabolomics: a promising new area for biomarker discovery
Metabolomics is the science of detecting small molecules, the result of metabolic pathways from biological specimens such as plasma, serum, urine, and tissues. Metabolomic studies in NEC remain limited to a few small case-control or cohort evaluations. The general conclusions are that no single metabolic biomarker or pathway will be sufficient to predict NEC susceptibility, disease staging, or disease management. Rather, most likely a panel of metabolites or a certain metabolomic signature will be required if a highly sensitive and specific biomarker is to be developed. Here, we highlight a handful of metabolomic studies over the past decade in **Table 5**.

SUMMARY AND FUTURE DIRECTIONS

NEC remains one of the most common causes of mortality and morbidity in preterm infants. Advances in large-scale -omics data and bioinformatic processing hold great promise for the future development of biomarkers for NEC. In addition to predicting NEC susceptibility, these biomarkers, together with the clinical data, have the potential to guide disease stratification, distinguishing NEC from non-NEC entities, and may even predict pharmacologic versus surgical management. Using the data and samples collected from the recently established NEC biorepository will likely facilitate and accelerate the basic and translational studies94. The data presented here is telling of the need for a combination approach in predicting NEC development, staging, and treatment. Probably, refined panels of proteins or genes in combination with clinical data will ultimately prevail as effective biomarkers for NEC instead of a single marker alone.

Best Practices

- Although investigations continue for biomarkers of NEC, widespread clinical application of these markers is limited.

- Clinicians should be aware of the limitation in using the current definitions for NEC including Bell's staging for the diagnosis of NEC, particularly its inability to differentiate classical/ preterm NEC from other neonatal intestinal injury or inflammation.

- Advances in the fields of transcriptomics, proteomics, and metabolomics, hold promised for the future. However, high-powered studies will be required to examine whether those newly discovered markers have a role in the diagnosis or prognosis of NEC.

DISCLOSURE

Hala Chaaban is supported by P20GM134973 from the National Institutes of Health. The content is solely the responsibility of the authors and does not represent the official views of the National Institutes of Health.

REFERENCES

1. Neu J, Walker WA. Necrotizing enterocolitis. N Engl J Med 2011;364(3):255–64.
2. Holman RC, Stoll BJ, Curns AT, et al. Necrotising enterocolitis hospitalisations among neonates in the United States. Paediatr Perinat Epidemiol 2006;20(6): 498–506.
3. Bazacliu C, Neu J. Necrotizing enterocolitis: long term complications. Curr Pediatr Rev 2019;15(2):115–24.

4. Federici S, De Biagi L. Long term outcome of infants with NEC. Curr Pediatr Rev 2019;15(2):111–4.

5. Stoll BJ, Hansen NI, Bell EF, et al. Neonatal outcomes of extremely preterm infants from the NICHD Neonatal Research Network. Pediatrics 2010;126(3):443–56.

6. Shah TA, Meinzen-Derr J, Gratton T, et al. Hospital and neurodevelopmental outcomes of extremely low-birth-weight infants with necrotizing enterocolitis and spontaneous intestinal perforation. J Perinatol 2012;32(7):552–8.

7. Eaton S, Rees CM, Hall NJ. Current research in necrotizing enterocolitis. Early Hum Dev 2016;97:33–9.

8. D'Angelo G, Impellizzeri P, Marseglia L, et al. Current status of laboratory and imaging diagnosis of neonatal necrotizing enterocolitis. Ital J Pediatr 2018;44(1):84.

9. Strimbu K, Tavel JA. What are biomarkers? Curr Opin HIV AIDS 2010;5(6):463–6.

10. Gordon PV, Swanson JR, Attridge JT, et al. Emerging trends in acquired neonatal intestinal disease: is it time to abandon Bell's criteria? J Perinatol 2007;27(11):661–71.

11. Biomarkers and surrogate endpoints: preferred definitions and conceptual framework. Clin Pharmacol Ther 2001;69(3):89–95.

12. Caplan MS, Underwood MA, Modi N, et al. Necrotizing enterocolitis: using regulatory science and drug development to improve outcomes. J Pediatr 2019;212:208–15.e201.

13. Giannone PJ, Luce WA, Nankervis CA, et al. Necrotizing enterocolitis in neonates with congenital heart disease. Life Sci 2008;82(7):341–7.

14. Torrazza RM, Li N, Neu J. Decoding the enigma of necrotizing enterocolitis in premature infants. Pathophysiology 2014;21(1):21–7.

15. Patel RM, Ferguson J, McElroy SJ, et al. Defining necrotizing enterocolitis: current difficulties and future opportunities. Pediatr Res 2020;88(Suppl 1):10–5.

16. Gordon PV, Swanson JR. Necrotizing enterocolitis is one disease with many origins and potential means of prevention. Pathophysiology 2014;21(1):13–9.

17. Lueschow SR, Boly TJ, Jasper E, et al. A critical evaluation of current definitions of necrotizing enterocolitis. Pediatr Res 2021. https://doi.org/10.1038/s41390-021-01570-y.

18. Ng PC, Ma TPY, Lam HS. The use of laboratory biomarkers for surveillance, diagnosis and prediction of clinical outcomes in neonatal sepsis and necrotising enterocolitis. Arch Dis Child Fetal Neonatal Ed 2015;100(5):F448–52.

19. Ng PC. Biomarkers of necrotising enterocolitis. Semin Fetal Neonatal Med 2014;19(1):33–8.

20. Ng PC. An update on biomarkers of necrotizing enterocolitis. Semin Fetal neonatal Med 2018;23(6):380–6.

21. Gordon PV, Swanson JR, Clark R, et al. The complete blood cell count in a refined cohort of preterm NEC: the importance of gestational age and day of diagnosis when using the CBC to estimate mortality. J Perinatology 2016;36(2):121–5.

22. Garg PM, O'Connor A, Ansari MAY, et al. Hematological predictors of mortality in neonates with fulminant necrotizing enterocolitis. J Perinatology 2021;41(5):1110–21.

23. Remon J, Kampanatkosol R, Kaul RR, et al. Acute drop in blood monocyte count differentiates NEC from other causes of feeding intolerance. J Perinatology 2014;34(7):549–54.

24. Ragazzi S, Pierro A, Peters M, et al. Early full blood count and severity of disease in neonates with necrotizing enterocolitis. Pediatr Surg Int 2003;19(5):376–9.

25. Pourcyrous M, Korones SB, Yang W, et al. C-reactive protein in the diagnosis, management, and prognosis of neonatal necrotizing enterocolitis. Pediatrics 2005;116(5):1064–9.
26. Cetinkaya M, Ozkan H, Köksal N, et al. Comparison of the efficacy of serum amyloid A, C-reactive protein, and procalcitonin in the diagnosis and follow-up of necrotizing enterocolitis in premature infants. J Pediatr Surg 2011;46(8):1482–9.
27. Turner D, Hammerman C, Rudensky B, et al. Low levels of procalcitonin during episodes of necrotizing enterocolitis. Dig Dis Sci 2007;52(11):2972–6.
28. Maheshwari A, Schelonka RL, Dimmitt RA, et al. Cytokines associated with necrotizing enterocolitis in extremely-low-birth-weight infants. Pediatr Res 2014;76(1): 100–8.
29. Benkoe T, Baumann S, Weninger M, et al. Comprehensive evaluation of 11 cytokines in premature infants with surgical necrotizing enterocolitis. PLoS One 2013; 8(3):e58720.
30. Terrin G, Stronati L, Cucchiara S, et al. Serum markers of necrotizing enterocolitis: a systematic review. J Pediatr Gastroenterol Nutr 2017;65(6):e120–32.
31. Cheng S, Yu J, Zhou M, et al. Serologic intestinal-fatty acid binding protein in necrotizing enterocolitis diagnosis: a meta-analysis. Biomed Res Int 2015;2015: 156704.
32. Luo J, Li HP, Xu F, et al. Early diagnosis of necrotizing enterocolitis by plasma RELMβ and thrombocytopenia in preterm infants: a pilot study. Pediatr Neonatol 2019;60(4):447–52.
33. Maheshwari A. Immunologic and hematological abnormalities in necrotizing enterocolitis. Clin Perinatol 2015;42(3):567–85.
34. Mohd Amin AT, Zaki RA, Friedmacher F, et al. C-reactive protein/albumin ratio is a prognostic indicator for predicting surgical intervention and mortality in neonates with necrotizing enterocolitis. Pediatr Surg Int 2021;37(7):881–6.
35. Edelson MB, Bagwell CE, Rozycki HJ. Circulating pro- and counterinflammatory cytokine levels and severity in necrotizing enterocolitis. Pediatrics 1999;103(4 Pt 1):766–71.
36. Tayman C, Tonbul A, Kahveci H, et al. C5a, a complement activation product, is a useful marker in predicting the severity of necrotizing enterocolitis. Tohoku J Exp Med 2011;224(2):143–50.
37. Chaaban H, Shin M, Sirya E, et al. Inter-alpha inhibitor protein level in neonates predicts necrotizing enterocolitis. J Pediatr 2010;157(5):757–61.
38. Shah BA, Migliori A, Kurihara I, et al. Blood level of inter-alpha inhibitor proteins distinguishes necrotizing enterocolitis from spontaneous intestinal perforation. J Pediatr 2017;180:135–40.e1.
39. Yang G, Wang Y, Jiang X. Diagnostic value of intestinal fatty-acid-binding protein in necrotizing enterocolitis: a systematic review and meta-analysis. Indian J Pediatr 2016;83(12–13):1410–9.
40. Heida FH, Hulscher JB, Schurink M, et al. Intestinal fatty acid-binding protein levels in Necrotizing Enterocolitis correlate with extent of necrotic bowel: results from a multicenter study. J Pediatr Surg 2015;50(7):1115–8.
41. Yakut I, Tayman C, Oztekin O, et al. Ischemia-modified albumin may be a novel marker for the diagnosis and follow-up of necrotizing enterocolitis. J Clin Lab Anal 2014;28(3):170–7.
42. Cetinkaya M, Ozkan H, Köksal N, et al. The efficacy of serial serum amyloid A measurements for diagnosis and follow-up of necrotizing enterocolitis in premature infants. Pediatr Surg Int 2010;26(8):835–41.

43. Sylvester KG, Moss RL. Urine biomarkers for necrotizing enterocolitis. Pediatr Surg Int 2015;31(5):421–9.
44. Harpole M, Davis J, Espina V. Current state of the art for enhancing urine biomarker discovery. Expert Rev Proteomics 2016;13(6):609–26.
45. Bakhoum CY, Basalely A, Koppel RI, et al. Acute kidney injury in preterm infants with necrotizing enterocolitis. J Matern Fetal Neonatal Med 2019;32(19):3185–90.
46. Schurink M, Kooi EM, Hulzebos CV, et al. Intestinal fatty acid-binding protein as a diagnostic marker for complicated and uncomplicated necrotizing enterocolitis: a prospective cohort study. PLoS One 2015;10(3):e0121336.
47. Coufal S, Kokesova A, Tlaskalova-Hogenova H, et al. Urinary intestinal fatty acid-binding protein can distinguish necrotizing enterocolitis from sepsis in early stage of the disease. J Immunol Res 2016;2016:5727312.
48. Evennett NJ, Hall NJ, Pierro A, et al. Urinary intestinal fatty acid–binding protein concentration predicts extent of disease in necrotizing enterocolitis. J Pediatr Surg 2010;45(4):735–40.
49. Reisinger KW, Derikx JPM, Thuijls G, et al. Noninvasive measurement of intestinal epithelial damage at time of refeeding can predict clinical outcome after necrotizing enterocolitis. Pediatr Res 2013;73(2):209–13.
50. Okada K, Sekino M, Funaoka H, et al. Intestinal fatty acid-binding protein levels in patients with chronic renal failure. J Surg Res 2018;230:94–100.
51. Coufal S, Kokesova A, Tlaskalova-Hogenova H, et al. Urinary I-FABP, L-FABP, TFF-3, and SAA can diagnose and predict the disease course in necrotizing enterocolitis at the early stage of disease. J Immunol Res 2020;2020:3074313.
52. Reisinger KW, Kramer BW, Van der Zee DC, et al. Non-Invasive Serum Amyloid A (SAA) measurement and plasma platelets for accurate prediction of surgical intervention in severe necrotizing enterocolitis (NEC). PLoS One 2014;9(3): e90834.
53. Niemarkt HJ, de Meij TG, van de Velde ME, et al. Necrotizing enterocolitis: a clinical review on diagnostic biomarkers and the role of the intestinal microbiota. Inflamm Bowel Dis 2015;21(2):436–44.
54. Blackwood BP, Wood DR, Yuan CY, et al. Urinary claudin-2 measurements as a predictor of necrotizing enterocolitis: a pilot study. J Neonatal Surg 2015;4(4):43.
55. Thuijls G, Derikx JPM, van Wijck K, et al. Non-invasive markers for early diagnosis and determination of the severity of necrotizing enterocolitis. Ann Surg 2010; 251(6):1174–80.
56. Konishi KI, Yoshida M, Nakao A, et al. Prostaglandin E-major urinary metabolite as a noninvasive surrogate marker for infantile necrotizing enterocolitis. J Pediatr Surg 2019;54(8):1584–9.
57. Arai Y, Matsuura T, Matsuura M, et al. Prostaglandin E-major urinary metabolite as a biomarker for inflammation in ulcerative colitis: prostaglandins revisited. Digestion 2016;93(1):32–9.
58. Gajda AM, Storch J. Enterocyte fatty acid-binding proteins (FABPs): different functions of liver and intestinal FABPs in the intestine. Prostaglandins Leukot Essent Fatty Acids 2015;93:9–16.
59. Guilmeau S, Niot I, Laigneau JP, et al. Decreased expression of Intestinal I- and L-FABP levels in rare human genetic lipid malabsorption syndromes. Histochem Cell Biol 2007;128(2):115–23.
60. van de Poll MC, Derikx JP, Buurman WA, et al. Liver manipulation causes hepatocyte injury and precedes systemic inflammation in patients undergoing liver resection. World J Surg 2007;31(10):2033–8.

61. Shores DR, Fundora J, Go M, et al. Normative values for circulating intestinal fatty acid binding protein and calprotectin across gestational ages. BMC Pediatr 2020;20(1):250.
62. Derikx JPM, Evennett NJ, Degraeuwe PLJ, et al. Urine based detection of intestinal mucosal cell damage in neonates with suspected necrotising enterocolitis. Gut 2007;56(10):1473–5.
63. Gollin G, Stadie D, Mayhew J, et al. Early detection of impending necrotizing enterocolitis with urinary intestinal fatty acid-binding protein. Neonatology 2014; 106(3):195–200.
64. Goldstein GP, Sylvester KG. Biomarker discovery and utility in necrotizing enterocolitis. Clin Perinatol 2019;46(1):1–17.
65. Aamann L, Vestergaard EM, Grønbæk H. Trefoil factors in inflammatory bowel disease. World J Gastroenterol 2014;20(12):3223–30.
66. Griffiths V, Al Assaf N, Khan R. Review of claudin proteins as potential biomarkers for necrotizing enterocolitis. Irish J Med Sci 2021;190(4):1465–72.
67. Ishida N, Miyazu T, Takano R, et al. Prostaglandin E-major urinary metabolite versus fecal immunochemical occult blood test as a biomarker for patient with ulcerative colitis. BMC Gastroenterol 2020;20(1):114.
68. Lehmann FS, Burri E, Beglinger C. The role and utility of faecal markers in inflammatory bowel disease. Ther Adv Gastroenterol 2015;8(1):23–36.
69. Aydemir O, Aydemir C, Sarikabadayi YU, et al. Fecal calprotectin levels are increased in infants with necrotizing enterocolitis. J Matern Fetal Neonatal Me 2012;25(11):2237–41.
70. Reisinger KW, Van der Zee DC, Brouwers HA, et al. Noninvasive measurement of fecal calprotectin and serum amyloid A combined with intestinal fatty acid-binding protein in necrotizing enterocolitis. J Pediatr Surg 2012;47(9):1640–5.
71. MacQueen BC, Christensen RD, Yost CC, et al. Elevated fecal calprotectin levels during necrotizing enterocolitis are associated with activated neutrophils extruding neutrophil extracellular traps. J Perinatol 2016;36(10):862–9.
72. Qu Y, Xu W, Han J, et al. Diagnostic value of fecal calprotectin in necrotizing enterocolitis: a meta-analysis. Early Hum Dev 2020;151:105170.
73. van Zoonen A, Hulzebos CV, Muller Kobold AC, et al. Serial fecal calprotectin in the prediction of necrotizing enterocolitis in preterm neonates. J Pediatr Surg 2019;54(3):455–9.
74. Däbritz J, Jenke A, Wirth S, et al. Fecal phagocyte-specific S100A12 for diagnosing necrotizing enterocolitis. J Pediatr 2012;161(6):1059–64.
75. Jenke AC, Postberg J, Mariel B, et al. S100A12 and hBD2 correlate with the composition of the fecal microflora in ELBW infants and expansion of E. coli is associated with NEC. Biomed Res Int 2013;2013:150372.
76. Garner CE, Ewer AK, Elasouad K, et al. Analysis of faecal volatile organic compounds in preterm infants who develop necrotising enterocolitis: a pilot study. J Pediatr Gastroenterol Nutr 2009;49(5):559–65.
77. Probert C, Greenwood R, Mayor A, et al. Faecal volatile organic compounds in preterm babies at risk of necrotising enterocolitis: the DOVE study. Arch Dis Child Fetal Neonatal Ed 2020;105(5):474–9.
78. Ng PC, Chan KYY, Lam HS, et al. A prospective cohort study of fecal miR-223 and miR-451a as noninvasive and specific biomarkers for diagnosis of necrotizing enterocolitis in preterm infants. Neonatology 2020;117(5):555–61.
79. de Meij TG, de Boer NK, Benninga MA, et al. Faecal gas analysis by electronic nose as novel, non-invasive method for assessment of active and quiescent

paediatric inflammatory bowel disease: proof of principle study. J Crohns Colitis 2014. https://doi.org/10.1016/j.crohns.2014.09.004.

80. Course CW, Watkins J, Muller C, et al. Volatile organic compounds as disease predictors in newborn infants: a systematic review. J Breath Res 2021. https://doi.org/10.1088/1752-7163/abe283.

81. Pinu FR, Beale DJ, Paten AM, et al. Systems biology and multi-omics integration: viewpoints from the metabolomics research community. Metabolites 2019; 9(4):76.

82. Liu H, Wang YB. Systematic large-scale meta-analysis identifies miRNA-429/200a/b and miRNA-141/200c clusters as biomarkers for necrotizing enterocolitis in newborn. Biosci Rep 2019;39(9). BSR20191503.

83. Ng PC, Chan KYY, Yuen TP, et al. Plasma miR-1290 is a novel and specific biomarker for early diagnosis of necrotizing enterocolitis-biomarker discovery with prospective cohort evaluation. J Pediatr 2019;205:83–90.e10.

84. Wu YZ, Chan KYY, Leung KT, et al. Dysregulation of miR-431 and target gene FOXA1 in intestinal tissues of infants with necrotizing enterocolitis. FASEB J 2019;33(4):5143–52.

85. Jiang P, Smith B, Qvist N, et al. Intestinal proteome changes during infant necrotizing enterocolitis. Pediatr Res 2013;73(3):268–76.

86. Murgas Torrazza R, Li N, Young C, et al. Pilot study using proteomics to identify predictive biomarkers of necrotizing enterocolitis from buccal swabs in very low birth weight infants. Neonatology 2013;104(3):234–42.

87. Sylvester KG, Ling XB, Liu GY, et al. Urine protein biomarkers for the diagnosis and prognosis of necrotizing enterocolitis in infants. J Pediatr 2014;164(3):607–12.e1-7.

88. Stewart CJ, Nelson A, Treumann A, et al. Metabolomic and proteomic analysis of serum from preterm infants with necrotising entercolitis and late-onset sepsis. Pediatr Res 2016;79(3):425–31.

89. Chatziioannou AC, Wolters JC, Sarafidis K, et al. Targeted LC-MS/MS for the evaluation of proteomics biomarkers in the blood of neonates with necrotizing enterocolitis and late-onset sepsis. Anal Bioanal Chem 2018;410(27):7163–75.

90. Morrow AL, Lagomarcino AJ, Schibler KR, et al. Early microbial and metabolomic signatures predict later onset of necrotizing enterocolitis in preterm infants. Microbiome 2013;1(1):13.

91. Sylvester KG, Kastenberg ZJ, Moss RL, et al. Acylcarnitine profiles reflect metabolic vulnerability for necrotizing enterocolitis in newborns born premature. J Pediatr 2017;181:80–5.e81.

92. Rusconi B, Jiang X, Sidhu R, et al. Gut sphingolipid composition as a prelude to necrotizing enterocolitis. Sci Rep 2018;8(1):10984.

93. Thomaidou A, Chatziioannou AC, Deda O, et al. A pilot case-control study of urine metabolomics in preterm neonates with necrotizing enterocolitis. J Chromatogr B Analyt Technol Biomed Life Sci 2019;1117:10–21.

94.. Chaaban Hala, Markel Troy, Canvasser Jenifer, et al. Biobanking for necrotizing enterocolitis: Needs and standards. J Pediatr Surg 2020;55(7):1276–9. https://doi.org/10.1016/j.jpedsurg.2019.05.002.

Prevention of Necrotizing Enterocolitis

Josef Neu, MD

KEYWORDS

- Gestational age • Necrotizing enterocolitis • Neonatal • Preterm

INTRODUCTION AND HISTORICAL PERSPECTIVE

Necrotizing enterocolitis (NEC) is considered to be one of the most devastating intestinal diseases seen in neonatal intensive care.[1–3] Measures to treat NEC are often too late, and we need effective preventative measures to alleviate the burden of this disease. The purpose of this review is to summarize currently used measures, and those showing future promise for prevention.

Any discussion related to preventative measures against NEC needs to take into account the caveat that what is termed "NEC" represents different forms of intestinal injury with different pathophysiology.[4] Preventative measures that would work for one may not work for others. Certainly spontaneous intestinal perforations, cardiogenic ischemic intestinal injury, and food protein intolerance are different entities but may present in a very similar manner with signs and symptoms of intestinal necrosis. The different "stages" of NEC[5] also may be readily misunderstood. Stage 1 represents a set of signs and symptoms that can be seen in most extremely-low-birth-weight infants, and hence does not actually represent a discrete disease process. Some of the signs of NEC that are seen in preterm infants, such as pneumatosis intestinalis and portal venous gas, can readily be misread[6] and also be seen in older children and adults,[7,8] thus they may not be as helpful in defining a specific intestinal disease largely seen in preterm infants. Nevertheless, when seen in older children or adults, these also usually represent some form of intestinal injury, but the inciting causes can be broad. It also needs mention that it remains controversial whether studies in animals have shed light on the pathophysiology of the versions of NEC that seem to be most common in preterm infants.[9,10] Thus extrapolation from studies in animals that involve prevention may often be misleading.

From this, the reader should be cognizant of the fact that what is termed "NEC" likely represents different disease entities. We are struggling with clear definitions. Although the different forms of intestinal injury referred to as "NEC" are likely to be differentiated using newly developing technologies such as artificial intelligence, machine learning, and multiomics, such delineations are currently not clearly available. Thus, herein, the "NEC" that we discuss likely represents an amalgamation of several

University of Florida, Gainesville, FL, USA
E-mail address: neuj@peds.ufl.edu

Clin Perinatol 49 (2022) 195–206
https://doi.org/10.1016/j.clp.2021.11.012
0095-5108/22/© 2021 Elsevier Inc. All rights reserved.

of these entities because it is difficult to separate these from within currently available databases or with readily available sensitive and specific biomarkers.

The information provided here, albeit crude because of the aforementioned short-comings, attempts to summarize some currently available issues related to the prevention of "NEC." These issues involve feeding practices, composition of feedings, use of antibiotics and acid suppressor therapies, transfusion practices, and manipulation of the intestinal microbial environment. There are numerous other inter-ventional strategies that have been proposed and studied including use of immuno-therapeutic agents, growth factors, and amino and fatty acids, which we will not be able to discuss in any detail. After summarizing some of the currently available mea-sures and those currently under investigation that show promise, we try to glimpse into the future where rapidly developing technologies may lead to earlier detection and prevention of various forms of intestinal injury that are now called "NEC."

FEEDING PRACTICES

A major factor in terms of feeding regimens requires consideration that not all preterm infants are the same—they are not "one size fits all"—or in other words, one nutritional regimen or guideline will be perfectly suited to every preterm infant. For example, an infant born at 24 weeks' gestation is very different in terms of intestinal maturity and metabolic capability than one born at 32 weeks' gestation. Furthermore, infants born at appropriate size for gestational age may differ markedly that those born intra-uterine growth restricted or large for gestational age.

One of the most vexing concerns of neonatologists caring for preterm infants is how fast to advance feedings in preterm babies.[12] Those born at less than approximately 34 weeks' gestation have uncoordinated suck swallow mechanisms and need to be fed by a tube. Because of various immaturities of the developing gastrointestinal (GI) tract, it is assumed that the immature intestine is not able to tolerate appreciable volumes or advancement of feeding volumes. Because of this, it was common practice in many neonatal intensive care units to withhold enteral feedings for several days and sometimes even weeks in these very preterm infants. Many excuses to withhold or use extremely slow advancement of enteral feedings are given. These excuses include the use of me-chanical ventilation, medications such as indomethacin, the presence of umbilical lines, and any form of instability in the infant. We have no solid evidence to support any of these reasons to not feed or stop feedings when they occur. The fact that parenteral nutrition is available does not mean it is a qualified substitute for enteral nutrition.[13]

While these practices were or still are ongoing in neonatal intensive care units, various studies show that the absence of nutrients in the GI tract, even with provision of parenteral nutrition, lead to intestinal mucosal atrophy, with a lack of bioactive in-testinal peptide production and liver injury.[14,15] Enteral feedings also stimulate various hormonal secretions as well as the motility of the GI tract that leads to propulsion of food and waste products aborally.[16–18]

Furthermore, studies suggest that a lack of enteral feeding was actually associated with decreased mesenteric artery blood flow[19] and a shift toward an intestinal micro-bial ecosystem during enteral fasting that is more like that seen before the develop-ment of intestinal injuries such as NEC.[20]

Furthermore, the fetal GI tract is not dormant. In utero, the fetus constantly swallows amniotic fluid; this along with sloughed epithelium, bile, and amniotic fluid solids con-tributes to the formation of meconium. The amniotic fluid also contains nutrients that may also play an important role in growth and development of GI tract.[21] Similarly, one would not expect the preterm infant intestinal tract to be dormant or inactive.

NEC in preterm infants usually occurs a few weeks after birth. The timing relates to gestational age at birth peaking at a corrected gestational age between 29 and 32 weeks.[22] At the time of diagnosis of NEC, most preterm infants have received enteral feeding. Owing to the concern that NEC may be associated with rapid advancement of enteral feeding[23] it was common practice for neonatologists to delay initiating enteral feedings and providing a very slow rate of advancement of enteral feeding.

Based on emerging evidence of the benefits of at least small quantities of enteral feedings, to minimize feeding intolerance and the risk of developing NEC in preterm infants, the practice of "minimal enteral nutrition" was developed. Considered as an alternative to complete fasting, minimal enteral nutrition, sometimes called "trophic feeds," "trickle feeds," or "priming," is usually started within the first few days after delivery.[15] Volumes can range from a few milliliters to approximately 20 mL/kg/d of milk given every 2 to 3 hours and continued for approximately the first week after birth.

A Cochrane systematic review of the literature compared the effect of minimal enteral nutrition to enteral fasting on feeding intolerance, growth, incidence of NEC, and mortality in 754 very-low-birth-weight infants. In this review, "enteral fasting" was nothing per mouth for at least 1 week after birth. This study showed no differences in the risk of developing NEC, time to achieve full feeds, or duration of hospital stay.[24] A subsequent Cochrane review compared fast versus slow rates of feeding advancement on the incidence of NEC, mortality, or other morbidities. This study did not provide evidence that advancing volumes at daily increments of 15 to 20 mL/kg compared with 30 to 40 mL/kg reduces the risk of NEC or death in this population of very-low-birth-weight or extremely-low-birth-weight infants. However, advancing the volume of enteral feeds at a slow rate also resulted in several days of delay in establishing full enteral feeds. The authors of this review[24] urged the need for randomized controlled trial to determine how trophic feeding compared with enteral fasting affects important outcomes in this population.

Such a randomized trial was completed in the United Kingdom. This trial showed that a more rapid advancement of feeds (30–35 mL/kg/d when compared with 15–20 mL/kg/d) does not increase the incidence of NEC in preterm infants.[25]

Other feeding practices have been evaluated to determine whether continuous versus intermittent tube feedings might decrease NEC. At this time, there is no evidence supporting continuous over intermittent tube feedings in preterm infants.[26]

Some studies showed potentially detrimental effects of delaying enteral feedings. In one such study, infants who had feedings initiated before 4 days after birth compared with greater than 4 days had greater adverse outcomes such as bronchopulmonary dysplasia, retinopathy of prematurity, and an increased trend toward the development of NEC. The infants also had higher concentrations of plasma proinflammatory mediators at 2 weeks after birth.[27]

Evaluation of feeding intolerance is considered an important marker for the development of NEC. However, at this time, there is no clear evidence-based definition of feeding intolerance. Even though the practice of routinely measuring gastric residuals before feedings was at one time a common practice in neonatal intensive care, this has been found to be an unnecessary practice.[28]

COMPOSITION OF FEEDINGS: HUMAN MILK, DONOR MILK, FORTIFICATION, MEDICATIONS

Several aspects of feeding composition relate to NEC. One of the most pertinent is the use of human milk. Since the studies of Lucas and Cole[29] several additional studies have supported the use of human milk in the prevention of NEC.[30] One meta-analysis of a large number of studies suggested that donor milk might only be effective in the prevention of NEC if some of the baby's own mother's milk is provided.[31] However, it has also become clear that some of the components of human milk may not meet the requirements of many preterm infants. Several studies have suggested better growth of preterm infants on formulas with higher concentrations of these components when compared with human milk. Human donor milk, especially, when pasteurized and banked loses many bioactive, including immunomodulatory, components[32,33] that are present in fresh baby's own mother's milk. Although prospective randomized controlled studies are lacking, the available evidence supports the use of the baby's own mother's milk over that of formula and pooled donor milk.

There are several fortifiers available for human milk to enhance the protein, mineral, and lipid composition.[34] Although several studies have suggested that a human milk-based fortifier may provide some advantages over a bovine-based fortifier, the evidence remains controversial.[35]

Most preterm formulas currently available attempt to mimic and even improve on the composition of human milk with respect to energy, protein, and lipids as well as micronutrients needed for the growth and development of preterm infants. However, there remain major differences. These formulas do not provide the highly bioactive components of human milk such as secretory IgA, lysozyme, lipase, alkaline phosphatase, human milk oligosaccharides, polyunsaturated fatty acids, and platelet-activating factor-acetyl hydrolase.[36] These components of human milk contribute to GI mucosal integrity and function and provide immunity against various infections, but their effect when administered without the overall human milk matrix needs elucidation. These components require evaluation as a system rather than as individual additives to nonhuman milk preparations.[37]

Data support that human milk also provides long-term benefits in term infants. These benefits include lowered sudden infant death syndrome; childhood infectious diseases such as respiratory tract infections, otitis media, and GI infection; as well as allergic diseases, celiac disease, inflammatory bowel disease, and obesity.[38] Preterm infants may also benefit from the nonnutritive bioactive components of human milk by reduced susceptibility to sepsis or to NEC.[39,40] These putative benefits for the most part are based on conjecture because there are currently no prospective randomized controlled studies comparing the effect of mother's own milk with formula on the incidence of NEC and mortality.

Several studies evaluated the effect of donor human milk versus formula on the incidence of NEC and mortality in preterm infants. Meta-analysis of trials comparing donor milk versus formula feeds in preterm infants showed that preterm infants fed with formula had a higher incidence of NEC.[41] Another retrospective analysis showed decreased NEC in babies fed donor milk or their own mothers' milk compared with formula.[42] These results seem to underscore the importance of human milk intake in preterm infants. However, these studies are fraught with confounders, and are not prospective randomized controlled trials adequately powered to evaluate NEC as the major outcome.

The American Academy of Pediatrics (AAP) policy statement in 2012 on breastfeeding and the use of human milk recommends human milk for term, preterm, and other high-risk infants, and this should be supplied either by direct breastfeeding and/or by expressed breast milk. The AAP statement also indicated that donor human milk might be a suitable alternative for infants whose mothers are unable or unwilling to provide their own milk.[43]

MILK FORTIFIERS AND NECROTIZING ENTEROCOLITIS

Even at full enteral feeds (200 mL/kg/d), the protein, calcium, and phosphorous content of human milk are not adequate to promote and sustain the tissue growth and bone mineralization in preterm infants.[44] Fortifiers are being used to enhance protein, calcium, and phosphorous concentrations of human milk. Studies of these fortified preparations show short-term improvements in weight gain and linear and head growth. However, these studies show a nonsignificant trend toward increased feeding intolerance in infants receiving fortified milk but no significant increase in NEC in infants receiving fortified human milk.[45]

Human milk fortification is with a human milk-based fortifier or a bovine milk-based fortifier. Early studies suggested advantages with the use of human milk-based fortifier,[46] but these had various limitations and were questionably not powered a priori to evaluate NEC. Meta-analysis and systematic review of several of these studies show a lack of benefit.[35,47] The systematic review concluded: "Given the low quality of evidence, adequately powered and well-designed RCTs without the influence of industry are required in this field."[35] A recent randomized controlled noninferiority trial conducted in India showed that fortification with preterm formula powder is not inferior to fortification with human milk fortifiers in terms of NEC or extrauterine growth restriction.[48]

OSMOLALITY

Osmolality is the concentration of a solution in terms of osmoles of solute per kilogram of solvent. Although there is concern about osmolality, no increase in adverse events occurs if the osmolality of enteral feeds is between 300 and 500 mOsm/kg.[49,50] However, the addition of drugs and especially supplements such as multivitamins markedly increase osmolality, with the exact magnitude depending on the amount of supplement and the volume of milk to which it is added.[51,52] The consequences of increased feed osmolality in human infants are not clear, but a retrospective study of infants born at less than 28 weeks' gestation receiving intakes that exceeded 450 mOsm/kg set by the AAP did not indicate an increased risk of NEC. From an intuitive perspective, feedings with very high osmolality should be associated with greater intestinal injury. However, convincing studies that relate osmolality causally to NEC are not yet available.

STANDARDIZED FEEDING PROTOCOLS

Reduction of the incidence of NEC by standardizing the care delivery approaches has been proposed and has suggested benefits.[53-55] Strategies that have been proposed by these investigators include "(1) a standardized feeding protocol, (2) early initiation of enteral feeding using human milk, (3) optimization of the osmolality of preterm milk feeds using standardized dilution guidelines for additives, and (4) promotion of healthy microbiome by use of probiotics, early oral care with colostrum and by restricting high-risk medications and prolonged use of empirical antibiotics."

NULLA PER OS DURING TRANSFUSIONS

Transfusions have been associated with NEC, and it has been proposed that withholding feedings during transfusion might reduce the risk of subsequent NEC development.[56] This proposal was addressed in a meta-analysis that did not demonstrate a reduction in transfusion-associated NEC with the implementation of feeding protocols that included withholding of feedings during packed red blood cell transfusions.[57]

H2 BLOCKERS

Gastric acidity is thought to protect infants against various pathogens from the environment. The histamine-2 receptor blockers (H2 blockers) are off-label drugs that are frequently prescribed in preterm neonates, and their impact on the development of NEC has been evaluated in several studies.[58–60] Ranitidine (an H2 blocker) therapy, commonly used in an attempt to protect from what in the past was thought to be reflux-related apnea, is associated with an increased risk of infections, NEC, and fatal outcomes in very-low-birth-weight infants.

The mechanism for the H2 blocker effect at least partially relates to alternations in the microbiome.[61] In a case-control, cross-sectional study, stool samples were compared between 25 infants receiving H2 blockers and 51 babies who had never received them. 16S sequencing showed that with H2 blockers, microbial diversity was lower and relative abundance of Proteobacteria (primarily of the family Enterobacteriaceae) was increased, whereas that of Firmicutes was decreased. It is thought that these alterations in fecal microbiota predispose the vulnerable immature gut to NEC and suggest prudence in the use of H2 blockers in the premature infant.

In summary, these studies support that H2 blocker should be only administered in strictly selected cases after careful consideration of the risk-benefit ratio.

ANTIBIOTICS

There is concern that the widespread use of antibiotics in the neonatal intensive care unit might play a role in the pathogenesis of NEC in preterm infants. Despite recent initiatives to limit antibiotic use,[62] most infants born at less than 33 weeks' gestation *who are likely uninfected* are exposed to a course of antibiotics. There are considerable retrospective, observational data that early antibiotic use in preterm infants predisposes to adverse clinical outcomes.[63–76] On the other hand, one large observational study suggests a lower incidence of NEC after early antibiotic use.[77] One pragmatic prospective randomized, but underpowered, pilot study showed no evidence of increased clinically detectable serious adverse events due to prospective randomization,[78] a fear thwarting previous randomized studies. However, in this study, detectable signals suggested differences in the microbiomes and metabolomes between the randomized groups[79,80] that require further investigation because of their implications for future health. The fact that microbiome-related metabolomics responses to antibiotics involved in the gut-brain axis, bile acid, and tryptophan and folate metabolism were discovered raises concern about longer-term effects of antibiotics.[79,80] Larger randomized prospective studies are needed because these outcomes, if validated, likely have major implications for future health of these individuals beyond their stay in the neonatal intensive care unit.[81–93] Antibiotic resistance with unnecessary antibiotic use is also a major concern.[94]

USE OF PROBIOTICS IN PRETERM INFANTS

Whether or not probiotics should be routinely provided to preterm infants to prevent NEC has become one of the more controversial questions in neonatology. Large collaborative databases in the United States report that approximately 10% of extremely low-gestational-age infants are treated with probiotics. Large meta-analyses of relatively small trials suggest efficacy of multiple-strain probiotics in reducing necrotizing enterocolitis, but single-strain preparations are less certain.[95,96] Furthermore, efficacy in infants having less than 1000 g birth weight has not been demonstrated.

Such probiotic use bypasses and does not meet the standards of the US Food and Drug Administration (FDA) approval process in safety, efficacy, and manufacturing standards.[97] Currently available probiotics lack FDA-approved drug labeling and cannot be marketed to treat or prevent disease in preterm infants, including necrotizing enterocolitis and late-onset sepsis. In a recent report by the AAP Committee of the Fetus and Newborn, it was stated that "current evidence does not support the routine universal administration of probiotics to preterm infants, particularly those with a birth weight < 1,000 g."[98]

OTHER FACTORS AND THE FUTURE

There are numerous other compounds including growth factors, amino acids, antimicrobial agents, and immune components that have been evaluated in animal models and humans. The studies in animals have been difficult to extrapolate to human preterm infants, and studies in humans have for the most part been underpowered and have shown variable results. It is beyond the scope of this review to summarize these in detail, but as mentioned at the beginning of this review, we need to first have better delineation of the entities we are calling NEC. This is similar to stating that we need to have better delineation of entities that we are calling respiratory distress. We obviously know that the latter consists of different entities, and therapies need to be targeted to subtypes of the overall category.

After nearly 60 years of lack of progress in what we have termed NEC,[3] there is progress in understanding the need to define the disease subtype.[11,99] Newly emerging technologies related to the microbiome and multiomics, and artificial intelligence techniques such as machine learning, now provide frameworks to better diagnose the subtypes[11,100–102] and evaluate these disease processes in humans using systems biology networks.[101,103]

This should open the field for precision-based preventative therapeutics. The future is exciting!

Best Practices
• Early enteral feeding enhances intestinal development and is not a clear risk factor for development of NEC.
• Many concerns related to transfusions and NEC and feeding have been alleviated.
• NEC is not a discrete entity and different forms of intestinal injury in the neonate need to be better defined.

DISCLOSURE

The author has nothing to disclose.

REFERENCES

1. Neu J, Walker WA. Necrotizing enterocolitis. N Engl J Med 2011;364(3):255–64.
2. Bazacliu C, Neu J. Necrotizing enterocolitis: long term complications. Curr Pediatr Rev 2019;15(2):115–24.
3. Caplan MS, Fanaroff A. Necrotizing: a historical perspective. Semin Perinatol 2017;41(1):2–6.
4. Neu J, Modi N, Caplan M. Necrotizing enterocolitis comes in different forms: historical perspectives and defining the disease. Semin Fetal Neonatal Med 2018; 23(6):370–3.
5. Bell MJ, Ternberg JL, Feigin RD, et al. Neonatal necrotizing enterocolitis:therapeutic decisions based upon clinical staging. Ann Surg 1978;187:1–7.

6. Rehan VK, Seshia MM, Johnston B, et al. Observer variability in interpretation of abdominal radiographs of infants with suspected necrotizing enterocolitis. Clin Pediatr (Phila) 1999;38(11):637–43.

7. Dibra R, Picciariello A, Trigiante G, et al. Pneumatosis intestinalis and hepatic portal venous gas: watch and wait or emergency surgery? a case report and literature review. Am J Case Rep 2020;21:e923831.

8. Lassandro G, et al. Intestinal pneumatosis: differential diagnosis. NY: Abdom Radiol; 2020.

9. Sulistyo A, Rahman A, Biouss G, et al. Animal models of necrotizing enterocolitis: review of the literature and state of the art. Innov Surg Sci 2018;3(2):87–92.

10. Ares GJ, McElroy SJ, Hunter CJ. The science and necessity of using animal models in the study of necrotizing enterocolitis. Semin Pediatr Surg 2018; 27(1):29–33.

11. Lueschow SR, et al. A critical evaluation of current definitions of necrotizing enterocolitis. Pediatr Res 2021.

12. Ramani M, Ambalavanan N. Feeding practices and necrotizing enterocolitis. Clin Perinatol 2013;40(1):1–10.

13. Neu J. Is it time to stop starving premature infants? J Perinatol 2009;29(6): 399–400.

14. Madnawat H, Welu AL, Gilbert EJ, et al. Mechanisms of parenteral nutrition-associated liver and gut injury. Nutr Clin Pract 2020;35(1):63–71.

15. Neu J. Gastrointestinal development and meeting the nutritional needs of premature infants. Am J Clin Nutr 2007;85(2):629S–34S.

16. Johnson LR. The trophic action of gastrointestinal hormones. Gastroenterology 1976;70(2):278–88.

17. Lucas A, Bloom SR, Aynsley-Green A. Gut hormones and 'minimal enteral feeding'. Acta Paediatr Scand 1986;75(5):719–23.

18. Berseth CL. Neonatal small intestinal motility: motor responses to feeding in term and preterm infants. J Pediatr 1990;117(5):777–82.

19. Elgendy MM, El Sharkawy HM, Elrazek HA, et al. Superior mesenteric artery blood flow in parenterally fed versus enterally fed preterm infants. J Pediatr Gastroenterol Nutr 2021;73(2):259–63.

20. Dahlgren AF, Pan A, Lam V, et al. Longitudinal changes in the gut microbiome of infants on total parenteral nutrition. Pediatr Res 2019;86(1):107–14.

21. Trahair JF, Harding R. Ultrastructural anomalies in the fetal small intestine indicate that fetal swallowing is important for normal development: an experimental study. Virchows Arch A Pathol Anat Histopathol 1992;420(4):305–12.

22. Neu J, Pammi M. Pathogenesis of NEC: impact of an altered intestinal microbiome. Semin Perinatol 2017;41(1):29–35.

23. Anderson DM, Kliegman RM. The relationship of neonatal alimentation practices to the occurrence of endemic necrotizing enterocolitis. Am J Perinatol 1991; 8(1):62–7.

24. Morgan J, Bombell S, McGuire W. Early trophic feeding versus enteral fasting for very preterm or very low birth weight infants. Cochrane Database Syst Rev 2013;(3):Cd000504.

25. Dorling J, Abbott J, Berrington J, et al. Controlled trial of two incremental milk-feeding rates in preterm infants. N Engl J Med 2019;381(15):1434–43.

26. Rövekamp-Abels LW, Hogewind-Schoonenboom JE, de Wijs-Meijler DP, et al. Intermittent bolus or semicontinuous feeding for preterm infants? J Pediatr Gastroenterol Nutr 2015;61(6):659–64.

27. Konnikova Y, Zaman MM, Makda M, et al. Late enteral feedings are associated with intestinal inflammation and adverse neonatal outcomes. PLoS One 2015; 10(7):e0132924.
28. Parker LA, Weaver M, Murgas Torrazza RJ, et al. Effect of gastric residual evaluation on enteral intake in extremely preterm infants. JAMA Pediatr 2019;173(6): 534–43.
29. Lucas A, Cole TJ. Breast milk and neonatal necrotising enterocolitis. Lancet 1990;336(8730):1519–23.
30. Zhang B, Xiu W, Dai Y, et al. Protective effects of different doses of human milk on neonatal necrotizing enterocolitis. Medicine (Baltimore) 2020;99(37):e22166.
31. Altobelli E, Angeletti PM, Verrotti A, et al. The impact of human milk on necrotizing enterocolitis: a systematic review and meta-analysis. Nutrients 2020; 12(5):1322.
32. Riskin A. Immunomodulatory constituents of human donor milk. Breastfeed Med 2020;15(9):563–7.
33. Colaizy TT. Effects of milk banking procedures on nutritional and bioactive components of donor human milk. Semin Perinatol 2021;45(2):151382.
34. Hair AB, Ferguson J, Grogan C, et al. Human milk fortification: the clinician and parent perspectives. Pediatr Res 2020;88(Suppl 1):25–9.
35. Ananthan A, Balasubramanian H, Rao S, et al. Response to comments by Prof Abrams and Prof Lucas on "human milk-derived fortifiers compared with bovine milk-derived fortifiers in preterm infants: a systematic review and meta-analysis". Adv Nutr 2020;11(5):1713–5.
36. Carr LE, Virmani MD, Rosa F, et al. Role of human milk bioactives on infants' gut and immune health. Front Immunol 2021;12:604080.
37. Christian P, Smith ER, Lee SE, et al. The need to study human milk as a biological system. Am J Clin Nutr 2021;113(5):1063–72.
38. Faucher MA. An updated scientific review of the benefits of breastfeeding with additional resources for use in everyday practice. J Midwifery Womens Health 2012;57(4):422–3.
39. Meinzen-Derr J, Poindexter B, Wrage L, et al. Role of human milk in extremely low birth weight infants' risk of necrotizing enterocolitis or death. J Perinatol 2009;29(1):57–62.
40. Sisk PM, Lovelady CA, Dillard RG, et al. Early human milk feeding is associated with a lower risk of necrotizing enterocolitis in very low birth weight infants. J Perinatol 2007;27(7):428–33.
41. Meinzen-Derr J, Poindexter B, Wrage L, et al. Role of human milk in extremely low birth weight infants' risk of necrotizing enterocolitis or death. J Perinatol 2009;29(1):57–62.
42. Sisk PM, Lambeth TM, Rojas MA, et al. Necrotizing enterocolitis and growth in preterm infants fed predominantly maternal milk, pasteurized donor milk, or preterm formula: a retrospective study. Am J Perinatol 2017;34(7):676–83.
43. Section on Breastfeeding. Breastfeeding and the use of human milk. Pediatrics 2012;129(3):e827–41.
44. Cohen RS, McCallie KR. Feeding premature infants: why, when, and what to add to human milk. JPEN J Parenter Enteral Nutr 2012;36(1 Suppl):20s–4s.
45. Kuschel CA, Harding JE. Multicomponent fortified human milk for promoting growth in preterm infants. Cochrane Database Syst Rev 2004;(1):Cd000343.
46. Sullivan S, Schanler RJ, Kim JH, et al. An exclusively human milk-based diet is associated with a lower rate of necrotizing enterocolitis than a diet of human milk and bovine milk-based products. J Pediatr 2010;156(4):562.e1.

47. Premkumar MH, Pammi M, Suresh G. Human milk-derived fortifier versus bovine milk-derived fortifier for prevention of mortality and morbidity in preterm neonates. Cochrane Database Syst Rev 2019;2019(11):CD013145.

48. Chinnappan A, Ghosh R, Ramanathan S, et al. Fortification of breast milk with preterm formula powder vs human milk fortifier in preterm neonates: a randomized noninferiority trial. JAMA Pediatr 2021;175(8):790–6.

49. Ellis ZM, Tan HSG, Embleton ND, et al. Milk feed osmolality and adverse events in newborn infants and animals: a systematic review. Arch Dis Child Fetal Neonatal Ed 2019;104(3):F333–40.

50. Pearson F, Johnson MJ, Leaf AA. Milk osmolality: does it matter? Arch Dis Child Fetal Neonatal Ed 2013;98(2):F166–9.

51. Willis DM, Chabot J, Radde IC, et al. Unsuspected hyperosmolality of oral solutions contributing to necrotizing enterocolitis in very-low-birth-weight infants. Pediatrics 1977;60(4):535–8.

52. Radmacher PG, Adamkin MD, Lewis ST, et al. Milk as a vehicle for oral medications: hidden osmoles. J Perinatol 2012;32(3):227–9.

53. Shah SD, Booth N, Nandula P, et al. Effects of standardized feeding protocol on growth velocity and necrotizing enterocolitis in extremely low birth weight infants. J Perinatol 2021;41(1):134–9.

54. Chandran S, Anand AJ, Rajadurai VS, et al. Evidence-based practices reduce necrotizing enterocolitis and improve nutrition outcomes in very low-birth-weight infants. JPEN J Parenter Enteral Nutr 2020;45(7):1408–16.

55. Gephart SM, Hanson CK. Preventing necrotizing enterocolitis with standardized feeding protocols: not only possible, but imperative. Adv Neonatal Care 2013; 13(1):48–54.

56. Killion E. Feeding practices and effects on transfusion-associated necrotizing enterocolitis in premature neonates. Adv Neonatal Care 2021;21(5):356–64.

57. Yeo KT, Kong JY, Sasi A, et al. Stopping enteral feeds for prevention of transfusion-associated necrotising enterocolitis in preterm infants. Cochrane Database Syst Rev 2019;2019(10):1–27.

58. Dalton J, Schumacher R. H2-blockers are associated with necrotizing enterocolitis in very low birthweight infants. J Pediatr 2012;161(1):168–9.

59. Terrin G, Passariello A, De Curtis M, et al. Ranitidine is associated with infections, necrotizing enterocolitis, and fatal outcome in newborns. Pediatrics 2012;129(1):e40–5.

60. Guillet R, Stoll BJ, Cotten CM, et al. Association of H2-blocker therapy and higher incidence of necrotizing enterocolitis in very low birth weight infants. Pediatrics 2006;117(2):e137–42.

61. Gupta RW, Tran L, Norori J, et al. Histamine-2 receptor blockers alter the fecal microbiota in premature infants. J Pediatr Gastroenterol Nutr 2013;56(4): 397–400.

62. Frymoyer A, Joshi NS, Allan JM, et al. Sustainability of a clinical examination-based approach for ascertainment of early-onset sepsis in late preterm and term neonates. J Pediatr 2020;225:263–8.

63. Torrazza RM, Ukhanova M, Wang X, et al. Intestinal microbial ecology and environmental factors affecting necrotizing enterocolitis. PLoS One 2013;8(12): e83304.

64. Mai V, Torrazza RM, Ukhanova M, et al. Distortions in development of intestinal microbiota associated with late onset sepsis in preterm infants. PLoS One 2013; 8(1):e52876.

65. Mai V, Young CM, Ukhanova M, et al. Fecal microbiota in premature infants prior to necrotizing enterocolitis. PLoS One 2011;6(6):e20647.
66. Pammi M, Cope J, Tarr PI, et al. Intestinal dysbiosis in preterm infants preceding necrotizing enterocolitis: a systematic review and meta-analysis. Microbiome 2017;5(1):31.
67. Wang Y, Hoenig JD, Malin KJ, et al. 16S rRNA gene-based analysis of fecal microbiota from preterm infants with and without necrotizing enterocolitis. ISME J 2009;3(8):944–954954.
68. Carl MA, Ndao IM, Springman AC, et al. Sepsis from the gut: the enteric habitat of bacteria that cause late-onset neonatal bloodstream infections. Clin Infect Dis 2014;58(9):1211–8.
69. Kuppala VS, Meinzen-Derr J, Morrow AL, et al. Prolonged initial empirical antibiotic treatment is associated with adverse outcomes in premature infants. J Pediatr 2011;159(5):720–5.
70. Ting JY, Roberts A, Sherlock R, et al. Duration of initial empirical antibiotic therapy and outcomes in very low birth weight infants. Pediatrics 2019;143(3): e20182286.
71. Fajardo C, Alshaikh B, Harabor A. Prolonged use of antibiotics after birth is associated with increased morbidity in preterm infants with negative cultures. J Matern Fetal Neonatal Med 2019 Dec;32(24):4060–6.
72. Cantey JB, Pyle AK, Wozniak PS, et al. Early antibiotic exposure and adverse outcomes in preterm, very low birth weight infants. J Pediatr 2018;203:62–7.
73. Asfour S, Al-Mouqdad M. Early initiation of broad-spectrum antibiotics in premature infants. Minerva Pediatr 2019.
74. Ting JY, Synnes A, Roberts A, et al. Association between antibiotic use and neonatal mortality and morbidities in very low-birth-weight infants without culture-proven sepsis or necrotizing enterocolitis. JAMA Pediatr 2016;170(12): 1181–7.
75. Firestein MR, Myers MM, Austin J, et al. Perinatal antibiotics alter preterm infant EEG and neurobehavior in the Family Nurture Intervention trial. Dev Psychobiol 2019;61(5):661–9.
76. Greenberg RG, Chowdhury D, Hansen NI, et al. Prolonged duration of early antibiotic therapy in extremely premature infants. Pediatr Res 2019;85(7):994–1000.
77. Li Y, Shen RL, Ayede AI, et al. Early use of antibiotics is associated with a lower incidence of necrotizing enterocolitis in preterm, very low birth weight infants: the NEOMUNE-NeoNutriNet Cohort Study. J Pediatr 2020;227:128–34.e2.
78. Ruoss JL, Bazacliu C, Russell JT, et al. Routine early antibiotic use in SymptOmatic Preterm Neonates (REASON): a pilot randomized controlled trial. J Pediatr 2020;229:294–8.e3.
79. Patton L, Li N, Garrett TJ, et al. Antibiotics effects on the fecal metabolome in preterm infants. Metabolites 2020;10(8):331.
80. Russell JT, et al. Antibiotics may influence gut microbiome signaling to the brain in preterm neonates. BioRxiv 2020.
81. Nobel YR, Cox LM, Kirigin FF, et al. Metabolic and metagenomic outcomes from early-life pulsed antibiotic treatment. Nat Commun 2015;6:7486.
82. Ruiz VE, Battaglia T, Kurtz ZD, et al. A single early-in-life macrolide course has lasting effects on murine microbial network topology and immunity. Nat Commun 2017;8(1):518.
83. Schokker D, Zhang J, Vastenhouw SA, et al. Long-lasting effects of early-life antibiotic treatment and routine animal handling on gut microbiota composition and immune system in pigs. PLoS One 2015;10(2):e0116523.

84. Livanos AE, Greiner TU, Vangay P, et al. Antibiotic-mediated gut microbiome perturbation accelerates development of type 1 diabetes in mice. Nat Microbiol 2016;1(11):16140.
85. Becattini S, Taur Y, Pamer EG. Antibiotic-Induced changes in the intestinal microbiota and disease. Trends Mol Med 2016;22(6):458–78.
86. Croswell A, Amir E, Teggatz P, et al. Prolonged impact of antibiotics on intestinal microbial ecology and susceptibility to enteric Salmonella infection. Infect Immun 2009;77(7):2741–53.
87. Dethlefsen L, Relman DA. Incomplete recovery and individualized responses of the human distal gut microbiota to repeated antibiotic perturbation. Proc Natl Acad Sci U S A 2011;108(Suppl 1):4554–61.
88. Jakobsson HE, Jernberg C, Andersson AF, et al. Short-term antibiotic treatment has differing long-term impacts on the human throat and gut microbiome. PLoS One 2010;5(3):e9836.
89. Jernberg C, Löfmark S, Edlund C, et al. Long-term impacts of antibiotic exposure on the human intestinal microbiota. Microbiology (Reading) 2010;156(Pt 11):3216–23.
90. Schubert AM, Sinani H, Schloss PD. Antibiotic-induced alterations of the murine gut microbiota and subsequent effects on colonization resistance against *Clostridium difficile*. mBio 2015;6(4):e00974.
91. Arboleya S, Sánchez B, Milani C, et al. Intestinal microbiota development in preterm neonates and effect of perinatal antibiotics. J Pediatr 2015;166(3):538–44.
92. Arboleya S, Sánchez B, Solís G, et al. Impact of prematurity and perinatal antibiotics on the developing intestinal microbiota: a functional inference study. Int J Mol Sci 2016;17(5):649.
93. Nogacka AM, Salazar N, Arboleya S, et al. Early microbiota, antibiotics and health. Cell Mol Life Sci 2018;75(1):83–91.
94. Ramirez CB, Cantey JB. Antibiotic resistance in the neonatal intensive care unit. Neoreviews 2019;20(3):e135–44.
95. Xiong T, Maheshwari A, Neu J, et al. An overview of systematic reviews of randomized-controlled trials for preventing necrotizing enterocolitis in preterm infants. Neonatology 2020;117(1):46–56.
96. Lenfestey MW, Neu J. Probiotics in newborns and children. Pediatr Clin North Am 2017;64(6):1271–89.
97. Caplan MS, Underwood MA, Modi N, et al. Necrotizing enterocolitis: using regulatory science and drug development to improve outcomes. J Pediatr 2019; 212:208–15.e1.
98. Poindexter B. Use of probiotics in preterm infants. Pediatrics 2021;147(6): e2021051485.
99. Neu J, Modi N, Caplan M. Necrotizing enterocolitis comes in different forms: historical perspectives and defining the disease. Semin Fetal Neonatal Med 2018; 23(6):370–3.
100. Kim JH, Sampath V, Canvasser J. Challenges in diagnosing necrotizing enterocolitis. Pediatr Res 2020;88(Suppl 1):16–20.
101. Thänert R, Keen EC, Dantas G, et al. Necrotizing enterocolitis and the microbiome: current status and future directions. J Infect Dis 2020;223(Suppl_3):S257–63.
102. Lure AC, Du X, Black EW, et al. Using machine learning analysis to assist in differentiating between necrotizing enterocolitis and spontaneous intestinal perforation: a novel predictive analytic tool. J Pediatr Surg 2020;56(10):1703–10.
103. Neu J. Necrotizing enterocolitis: a multi-omic approach and the role of the microbiome. Dig Dis Sci 2020;65(3):789–96.

Differences of Sex Development

What Neonatologists Need to Know

Natalie G. Allen, MD*, Kanthi Bangalore Krishna, MD,
Peter A. Lee, MD, PhD

KEYWORDS

- Differences of sex development (DSD) • Atypical genitalia
- Variations of sex development

KEY POINTS

- Initial evaluation of DSD should be carefully completed with open discussion and shared decision making between the medical staff and family.
- The assessment of atypical genitalia must be individualized because the spectrum of findings and severity vary considerably.
- The initial evaluation must assess whether there is a medical emergency, such as adrenal insufficiency, renal failure, or other life-threatening illness.

INTRODUCTION

The term disorders of sex development (DSD) was proposed at the first international consensus in 2005[1] that was organized to review the diagnosis and care of individuals having intersex, including those born with ambiguous genitalia. This proposal was in part a response to the dissatisfaction regarding past care expressed by patients and support groups. The DSD designation was adopted to avoid use of previous terminology, including intersex, because of what this term was interpreted to imply. Although full disclosure was already being adopted before this conference, this was endorsed, as well as the need for the establishment of multidisciplinary groups consisting of available experts among psychologists, surgeons, endocrinologists, neonatologists, and patient advocates. Such groups were envisioned to function by informing parents regarding the diagnosis and care of their child and, together with the parents, making decisions regarding all aspects of care. However, it was recognized that experts in each of these disciplines are not available at many of the tertiary medical centers to which infants with DSD are referred. Conversely, it was recognized

All authors declare no commercial or financial conflicts of interest.
Division of Endocrinology and Diabetes, Department of Pediatrics, Penn State Health Milton S. Hershey Medical Center, Hershey, PA 17033, USA
* Corresponding author. 12 Briarcrest Square, Hershey, PA 17033
E-mail address: nallen4@pennstatehealth.psu

Clin Perinatol 49 (2022) 207–218
https://doi.org/10.1016/j.clp.2021.11.013
perinatology.theclinics.com

that although many centers lacked the full components of a multidisciplinary team, there were excellent, experienced surgeons, endocrinologists, mental health professionals, and others capable of appropriate interactions with individuals and families with DSDs. This article focuses on those with DSDs born with genital ambiguity/atypia or nonbinary external genitalia. The impact of the 2005 consensus was summarized in 2014 and 2016.[2,3] The latter included those from advocacy and support groups in a concerted effort to provide a voice for all involved.

During the critical time right after birth, education is crucial so that parents understand enough embryology to understand how this genital atypia can develop. The impact of this first interaction is long remembered by parents, and its importance should not be underestimated. Such background should be presented together with an introduction to all aspects of care including sex assignment if appropriate, gender identity, surgical options and associated controversies, as well as need for psychological counseling now and likely throughout the lifetime of persons with DSD.[4]

The 3 most common presentations to the neonatologist are (1) the newborn with genitalia outside a broad range of normal for female or male external genitalia, (2) the newborn with physical presentation (external genitalia) inconsistent with karyotype obtained prenatally or results of prenatal ultrasonography, and (3) newborns with a risk of DSD because of a family history. The initial evaluation must assess whether there is a medical emergency, such as adrenal insufficiency, renal failure, or other life-threatening illness. Adrenal insufficiency may occur in severe congenital adrenal hyperplasia (CAH), whereas some genital atypia may present with other developmental defects.

Those presenting with atypical genitalia basically involve virilization of female genitalia or undervirilization of male genitalia (note that this categorization accepts the traditional bimodal physical development of genitalia as male and female, as separate from development of gender). The 2 most common diagnoses involving external genital atypia are CAH (most frequently 21-hydroxylase deficiency) associated with 46,XX karyotype and testicular dysgenesis associated with 46,XY karyotype. The diagnosis of CAH among those with symmetrically virilized genitalia is made by baseline hormone profiles and clinical presentation such as evidence of salt loss (after the first 3–5 days of life) and often can be verified by molecular genetic mutations.[5] Testicular dysgenesis usually cannot be further categorized by etiologic diagnostic category or by a genetic mutation. Both these categories are discussed later. It is the perspective of the authors that the assessment of atypical genitalia must be individualized, even within etiologic diagnoses such as CAH, because the spectrum of findings and severity vary considerably, and shared decision making after careful review of available outcome data can guide this process.

TERMINOLOGY AND FULL DISCLOSURE

It is important to realize that the term DSD and the DSD classification were proposed to provide a framework for the approach to an etiologic diagnosis and for research endeavors. It was intended that this term should only be used until an etiologic diagnosis could be made (realizing that an etiologic diagnosis may not be possible in a large percentage of individuals, particularly those with a 46,XY karyotype).

Actually, the DSD term was proposed in response to complaints concerning use of terms such as intersex, hermaphroditism, and pseudohermaphroditism and the guilt and shame that some associated with these. Furthermore, the word sex was intentionally used as the middle word in DSD rather than sexual in an effort to avoid implications regarding sexuality.

Dissatisfaction with DSD has resulted in different suggested terminology including substitution of the word Differences for Disorders and VSD (Variations of Sex Development).[6] Complaints of the term Disorder involve the implication that there are pathologic differences among these individuals. On the other hand, full disclosure is somehow denied when terms such as differences and variations are used unless it is clearly defined what is a pathologic difference or variation beyond the broad variation of normal. A broad variation of normal recognizes that normal variation of penis and clitoris length may be beyond $\pm$ 2 or even 2.5 SD. Such definitions do not imply that any treatment, including surgery, is indicated.

It has also been stated that individuals with DSDs should not perceive that they have a defect because such would imply guilt and shame. The basis of full disclosure is truth, and having a medical diagnosis should not imply a basis for guilt and shame. This concern should be addressed by skillful counseling. Inherent as part of full disclosure are ethical principles focused on fostering the well-being of the child and future adult. The rights of children and adolescents considering decision making[7] must be balanced with the rights respecting family and parent-child relationships.[8] Ethical principles critical for the appropriate management of DSD are presented in **Box 1**.

Regarding the term to be used for genitalia that are beyond the long-term accepted wide range of female or male development, complaints involve the term ambiguous genitalia (sometimes citing the nonbinary perception of gender). However, basic to biology is binary male and female physical development and the fact that genitalia that develop prenatally beyond the broad range of normal male and female development should be evaluated for an underlying physiologic problem or defect. Because there is not another term that describes this physical situation, in this article atypical genitalia is used.

GENDER IDENTITY AND GENDER FLUIDITY: DEVELOPMENT, DEFINITION, AND CHANGING PERCEPTIONS

The multiple determinants of gender identity development are not understood, even though it is clear that prenatal factors likely genetic as well as differentiation of the brain play a major role; this is dramatically different than a predominant theory especially in the 1960s and the 1970s that environment was a major overriding factor. Based on this approach, it was considered, for example, that if an infant was assigned male and treated by his family as a male, he would develop a male gender identity. However, sadly the outcome was not always as predicted, especially when a child was assigned female who had had normal testicular function during fetal life. Traditionally it is understood that gender development is initially manifested during infancy. It is suggested by a child's behavior and usually indicated by their self-identification as a boy or a girl by 18 to 24 months of age. Indeed, gender identity has been defined when each person self-identifies as male or female. Such is not necessarily concordant with sexual orientation, which will become manifest later. At present, it seems

---

Box 1
Ethical principles

1. Foster the well-being of the child and future adult
2. Uphold the rights of children and adolescents to participate in and/or self-determine decisions that affect them now or later
3. Respect family and parent-child relationship

that gender identity is perceived differently, particularly among young adolescents who seem to be focused on an external, social definition of how others perceive them. This, together with the current social acceptance of gender dysphoria or gender fluidity, may be related to the dramatically increased percentage of those presenting having or being diagnosed with gender dysphoria.[9,10]

Regarding those children born with atypical genitalia, almost all parents want to assign a gender, although some will not. The goal is to assign the gender that the child will most likely develop, which cannot be done with certainty. The right and responsibility for gender assignment is primarily that of the parents, together with and after extensive discussions with experts, who are ideally part of a multidisciplinary task force. Of course, parents must realize that there is always a risk that gender will not develop as assigned and be prepared to accept the situation if the opposite or neutral gender develops. If that occurs, future discussions and decisions must be directed to whatever should result in the best overall quality of life as an adult. The individual should play an appropriate role, based on ability to assent or consent.

Among 46,XX individuals with CAH, data report a higher percentage having discordant gender identity at 11.3% and homosexual orientation at 23.8%.[11] The report also cites variable outcomes concerning sexual function, finding that most, in contrast to previous reports, are sexually active and indicate satisfaction with surgical outcomes. The rate of homosexual orientation in 46,XX CAH is found after meta-analysis and seems to be a valid estimate of those treated a generation ago, whereas determining factors (innate and environmental) may differ for younger individuals.[12] Although this is evidence of an impact on the central nervous system (CNS) of prenatal and postnatal androgen excess, sexual orientation in contrast to gender identity should not be judged as evidence of incorrect assignment.

It is important to recognize that the common current broader perception of gender is not necessarily tied to either internal or external genital development or to physical expression of sexuality. The vast majority of humans have binary physical reproductive system development, whereas gender may, particularly at certain stages of life, not appear binary. Early adolescence is likely such a stage, a time when gender confusion always has been prevalent. Although the approach to the care of those with DSDs must be open to each individual's gender choice and expression, it is just as important to realize that most will eventually arrive at a male or female gender consistent with their genitalia.

EMBRYOLOGY OF INTERNAL AND EXTERNAL SEXUAL DIFFERENTIATION

Gonadal differentiation in the fetus begins within the urogenital ridges that form the gonads and reproductive tract and are present around 6 weeks of gestation. By 6 to 7 weeks of gestation, the bipotential gonads have been committed to development into ovaries or testes and by 14 weeks of gestation the external genitalia have differentiated. Critical to the process of sexual differentiation is the sex-determining region on the Y chromosome (SRY), which triggers male sexual differentiation through a cascade of transcription factors including SOX9.[13] In the female, typical ovarian development requires absence of the SRY as well as the presence of transcription factors that specifically support ovarian development including WNT 4 and DAX1.[14]

Initially in the embryo, both Wolffian and Müllerian ducts develop. In fetal testis anti-Müllerian hormone production begins in the Sertoli cells by the seventh week of gestation leading to regression of Müllerian duct development. Testosterone production, initially stimulated by placental human chorionic gonadotropin allows for further development of the Wolffian ducts, which subsequently develop into the epididymis, vas deferens, ejaculatory duct, and seminal vesicle. Testosterone also serves to promote testicular descent from the abdomen to the scrotum later in gestation around 35 weeks. In the female fetus, without the presence of testosterone or dihydrotestosterone (DHT) the Wolffian ducts regress and, without anti-Müllerian hormone, Müllerian ducts develop into fallopian tubes, uterus, cervix, and the upper one-third of the vagina. Internal sexual differentiation is depicted in **Fig. 1**.

Phenotypic development of external genitalia depends on the presence or absence of androgens. In the male fetus, testosterone is produced by the testes and converted to DHT that promotes differentiation of male external genitalia. By about 14 weeks of gestation, the genital tubercle develops into the corpora cavernosa of the penis, the urethral folds fuse, and the labioscrotal folds fuse to form the scrotum. When

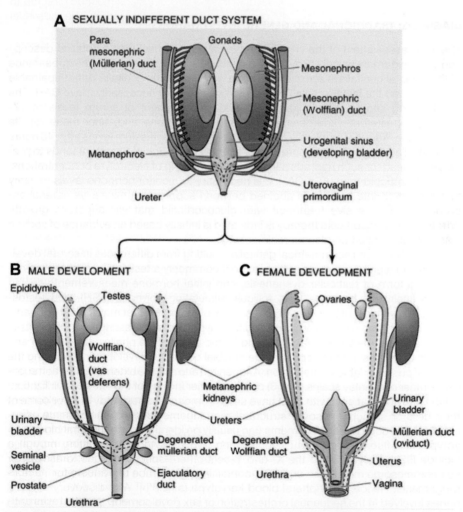

Fig. 1. Internal sexual differentiation. Differentiation of the bipotential gonad is typically complete by week 7 of gestation with subsequent development of the typical male or female internal structures from Wolffian and Müllerian ducts. (*From* Boron WF, Boulpaep EL. Medical Physiology, 3rd edition. Elsevier; 2016. Figure 53-5; with permission.)

androgens are not present, the external genital structures develop into the clitoris, labia, and vagina. External sexual differentiation is represented in **Fig. 2**.

DHT, which is critical to the development of male external genitalia, was originally thought to be produced only by the classical pathway in which testosterone is converted to DHT by 5α-reductase. DHT is also produced by an alternative "backdoor" pathway from 17-hydroxyprogesterone through steroid metabolites to androstanediol. Androstanediol is converted to DHT primarily in peripheral tissues. In 46XX patients with 21-hydroxylase deficiency, the backdoor pathway contributes to significant virilization.[15] In 46XY individuals, mutations in the backdoor pathway have been found to cause undervirilization.

Disruption at any step in fetal genital differentiation and development can result in DSD and atypical genitalia.

DIAGNOSIS: TRADITIONAL AND GENETIC INVESTIGATIONS

The initial assessment of the child with atypical genitalia includes a detailed description of the external genitalia (**Box 2**). This description includes whether the appearance of the external genitalia is symmetric. Those with symmetric genitalia without palpable masses within the labial-scrotal folds most likely, but not necessarily, have CAH. The initial testing should include karyotype and measurement of serum levels of 17-hydroxyprogesterone, androstenedione, and testosterone and, until these results are available, frequent monitoring of serum sodium and potassium levels after 48 hours of life. Availability of newborn screening with early institution of treatment tends to preclude the need for such rigorous serial laboratory testing of electrolyte concentrations. For glucocorticoid therapy in CAH, it is necessary to monitor hormone levels to verify that an appropriate balance is attained between suppressing excessive adrenal androgens and excessive treatment with glucocorticoid that will suppress growth. Whether mineralocorticoid therapy is indicated is initially based on evidence of sodium loss and later based on plasma renin activity.

Among those with asymmetrical genitalia resulting from differences in scrotal development and a unilateral mass, which is most commonly a testis, the most likely diagnosis is a form of testicular dysgenesis, and initial hormone measurements should include luteinizing hormone (LH), follicle-stimulating hormone (FSH), and testosterone. This window of time allows assessment of the profile that may indicate gonadal failure or suggest hypothalamic or pituitary hypofunction. Descriptions of genitalia should also include the appearance, length, and width of the phallus; the number and location of orifices; and the appearance of labial or scrotal development including the extent of posterior labioscrotal fusion. Anogenital ratio and the external virilization score with Prader or Quigley scales (**Fig. 3**) provide further indices of the extent of virilization.

Up to 15% of patients with DSD have sex chromosome aneuploidy in all or some of their cells or sex chromosome structural rearrangements. Sex chromosome aneuploidy and structural rearrangements can usually be identified by peripheral blood karyotype with fluorescent in situ hybridization (FISH). Cytogenetic testing may also include FISH analysis using the X- and Y-centromere-specific probes to assess for sex chromosome mosaicism and SRY-containing FISH probe to evaluate for Yp rearrangements. Hence, a peripheral blood karyotype is helpful. With discovery of novel genes involved in the sequential orchestration of sex development, the ideal approach to each patient involves use of increasingly sophisticated technology to identify the specific genetic variant. DNA microarrays and next-generation sequencing techniques have identified multiple genetic variations associated with DSD. Investigations into these genetic variations have elucidated novel genetic mechanisms leading to DSD.[17]

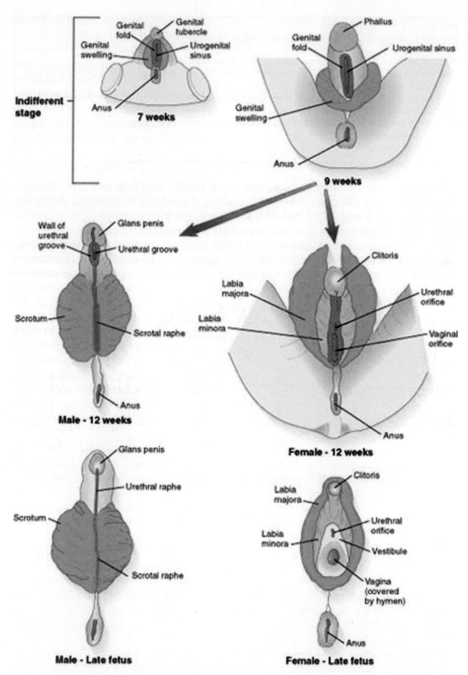

Fig. 2. Development of external genitalia. By 14 weeks' gestation, external genitalia are differentiated. Critical to this process are the sex-determining region of the Y chromosome (SRY) and multiple transcription factors that support either male or female genital development. (*From* Carlson BM. Human embryology and developmental biology, 4th edition. St. Louis: Mosby; 2009; with permission.)

Box 2
Physical examination of the infant with atypical genitalia

Physical examination: genital examination and description
- External genitalia: symmetric versus asymmetric. Include presence or absence of palpable gonadal structures on both sides
- Measure phallic/corporeal length and diameter (exclude clitoral hood measurement)
- Examine number of perineal openings
- Examine the extent of fusion and rugation of the labial/scrotal area
- Obtain anogenital ratio[16]
- Genital pigmentation

Molecular genetic testing has become more readily available and cost-efficient. When such testing identifies a known mutation, it confirms an etiologic diagnosis, whereas the lack thereof does not necessarily rule out the diagnosis. This is particularly true for 21-hydroxylase adrenal hyperplasia and androgen insensitivity syndrome, both having numerous mutations some of which have not yet been identified. A mutation confirms the diagnosis, but the traditional approach is needed to determine medical therapy. A specific mutation may not be associated with genotype-phenotype

Quigley Scale

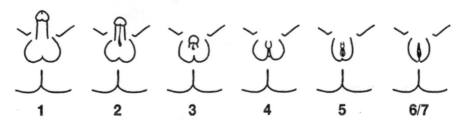

Adapted from Quigley, et. Al. Androgen Receptor Defects: Historical, clinical and Molecular Perspectives; Endocrine Reviews 16(3): 271-321; 1995and re-printed with permission.

Prader Scale

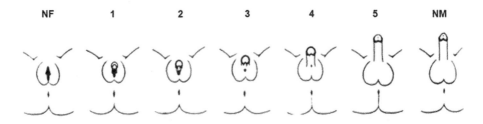

From NICHD, adapted from White and Speiser; Congenital Adrenal Hyperplasia due to 21-Hydroxylase Deficiency; Endocrine Reviews 21(3): 245-291; 2000)

Fig. 3. The Quigley and Prader Scales. These tools are used to describe genital atypia and degrees of virilization. (*From* Nokoff NH, Palmer B, Mullins AJ, et al. Prospective assessment of cosmesis before and after genital surgery. J Pediatr Urol 2017;13(1): 28e1–28e6; with permission.)

correlation,[18] except for the null mutation, which is associated with no enzyme activity, hence always a severe condition. An algorithm to approach the clinical evaluation of an infant born with atypical genitalia is shown in **Fig. 4.**

GUIDELINES FOR PSYCHOLOGICAL COUNSELING

Screening questions are available to help understand individual families' background and outlook to provide appropriate counseling.[19] Because having a DSD involving atypical genitalia impacts all of life, the basics regarding psychological support should be reviewed with the parents and later as age-appropriate with each individual. This interaction should also assess the need for further counseling. Counseling is tailored to the age of the individual and from adolescence onward should include all aspects of life, including indicated health care, occupation, and general and intimate social activities, including sexuality. The goal is a good quality of life, considering all these domains.

GENITAL SURGERY DURING INFANCY

A generation or longer ago, the approach to the infant with genitalia that were atypical was to "correct" this surgically to conform to the assigned sex. It was considered that if a child grew up being treated as a girl having female genitalia, she would develop a female

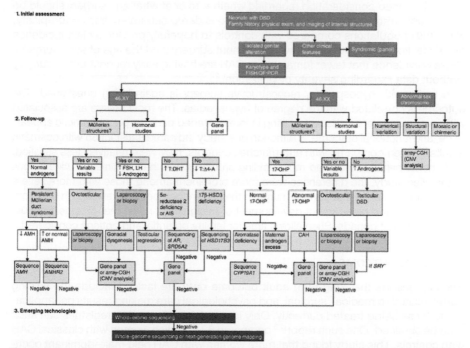

Fig. 4. Approach to the initial evaluation of an infant born with atypical genitalia. The flowsheet goes through stepwise testing to help identify the cause of a DSD. CNV, copy number variant; AIS, androgen insensitivity syndrome; CGH, comparative genomic hybridization; AMH, Anti Mullerian Hormone; FSH, Follicle Stimulating Hormone; LH, Leutenizing Hormone; OHP, is part of a substance; QF-PCR, Quantitative fluorescent polymerase chain reaction; DHT, Di hydrotestosterone. (*Adapted from* León NY, Reyes AP, Harley VR. A clinical algorithm to diagnose differences of sex development. Lancet Diabetes Endocrinol. 2019;7(7):560–74; with permission.)

gender identity. As discussed in the section regarding gender identity, this approach involved the incorrect presumption that humans are born with the potential of developing either a female or male gender identity. The situation in which this failed most dramatically was among those assigned female who had functional testes during fetal life and whose CNS had been exposed to androgen levels typical of the male fetus, such as 46,XY individuals with cloacal extrophy. It has become evident that most such individuals develop a male gender identity, and this is particularly problematic after feminizing surgery has been done and is a reason to carefully consider consequences of genital surgery.

Among those raised female, primarily those with CAH, feminizing genital surgery decades ago often resulted in cosmetically unacceptable genitalia with lack of neurologic sensitivity. Individuals and advocacy groups have expressed dissatisfaction especially in relation to sexual function. Even more recent outcome data from those having surgery 2 decades ago do not necessarily apply to the cosmetic appearance and neurologic responsiveness for those having surgery today.[20] Although over recent decades, genital surgery has become progressively more and more refined, current reports vary in relation to sexual function. In contrast to earlier impressions, more recent reports[21] find that most individuals are sexually active, with some complaining of clitoral insensitivity, although ability to experience orgasm has been reported not to correlate with this complaint. Furthermore, it is likely that poorer anatomic outcome is correlated with extent of virilization at birth. Detailed outcome information is crucial to have a balanced consideration regarding whether to or at what age surgery should be done. Furthermore, vaginoplasty should be considered separately from clitoroplasty, with study populations compared with controls to hopefully provide a clear incidence of satisfaction or dissatisfaction with or without surgery (and the age of such surgery). There is evidence that fewer females with CAH are having early reconstructive surgery (without data regarding severity of virilization).[22]

In males with hypospadias, reconstructive surgery is again being questioned. The outcome is correlated with the degree of hypospadias. The most severe are associated with inadequate genital tissue, resulting in foreshortened penises, poor cosmetic appearance, and functional outcome.[23] Although one study indicated satisfaction with cosmetic results,[24] when compared with age-matched controls, they were relatively less satisfied, had shorter penile length, had more voiding problems, and had diminished urinary flow. In the cited study, the differences were more prominent among those with more severe hypospadias. In regard to gonadal surgery, the current perspective, resulting in part from the lower risk and older age of development of malignancy, notes that providers should delay removal of gonads. Such allows time for fertility potential and options considered.

LONG-TERM OUTCOME

Primary reasons that long-term adult outcome data are lacking include the shifting norms related to medical, surgical, and psychological care making results nonapplicable to those being treated currently. Only in countries with central registries can such data be obtained. One such report[25] compared 62 Swedish women with classical CAH with controls. This study found that more women with CAH held male-dominant occupations, had a greater interest in 'rough sports', reported a prime interest in motor vehicles and had non-heterosexual orientation among 19% noted this was more common among those with null genotype. These investigators suggest dose-dependent effects of prenatal androgens on CNS function. Future outcome data, related to societal changes, are expected to show further broadening of careers and occupations, less gender dysphoria, and also hopefully more cosmetically and functionally satisfying genitalia as the result of refined surgical techniques.

SUMMARY

The goal of treatment of DSD is to provide for a good quality of life. To attain this, psychological support is of primary importance. The aim of such support involves full disclosure, which should remove any guilt or shame, provide for adaption to gender development, and enable the individuals and their families to envision and enhance a balanced, fulfilling life. Crucial to this is recognition of the impact that hormones and environment have on outcome. Molecular genetics will continue to provide etiologic diagnoses while still more refined and cost-effective techniques are evolving. Surgical techniques on genitalia can be expected to improve and provide better results, although the dilemma of how to avoid surgery resulting in elimination of crucial structures (clitoris or penis) will persist. Given the lower risk of gonadal malignancy at a young age, removal of gonads should be delayed to allow time for fertility potential and options considered. Individuals with DSD should grow up expecting the same positive experiences in life as anyone else, concomitantly with a lifelong condition. Initial evaluation should be carefully completed with open discussion between the medical staff and family.

Best Practices

Initial evaluation should be carefully completed with open discussion between the medical staff and family.

Molecular genetic studies can be used to confirm the etiologic diagnosis.

Given the lower risk of gonadal malignancy at a young age, removal of gonads should be delayed, to allow time for potential fertility preservation.

Full disclosure and ongoing psychological support for individuals with DSD and their families are key to provide for a good quality of life.

REFERENCES

1. Lee PA, Houk CP, Ahmed SF, et al, Endocrinology ICColobtLWPESatESfP. Consensus statement on management of intersex disorders. International Consensus Conference on Intersex. Pediatrics 2006;118(2):e488–500.
2. Lee PA, Nordenström A, Houk CP, et al. Global disorders of sex development update since 2006: perceptions, approach and care. Horm Res Paediatr 2016; 85(3):158–80.
3. Lee PA, Wisniewski A, Baskin L, et al. Advances in diagnosis and care of persons with DSD over the last decade. Int J Pediatr Endocrinol 2014.
4. Ernst MM, Gardner M, Mara CA, et al. The DSD-Translational Research Network Leadership Group and Psychosocial Workgroup. Psychosocial screening in disorders/differences of sex development: Psychometric evaluation of the psychosocial assessment tool. Horm Res Paediatr 2018;90(6):368–80.
5. Parivesh A, Barseghyan H, Délot E, et al. Translating genomics to the clinical diagnosis of disorders/differences of sex development. Curr Top Dev Biol 2019;134:317–75.
6. Bennecke E, Köhler B, Röhle R, et al. Disorders or differences of sex development? Views of affected individuals on DSD terminology. J Sex Res 2021;58(4):522–31.
7. Health VGDo. Victorian Department of Health. Decision-making principles for the care of infants, children and adolescents with intersex conditions. Melbourne, Australia: Victorian Government Department of Health; 2013. Available at: http://docs.health.vic.gov.au/docs/doc/Decision-making-principles-for-the-care-of-infants-children-and-adolescents-with-intersex-conditions.

8. Wiesemann C, Ude-Koeller S, Sinnecker GH, et al. Ethical principles and recommendations for the medical management of differences of sex development (DSD)/intersex in children and adolescents. Eur J Pediatr 2010;169(6):671–9.

9. Byne W, Karasic DH, Coleman E, et al. Assessment and treatment of gender dysphoria and gender variant patients: a primer for Psychiatrists. Am J Psychiatry 2018;175(10):1046.

10. Steve J. Langdon. Native People of Alaska, Traditional Living in a Northern Land, 5th Edition. Anchorage January 1, 2013.

11. Almasri J, Zaiem F, Rodriguez-Gutierrez R, et al. Genital reconstructive surgery in females with congenital adrenal hyperplasia: a systematic review and meta-analysis. J Clin Endocrinol Metab 2018;103(11):4089–96.

12. Daae E, Feragen KB, Waehre A, et al. Sexual orientation in individuals with congenital adrenal hyperplasia: a systematic review. Front Behav Neurosci 2020;14:38.

13. Capel B. Sex in the 90s: SRY and the switch to the male pathway. Annu Rev Physiol 1998;60:497–523.

14. Bernard P, Ryan J, Sim H, et al. Wnt signaling in ovarian development inhibits Sf1 activation of Sox9 via the Tesco enhancer. Endocrinology 2012;153(2):901–12.

15. Kamrath C, Hochberg Z, Hartmann MF, et al. Increased activation of the alternative "backdoor" pathway in patients with 21-hydroxylase deficiency: evidence from urinary steroid hormone analysis. J Clin Endocrinol Metab 2012;97(3): E367–75.

16. Castets S, Nguyen KA, Plaisant F, et al. Reference values for the external genitalia of full-term and pre-term female neonates. Arch Dis Child Fetal Neonatal Ed 2021; 106(1):39–44.

17. Yatsenko SA, Witchel SF. Genetic approach to ambiguous genitalia and disorders of sex development: what clinicians need to know. Semin Perinatol 2017;41(4): 232–43.

18. Khattab A, Yuen T, Al-Malki S, et al. A rare CYP21A2 mutation in a congenital adrenal hyperplasia kindred displaying genotype-phenotype nonconcordance. Ann N Y Acad Sci 2016;1364:5–10.

19. Bangalore Krishna K, Kogan BA, Ernst MM, et al. Individualized care for patients with intersex (disorders/differences of sex development): Part 3. J Pediatr Urol 2020;16(5):598–605.

20. Schober J, Cooney T, Pfaff D, et al. Innervation of the labia minora of prepubertal girls. J Pediatr Adolesc Gynecol 2010;23(6):352–7.

21. Strandqvist A, Falhammar H, Lichtenstein P, et al. Suboptimal psychosocial outcomes in patients with congenital adrenal hyperplasia: epidemiological studies in a nonbiased national cohort in Sweden. J Clin Endocrinol Metab 2014;99(4): 1425–32.

22. Sturm RM, Durbin-Johnson B, Kurzrock EA. Congenital adrenal hyperplasia: current surgical management at academic medical centers in the United States. J Urol 2015;193(5 Suppl):1796–801.

23. van der Zwan YG, Callens N, van Kuppenveld J, et al. DSD DSGo. Long-term outcomes in males with disorders of sex development. J Urol 2013;190(3):1038–42.

24. Örtqvist L, Fossum M, Andersson M, et al. Long-term followup of men born with hypospadias: urological and cosmetic results. J Urol 2015;193(3):975–81.

25. Frisén L, Nordenström A, Falhammar H, et al. Gender role behavior, sexuality, and psychosocial adaptation in women with congenital adrenal hyperplasia due to CYP21A2 deficiency. J Clin Endocrinol Metab 2009;94(9):3432–9.

Novel Ventilation Strategies to Reduce Adverse Pulmonary Outcomes

Martin Keszler, MD

KEYWORDS

- Mechanical ventilation • Lung injury • Bronchopulmonary dysplasia
- Noninvasive respiratory support • Less invasive surfactant administration
- Volutrauma • Volume-targeted ventilation

KEY POINTS

- The pathogenesis of chronic lung disease is multifactorial and consequently strategies to prevent bronchopulmonary dysplasia must be equally comprehensive.
- Less invasive approaches to initial stabilization and surfactant administration are based on sound evidence and generally accepted. Various modalities of noninvasive respiratory support are widely practiced, but evidence of superiority of one over another is incomplete.
- Optimal lung aeration and avoidance of atelectrauma is an essential element of any lung-protective ventilation strategy.
- Volume-targeted ventilation is the most evidence-based approach to invasive mechanical ventilation; other novel modalities are potentially attractive, but insufficiently studied.

Advances in obstetric and neonatal intensive care have led to the survival of smaller and more immature infants born at earlier stages of lung development. Although the survival of very premature infants improved, the rate of bronchopulmonary dysplasia (BPD) has remained the same, or even increased.[1,2] Extremely premature survivors who are most likely to develop BPD after a prolonged hospitalization suffer from chronic cardiopulmonary impairment, growth failure, neurodevelopmental impairment, and difficulties with social functioning, all of which can have a profound impact on the entire family, financially and emotionally.[3,4] Efforts to prevent or mitigate the severity of BPD must take into account the multifactorial nature of the condition and the substantial individual differences in susceptibility. Well known factors that increase the risk of BPD include intrauterine factors, such as chorioamnionitis, maternal smoking, and intrauterine growth restriction; perinatal factors, the most prominent of which

Department of Pediatrics, Women & Infants Hospital of Rhode Island, Alpert Medical School of Brown University, 101 Dudley Street, Providence, RI 02905, USA
E-mail address: Martin_Keszler@Brown.edu

Clin Perinatol 49 (2022) 219–242
https://doi.org/10.1016/j.clp.2021.11.019
0095-5108/22/© 2021 Elsevier Inc. All rights reserved.

is prematurity; and postnatal factors including exposure to relative hyperoxia and mechanical ventilation.[5–7] Suboptimal initial stabilization and postnatal infections further increase the risk. Some of the postnatal factors are within control, but most of the intrauterine factors are not easily modifiable. Gestational age remains the most important risk factor for BPD and prevention of prematurity remains an elusive goal. Impairment of normal pulmonary development is likely unavoidable when a fetus in the early saccular stage of lung development finds himself or herself in the hyperoxic environment (relative to the intrauterine oxygen level) and is required to support his or her gas exchange with lungs that are inadequately developed. Nonetheless, the substantial variation in the incidence of BPD among different institutions not explainable by differences in patient population strongly suggests that postnatal management can influence the degree of lung injury.[2,8]

Detailed discussion of the mechanisms of ventilator-associated lung injury (VALI) and cause of BPD is beyond the scope of this article, but is discussed elsewhere.[9–11] In this article, we briefly discuss the mechanisms of lung injury and review the available evidence for possible benefits of various newer strategies of respiratory support.

VENTILATOR-ASSOCIATED LUNG INJURY

Lung injury and subsequent repair that ultimately leads to BPD is a complex process with no single element being able to fully account for its development. However, several aspects are generally believed to be central to its development. (1) Excessive tissue stretch (volutrauma) is the key determinant of VALI. Inflation pressure by itself, without generating an excessively large tidal volume (V_T), has been shown to not result in acute lung injury.[12,13] (2) Positive-pressure ventilation in lungs that are partially atelectatic predisposes to VALI by a variety of mechanisms collectively known as atelectrauma. Maintenance of alveolar stability at end-expiration by using adequate positive end-expiratory pressure (PEEP) mitigates lung injury.[9,14] (3) Both antenatal and postnatal infection can initiate the cascade of lung injury and repair,[15] a process sometimes referred to as biotrauma.

INITIAL STABILIZATION AND STRATEGIES TO OPTIMIZE LUNG AERATION AT BIRTH

Avoidance of practices that can potentiate lung injury must start during initial stabilization of the preterm infant during the "golden first hour."[16] Even a brief period of manual ventilation with excessive V_T can rapidly injure the immature lung in the delivery room.[17] The best strategy aimed at helping the preterm infant with insufficient chest wall rigidity to establish functional residual capacity (FRC) and facilitating lung fluid clearance is the subject of ongoing studies. There is strong physiologic rationale and substantial preclinical data to support the use of PEEP in the delivery room, but paucity of clinical evidence from randomized trials. Sustained inflation became widespread in Europe based on encouraging preclinical studies and several modest-sized clinical trials,[18–20] but the largest study to date, the Sustained Aeration of Infant Lungs (SAIL) trial, failed to substantiate its presumed benefit.[21] Although there was no overall difference in the primary outcome of death or BPD, there was a signal of increased early mortality in this highly vulnerable population of infants less than 27 weeks gestational age and no hint of benefit. An updated meta-analysis clearly indicates caution, because the cumulative evidence shows a strong, although not statistically significant trend to higher mortality with sustained inflation (**Fig. 1**).[22] A large multicenter trial to explore a titrated PEEP strategy that seeks to tailor the level of distending pressure to each infant's need based on initial response is underway (Australian New Zealand Clinical Trials Registry ACTRN12618001686291).

Current evidence, although incomplete, suggests that sustained inflation should be avoided in favor of sufficient PEEP, and gentle positive-pressure inflations, if needed, and early application of continuous positive airway pressure (CPAP). A T-piece resuscitator is preferred to self-inflating bag, because it achieves more consistent inflation pressure and effective PEEP delivery.[23,24] Estimation of V_T by observation of chest wall movement is inaccurate and tends to substantially underestimate the actual V_T.[25] Therefore the goal is to use just enough pressure to achieve a barely perceptible chest rise. V_T measurement during manual ventilation is feasible, but seldom used clinically. A prototype volume-targeted resuscitation device has been developed,[26] a tool that is highly desirable, because of sound evidence that volutrauma is the key factor in lung injury and that respiratory system compliance changes rapidly soon after birth. Clinical studies are needed to determine if this device results in reduction of lung injury.

Neonatal Resuscitation Program (NRP) recommends that the initial fraction of inspired oxygen (F_{IO_2}) should be between 0.21 and 0.30 for preterm infants and 0.21 for term infants.[27] However, all preterm infants who were started with F_{IO_2} of 0.21 required increased F_{IO_2} to reach adequate saturation levels[28]; therefore, most clinicians begin with F_{IO_2} around 0.30. Avoidance of excessive oxygen exposure should be part of any lung-protective ventilation strategy. F_{IO_2} should be promptly titrated to maintain target saturation according to published nomograms.[29] Intubation solely for the purpose of administering prophylactic surfactant is no longer recommended, but if intubation is required for initial stabilization, surfactant should be administered promptly, once the endotracheal tube (ETT) position has been confirmed.[30]

NONINVASIVE RESPIRATORY SUPPORT/LESS INVASIVE SURFACTANT ADMINISTRATION

Noninvasive support with CPAP is successful in most infants greater than 26 weeks gestation.[31] Although the effect on BPD seen in a series of large randomized controlled trials comparing CPAP with routine intubation and surfactant administration was smaller than anticipated, the cumulative evidence clearly supports the role of CPAP in reducing the need for mechanical ventilation and the risk of BPD.[32,33] Less invasive approaches to surfactant administration via a thin catheter or laryngeal mask airway are gaining acceptance based on accumulating evidence of the potential benefit of surfactant administration without the need for mechanical ventilation.[34–36] Until recently, the use of laryngeal mask airway was limited by lack of sufficiently small devices, but newer laryngeal mask airways are adequate down to 1000-g infants. Nebulized surfactant administration, the only truly noninvasive strategy, is another attractive option, but its use remains investigational.[37,38]

In the absence of adequately powered prospective trials controversy persists regarding relative merits of various forms of CPAP. A preclinical study in preterm lambs showed that bubble CPAP improved gas exchange and decreased markers of lung injury.[39] Clinical data are limited to a series of small single-center studies, but a recent meta-analysis indicated that bubble CPAP reduced the incidence of CPAP failure compared with ventilator CPAP.[40]

Bilevel CPAP was touted as a better approach than static CPAP, but the cyclic pressure swings do not produce a measurable V_T[41,42] and when applied at equivalent mean airway pressure (MAP), bilevel CPAP did not seem to offer any advantage over constant pressure CPAP.[43,44]

Nasal intermittent positive-pressure ventilation (NIPPV) has rapidly gained acceptance as an effective modality of noninvasive support based on a handful of

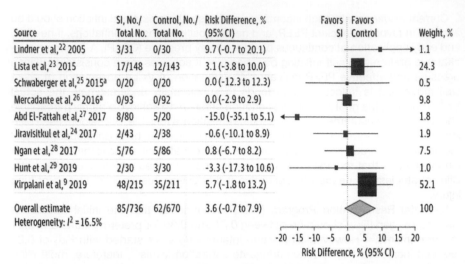

Source	SI, No./ Total No.	Control, No./ Total No.	Risk Difference, % (95% CI)	Favors SI	Favors Control	Weight, %
Lindner et al,[22] 2005	3/31	0/30	9.7 (-0.7 to 20.1)			1.1
Lista et al,[23] 2015	17/148	12/143	3.1 (-3.8 to 10.0)			24.3
Schwaberger et al,[25] 2015[a]	0/20	0/20	0.0 (-12.3 to 12.3)			0.5
Mercadante et al,[26] 2016[a]	0/93	0/92	0.0 (-2.9 to 2.9)			9.8
Abd El-Fattah et al,[27] 2017	8/80	5/20	-15.0 (-35.1 to 5.1)			1.8
Jiravisitkul et al,[24] 2017	2/43	2/38	-0.6 (-10.1 to 8.9)			1.9
Ngan et al,[28] 2017	5/76	5/86	0.8 (-6.7 to 8.2)			7.5
Hunt et al,[29] 2019	2/30	3/30	-3.3 (-17.3 to 10.6)			1.0
Kirpalani et al,[9] 2019	48/215	35/211	5.7 (-1.8 to 13.2)			52.1
Overall estimate Heterogeneity: I^2 = 16.5%	85/736	62/670	3.6 (-0.7 to 7.9)			100

-20 -15 -10 -5 0 5 10 15 20
Risk Difference, % (95% CI)

Fig. 1. Updated meta-analysis of available randomized controlled trials of sustained inflation (SI) for in-hospital mortality. The size of each trial is reflected by the size of the *box* representing the point estimate. The total number of subjects included is 1406 with an overall mortality risk difference, represented by the *diamond*, of +3.6% (95% confidence interval [CI], −0.7 to 7.9). (*From* Foglia EE, Te Pas AB, Kirpalani H, Davis PG, Owen LS, van Kaam AH, et al. Sustained Inflation vs Standard Resuscitation for Preterm Infants: A Systematic Review and Meta-analysis. *JAMA Pediatr.* 2020;174(4):e195897.)

randomized trials, whereas the largest randomized trial did not show any benefit.[45,46] The widely held belief that NIPPV is able to provide effective ventilation via a nasal interface is not supported by evidence. Only a fraction of ventilator inflations achieve a measurable V_T with unsynchronized NIPPV (the only kind currently available in the United States) because in newborn infants the glottis is closed unless the infant is actively inspiring.[47,48] Thus, the benefit of NIPPV, primarily in reducing postextubation failure documented in the most recent Cochrane review,[45] seems to derive from the higher MAP used with NIPPV, compared with CPAP in most of the published studies. Buzzella and colleagues[49] demonstrated that the use of higher, as opposed to lower CPAP level following extubation significantly reduced CPAP failure, providing the plausible explanation for the apparent superiority of NIPPV over CPAP. Studies are underway to test the hypothesis that CPAP and NIPPV are equivalent when used at the same MAP (ClinicalTrials.gov Identifier: NCT03512158 and NCT03670732).

The importance of patient interface has not received adequate attention until recently. The RAM cannula (Neotech, Valencia, CA) was designed and approved by the Food and Drug Administration as a nasal cannula for delivery of low- or high-flow oxygen, but has been promoted for off-label use as a device to deliver CPAP and NIPPV. The cannula rapidly gained popularity because of the ease of application and less need for skilled nursing attention. However, it has become clear that such off-label use is problematic. Extensive evidence indicates that short binasal prongs are superior to the RAM cannula for delivery of CPAP and NIPPV, because of the large loss of pressure across the high resistance of the RAM cannula (**Fig. 2**).[50–55]

NOVEL APPROACHES TO NONINVASIVE RESPIRATORY SUPPORT

A proprietary variant of NIPPV known as noninvasive neurally adjusted ventilatory assist (NIV NAVA) seems to overcome the limitations of nonsynchronized NIPPV.

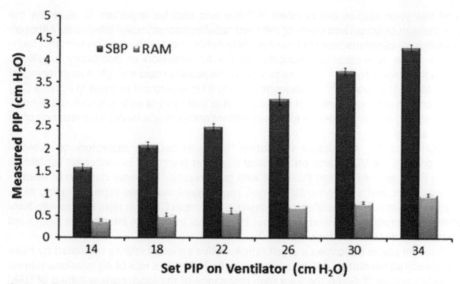

Fig. 2. Transmitted peak inflation pressure (measured at the distal airway) during NIPPV via small RAM cannula, compared with small binasal prongs (SBP) in a bench study. There is a large drop across both interfaces, with minimal pressure being transmitted via the RAM cannula. PIP, peak inflation pressure. (*From* Mukerji A, Beli, k J. Neonatal nasal intermittent positive pressure ventilation efficacy and lung pressure transmission. *Journal of perinatology : official journal of the California Perinatal Association.* 2015;35(9):716-719.)

This unique method of noninvasive ventilation uses the electrical activity of the diaphragm (EAdi) to synchronize inflation with the infant's respiratory effort and therefore is able to synchronize effectively with the open interface of NIV. The evidence for superiority of NIV NAVA is limited to a few small single-center studies demonstrating improved synchrony, lower peak pressures, greater patient comfort, and lower rate of extubation failure.[56–60] A large National Institutes of Health–funded multicenter trial, the Diaphragmatic Initiated Ventilatory Assist (DIVA) trial (Clinicaltrials.gov registration pending) seeks to provide more definitive evidence of benefit of this promising approach. Currently NIV NAVA is only available on the Maquet SERVO ventilators (Getinge, Solna, Sweden). A prototype of NIV NAVA-dedicated device termed "Neuro-PAP" that not only supports spontaneous respiratory effort of the infant with inflation pressure proportional to the magnitude of the EAdi like regular NIV NAVA, but also uses the resting tonic activity of the diaphragm to actively modulate the PEEP, performed well in a small crossover trial in preterm infants. Despite being actively modulated, the average PEEP was similar as the set PEEP during NIPPV.[61]

Interest in improving noninvasive respiratory support by using high-frequency oscillatory ventilation (HFOV) via the nasal route dates back a couple of decades.[62] More recently, several small and medium-sized single-center randomized studies reported encouraging findings when comparing nasal HFOV with biphasic CPAP,[63] or static nasal CPAP.[64–67] These studies varied widely in terms of the population and the specific settings. Some studies did not match the MAP between the groups. Two meta-analysis sum up the findings and acknowledge the heterogeneity; nonetheless, the overall effect was a significant reduction in the need for invasive mechanical ventilation.[68,69] Some of the studies also reported lower P_{CO_2} in the nasal HFOV arm. Larger randomized trials are needed to establish the safety and effectiveness of nasal HFOV and two such studies are planned.[70,71] It would also be important to elucidate the mechanism of action and effect of different nasal/nasopharyngeal interfaces. Although anecdotally clinicians report observing detectable chest wall vibration with this technique, there is substantial reduction in the transmission of oscillatory amplitude through narrow prongs.[72] For this reason some studies used a single nasopharyngeal tube as the interface.[62,73,74] Frequency of 6 to 8 Hz was found to result in optimal CO_2 clearance in a bench study.[75] It is also possible that there is an increase in distal pressure leading to more effective lung recruitment and perhaps better maintenance of an open airway.

High-frequency percussive ventilation has been used in laboratory on preterm sheep using the VDR4 and on neonatal transport using the Bronchotron ventilators (both Percussionaire, Sand Point, ID) with good results.[76] Shorter duration of respiratory support and supplemental oxygen requirement was also reported using high-frequency percussive ventilation, compared with nasal CPAP in term infants with transient tachypnea of the newborn,[77] but larger trials in preterm infants with significant respiratory distress are lacking.

A recent paper described a small retrospective series of infants ventilated by high-frequency jet ventilation (HFJV) combined with NIPPV at a rate of 40 inflations/min via a RAM cannula.[78] Given the very high resistance of the long, narrow tubing of RAM cannula, it is questionable whether this approach could result in anything but a substantially increased (and unmeasured) distending airway pressure as the high gas flow from the jet ventilator acts like a very high-flow nasal cannula. In the laboratory setting nasal HFJV is effective when applied via a nasopharyngeal tube in preterm lambs (K. Albertine, personal communication). Clearly, more data are needed regarding nasal HFJV safety and efficacy of nasal HFJV and the pressure and flow transmission through various interfaces. A prospective trial has been registered in ClinicalTrials.gov (NCT03558737) proposing to use a nasopharyngeal interface for the delivery of nasal HFJV.

It remains to be seen if any of these noninvasive high-frequency modalities can improve overall outcome when compared with bubble CPAP at similar distending pressures.

INCREASED DURATION OF CONTINUOUS POSITIVE AIRWAY PRESSURE

It is well known that the distending pressure exerted on fetal lungs in utero is critical for normal lung growth and that prolonged oligohydramnios is associated with lung hypoplasia. Animal models have demonstrated that lung growth is induced by continuous distending pressure.[79,80] Occlusion of fetal trachea in fetuses with congenital diaphragmatic hernia results in significant lung growth.[81,82] Therefore, it is conceivable that infants born extremely preterm might benefit from continuation of distending airway pressure until lung development is near-complete. Continuation of CPAP beyond the traditional criteria has long been the practice at Morgan Stanley Children's Hospital in New York and seems to be associated with a remarkably low incidence of BPD.[83] However, this approach has never been subjected to a randomized controlled trial. The first evidence supporting the concept that prolonged CPAP use may improve lung function in preterm infants was a clinical trial that randomly assigned infants less than 32 weeks gestation who reached traditional criteria for discontinuation of CPAP to be weaned to room air or to continue on CPAP for 2 additional weeks.[84] Infants randomized to extended CPAP had a significantly greater increase in FRC from baseline through 2 weeks of treatment (12.6 mL vs 6.4 mL; $P = 0.03$) and this benefit was still evident at discharge (FRC, 27.2 mL vs 17.1 mL; $P = 0.01$). The longer duration of

CPAP did not affect initiation of oral feeding or prolong hospitalization. These data are certainly encouraging but whether this increased lung growth translates into a reduction in the rate of BPD or long-term respiratory morbidity in the most vulnerable infants requires a larger randomized trial with important clinical outcomes. It is unlikely that this intervention alone could affect the rate of type II severe BPD, because these infants generally receive positive-pressure support throughout their hospitalization,[85-] but less severe degrees of BPD may well be preventable.

PREVENTION OF ATELECTRAUMA

Prevention of atelectrauma is not a new concept, but is not rigorously applied in neonatal respiratory support. Reluctance to use sufficiently high PEEP, known as "PEEP-o-phobia," remains pervasive, despite evidence that sufficient PEEP mitigates lung injury.[86–88] Ventilation of injured lungs using insufficient PEEP results in repeated alveolar collapse and expansion with each inflation, leading rapidly to injury of the immature lung. When the lungs remain partially atelectatic, the gas that enters the lungs preferentially distends the more compliant aerated portion of the lung, whereas the atelectatic portion with its high critical opening pressure remains collapsed. This fact is evident from Laplace's law and is corroborated by experimental evidence, showing that the most injured portion of the lung was the aerated, nondependent lung.[89] Because of this maldistribution of V_T, volutrauma can occur even with normal physiologic V_T and this may explain why high oxygen requirement in infants on CPAP, a marker of ventilation/perfusion mismatch (i.e., atelectasis), was associated with increased risk of pneumothorax.[90] Studies exploring the use of substantially higher PEEP suggest that this approach is safe and effective, but more data are needed from larger studies.[91]

Thus the key elements in minimizing lung injury include: (1) minimizing alveolar overdistention (volutrauma), (2) optimizing end-expiratory lung volume by reversing atelectasis by means of some form of lung recruitment, and (3) stabilizing lung units throughout the ventilatory cycle (avoiding repeated collapse and re-expansion). Applying this strategy also improves ventilation/perfusion matching and thus oxygenation, allowing reduction of supplemental oxygen concentration (less oxygen toxicity). This lung-protective ventilation strategy is referred to as an open lung strategy.[14,92]

Lung volume recruitment seems to be more easily achieved with HFOV,[93] but is also feasible with conventional ventilation.[94] With either approach, the critical opening pressure of the atelectatic saccules needs to be reached and then maintained with sufficiently high end-expiratory pressure.[95] With HFOV, lung volume recruitment is performed by inflating the lungs to close to their maximum volume with stepwise increases in MAP. Electrical impedance tomography is a promising tool to visualize lung aeration in real time, but is not yet widely available.[96,97] Therefore, oxygen requirement as a reflection of ventilation/perfusion matching is used to guide this strategy. The lungs are considered to be fully inflated when F_{IO_2} is weaned to less than 0.30. The lungs are then deflated to the closing volume that is indicated by deterioration in oxygen saturation on pulse oximetry. The lungs are subsequently reinflated and the final MAP is set at a point just above closing volume.[93] This technique allows ventilation to move from the inspiratory limb of the pressure-volume curve to the expiratory limb, allowing effective ventilation and oxygenation at lower pressures.[98] Surfactant distribution is improved when it is administered into an adequately aerated lung.[99] Aggressive lung recruitment is seldom necessary in infants with uncomplicated respiratory distress syndrome after surfactant treatment, but if high oxygen requirement persists, optimization of lung volume should be attempted. However, not all lungs are recruitable; some infants may have neonatal pneumonia or other conditions that preclude effective recruitment. Consequently, if two consecutive increases in MAP fail to produce an improvement in oxygenation, further efforts should be abandoned. It is important to recognize that once the lungs are adequately recruited, lung compliance improves and the pressure needed to maintain that recruitment is less than the pressure that was initially required to open the atelectatic portions of the lungs. Thus, it is important to reduce the distending pressure once lung volume is optimized. With conventional ventilation, recruitment is achieved by stepwise increases in PEEP, while maintaining adequate peak inflation pressure to avoid hypoventilation and reach the critical opening pressure of atelectatic saccules.[94]

AVOIDANCE OF VOLUTRAUMA

Several meta-analyses have documented the benefits of volume-controlled and volume-targeted ventilation (VTV) in newborn infants, including significant decrease in the rate of BPD, pneumothorax, severe intraventricular hemorrhage, periventricular leukomalacia, less hypocapnia and shorter duration of mechanical ventilation **(Table 1)**.[100,101] Volume-controlled ventilation, where a user-set volume of gas is injected into the proximal (ventilator) end of the circuit, is routinely used in pediatric and adult intensive care units, because direct control of minute ventilation and avoidance of volutrauma is recognized as an important goal. However, early attempts at volume-controlled ventilation in neonates using ventilators designed for large patients were a dismal failure because of loss of V_T to compression of gas within the circuit and leak around uncuffed ETT. This experience resulted in the adoption of pressure-controlled ventilation in the neonatal intensive care unit, a situation that persists to a significant degree in the United States.[102] The major problem with pressure-controlled ventilation is that V_T changes with changes in lung compliance, which can occur rapidly and often results in lung overexpansion, volutrauma, and hypocapnia.

Modern ventilators now make it possible to use volume-controlled ventilation in newborn infants by allowing for measurement of exhaled V_T at the airway opening, so that manual adjustment of set V_T at the ventilator end of the patient circuit is

Table 1
Metaanalysis of studies comparing volume controlled/targeted ventilation modalities with pressure controlled ventilation.[101]

	Relative Risk or Mean Difference	95% CI	NNTB (95% CI)
Death or BPD at 36 wk	0.75	0.53 to 1.07	NA
BPD at 36 wk PMA	0.73	0.59 to 0.89	8 (5 to 20)
Grade 3-4 IVH	0.53	0.37 to 0.77	11 (7 to 25)
PVL ± severe IVH	0.47	0.27 to 0.80	11 (7 to 33)
Pneumothorax	0.52	0.31 to 0.87	20 (11 to 100)
Hypocapnia	0.49	0.33 to 0.72	3 (2 to 5)
Days of MV	−1.35	−1.83 to −0.86	

Abbreviations: CI, confidence interval; IVH, intraventricular hemorrhage; MV, mechanical ventilation; PVL, periventricular leukomalacia; NA, not applicable; NNTB, number needed to benefit; PMA, postmenstrual age.

made to achieve a desired exhaled V_T.[103] More convenient are volume-targeted modes that are modifications of pressure-controlled ventilation that automatically adjust inflation pressure to achieve a target V_T.[104] With V_T as the primary control variable, peak inflation pressure is automatically reduced as lung compliance and patient inspiratory effort improve, resulting in real-time weaning, in contrast to intermittent manual lowering of peak inflation pressure in response to blood gas measurement. Volume guarantee (VG) is the most extensively studied form of VTV and the basic control algorithm is increasingly being adopted by other ventilator manufacturers. The key to successful use of VTV is recognition of the importance of choosing the appropriate V_T target. A series of observational studies defined the typical V_T requirement in various conditions and patient categories.[105–108] However, it is important to recognize that these values are population means, which are a good starting point, but clinical assessment of the patient's response to these initial settings should be promptly assessed and adjustments made as indicated based on patient's respiratory effort (tachypnea, retractions, or apnea) and of ventilator waveforms.[109] VG ventilation has been clinically available for more than 20 years, but despite strong evidence of benefit, it has not been universally accepted. Reasons for this include simple inertia, but also lack of suitable equipment in many neonatal intensive care units and a lack of understanding of the complexities of the approach.[102] For more detailed discussion of VTV the interested reader is referred to the latest article on the subject.[110]

HIGH-FREQUENCY VENTILATION WITH VOLUME TARGETING

High-frequency ventilation is not novel and the evidence for its benefit as first-line therapy for infants with uncomplicated RDS is weak.[111] HFOV facilitates lung volume recruitment and HFJV is an effective rescue therapy for air leak.[112] The novel aspect of HFOV, which is already widely available in the rest of the world and may soon become available in the United States, is the ability to combine VG with HFOV.[113–115] The volume-targeting concept is similar to conventional VG, but because of the high frequency, V_T is averaged over several cycles to guide automatic adjustment of pressure amplitude within user-preset limits. This technological advance should reduce the risk of inadvertent overventilation that readily occurs with high-frequency ventilation because even modest change in V_T has a large impact on CO_2 elimination because of the geometric relationship between V_T and ventilation efficiency. A multicenter clinical trial to document safety and efficacy of HFOV combined with VG has been completed (ClinicalTrials.gov Identifier: NCT02445040) with the goal of obtaining Food and Drug Administration approval.

PROPORTIONAL ASSIST MODALITIES

Giving the patient more complete control of the entire respiratory cycle is an attractive concept that has the potential to achieve more complete synchrony, greater patient comfort, improved gas exchange, and lower ventilator pressures.[116] Two such approaches have been available for more than a decade, although their use remains limited, in part because they are both proprietary technologies. Proportional assist ventilation (PAV) is available on the Stephanie ventilator (Stephan, Gackenbach, Germany) and is not available in the United States. The NAVA modality is only available on the Maquet SERVO ventilators (Getinge, Solna, Sweden).

PAV is a sophisticated modality that senses the patient's effort throughout the respiratory cycle by means of a high-fidelity pneumotachograph with a rapid sampling rate and generates inflation pressure in proportion to the inspired volume and flow. The gain applied to the patient's effort is designed to keep the inspiratory effort needed to generate a given volume stable to the preset degree of unloading of the total respiratory system elastance, including the ventilator and circuit. This is referred to as elastic unloading and the gain is denominated in cm H_2O/mL of V_T measured at the airway opening. The resistance is unloaded in a similar fashion by keeping the effort needed to generate a given airflow constant, a process known as resistive unloading and is denominated in cm H_2O/mL/s. The estimated ETT resistance is usually included in the calculation.

PAV has been evaluated in animal models[117] and a handful of small clinical studies with short-term outcomes, demonstrating lower work of breathing, lower MAPs, and no apparent complications.[118–121] There are several impediments to widespread acceptance of PAV. The technique is complex and presents several unique challenges. The choice of appropriate gain setting for elastic and resistive unloading is not intuitive and normative data are not readily available for different patient conditions. Excessive gain setting can result in oscillation of the system, lack of respiratory muscle training, and prolonged ventilator dependence. The method requires the use of inspiratory flow and volume measurement, which presents a problem if there is a substantial leak around the uncuffed ETT. Water condensation in the pneumotachograph can affect performance and lead to oversupport or undersupport. Finally, the immature respiratory control in very preterm infants requires a backup ventilation mode and appropriate pressure limits to deal with periodic breathing and apnea, and brief bursts of vigorous respiratory effort with handling or stimulation. Larger randomized trials with important clinical outcomes are needed to determine if the effort of mastering this modality is warranted.

NAVA is a modality developed for use in adult patients but now more widely used in newborn infants. As with PAV, the goal is to give the patient full control of the respiratory cycle, including onset of inflation, peak inflation pressure, and onset of exhalation. EAdi is measured by an array of electrodes mounted on a special catheter that can simultaneously serve as a feeding tube. When the infant initiates inspiration by activating his or her phrenic nerve, the EAdi is sensed by the EAdi catheter and this signal triggers inflation pressures in proportion to the voltage (measured in μV), and multiplied by the "NAVA level," measured in cm H_2O/μV, which is the gain, or degree of unloading of the patient's respiratory work. The ventilator displays the maximal EAdi and the minimal EAdi, the former being the maximal EAdi reached at peak inspiration and the latter being the EAdi at end-expiration and represents the tonic activity of the diaphragm activity. Monitoring the peak EAdi lets the clinician monitor how much work of breathing the infant is generating. High or rising peak EAdi suggests a need for increasing the NAVA level. Patients with significant lung disease and intact respiratory control typically generate strong inspiratory effort, but are unable to achieve adequate V_T. With progressive increases in the NAVA level, the EAdi initially remains stable while the inflation pressure and resulting V_T increase. At some point, the degree of unloading becomes sufficient to achieve adequate minute ventilation and the infant's respiratory effort, as measured by the EAdi, comes down, indicating lower work of breathing. This point is referred to as the "break point" (**Fig. 3**).[122] Further increases in EAdi do not increase the V_T or minute ventilation, but simply result in lower work of breathing for the infant. However, a recent study demonstrated that in premature infants, this response is not always reliable. They observed that as the NAVA level increased, a higher proportion of excessive V_T was delivered, with 20% to 25% of V_T greater than 10 mL/kg (measured at the airway opening) at NAVA level of 2.5 cm H_2O/μV (**Fig. 4**).[123] This is likely because preterm infants often respond to external stimuli and may briefly generate large inspiratory effort, when disturbed, which is potentiated by the positive feedback of NAVA (**Fig. 5**).

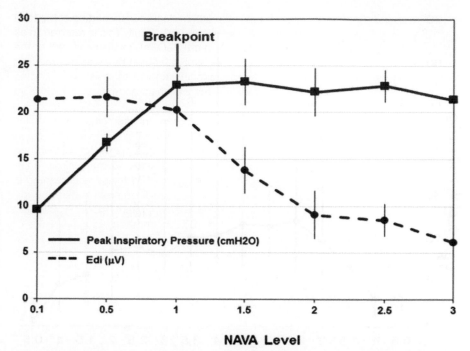

Fig. 3. The breakpoint in a subject with a mature respiratory pattern. Increasing the NAVA level, the gain applied to EAdi initially results in higher peak inflation pressure, but once the unloading of the diaphragm is sufficient, further increases in the NAVA level result in no further increase in peak inflation pressure, as the patient's respiratory effort decreases to maintain stable minute ventilation. (*From* Firestone KS, Fisher S, Reddy S, White DB, Stein HM. Effect of changing NAVA levels on peak inspiratory pressures and electrical activity of the diaphragm in premature neonates. *Journal of perinatology : official journal of the California Perinatal Association.* 2015;35(8):612-616.)

Elevated minimum EAdi level indicates tonic activity of the diaphragm is increased, which reflects the patient's effort to maintain FRC by not completely exhaling and suggests the need to increase PEEP, which is set manually, not controlled by the patient. The feedback available to the clinician is an attractive feature of NAVA and allows physiologic monitoring and appropriate adjustments of respiratory support. The EAdi signal has minimal trigger delay and is unaffected by movement, airflow artifacts, or air leak around uncuffed ETT. Unlike pneumatic triggers the EAdi signal is unaffected by leakage in an open system, making NAVA attractive for noninvasive ventilation with a high degree of synchrony.

The key disadvantage is that NAVA requires sustained spontaneous respiratory drive and thus is best suited for more physiologically mature subjects. For preterm infants with frequent apnea and periodic breathing the device provides flow or pressure-triggered pressure support ventilation mode and backup ventilation in case of inadequate EAdi signal. In some circumstances, the device switches in and out of backup ventilation frequently, which is undesirable. In addition to immature respiratory system, it is also important to consider the immaturity of other organs, such as the kidneys, which commonly leads to transient renal tubular acidosis in the first few days of life. Because respiratory control is driven by pH, not simply Pco_2, clinicians must

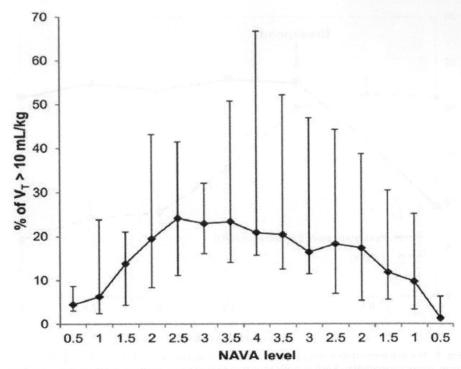

Fig. 4. In preterm infants with immature respiratory control, external stimuli often affect the immature respiratory pattern of the infant and result in a substantial proportion of potentially dangerous tidal volumes. Some 20% to 25% of tidal volumes were greater than 10 mL/kg at NAVA levels greater than or equal to 2.5 cm H_2O/mV. (*From* Nam SK, Lee J, Jun YH. Neural feedback is insufficient in preterm infants during neurally adjusted ventilatory assist. Pediatric pulmonology. 2019;54(8):1277-1283.)

not focus solely on Pco_2 targets but rather evaluate the patient's respiratory drive in the context of pH.

Several small clinical studies of NAVA have compared NAVA with various modalities of synchronized ventilation and have demonstrated improved synchrony, lower peak pressure, and comparable gas exchange.[124–128] One study reported lower V_T and lung compliance with NAVA, compared with pressure-support ventilation.[129] However, V_T measurement with the SERVO-i in small infants is inaccurate (the reported values were barely above anatomic dead space) and lung compliance derived from the ventilator fails to take into account the patient's spontaneous respiratory effort. The single randomized trial failed to demonstrate any benefit of NAVA in terms of duration of ventilation, rate of pneumothorax, intraventricular hemorrhage, or BPD.[130] More recently, interest has shifted to using NAVA in olderinfants with evolving or established BPD, an application that may be better suited for NAVA. The findings were encouraging, but the studies were small and observational or crossover design in nature.[131–134]

The approach of positive feedback mechanism used by these proportional modalities would seem more appropriate for more mature subjects with reliable respiratory effort. There are limited data regarding the stability of V_T delivered with these devices and the potential exists for inadequate support and potentially dangerously large V_T

Infant

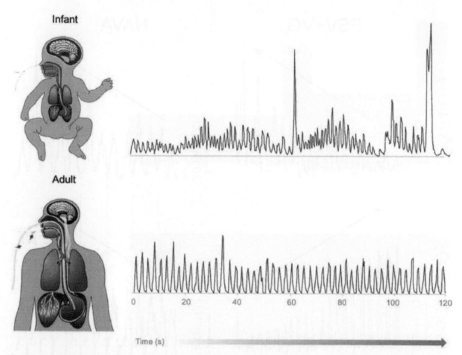

Adult

Time (s)

Fig. 5. In contrast to the adult or child with mature respiratory control (*bottom*), the pre-term infant's breathing pattern, as reflected by the EAdi, is erratic with bursts of vigorous breathing interspersed with periods of hypoventilation and short apneas (*top*). (*From* Firestone KS, Fisher S, Reddy S, White DB, Stein HM. Effect of changing NAVA levels on peak inspiratory pressures and electrical activity of the diaphragm in premature neonates. *Journal of perinatology: official journal of the California Perinatal Association.* 2015;35(8):612-616.)

with the sometimes erratic respiratory effort of the preterm infant.[123] VG, a modality developed specifically for preterm infants is, by contrast, a negative feedback approach, which generates less inflation pressure when the V_T exceeds the target and more when it is less than target, aiming to maintain a stable V_T (**Fig. 6**). Although NAVA and PAV are interesting modalities with obvious potential benefits, larger randomized trials are needed to establish safety and efficacy in preterm infants with immature respiratory control.

AIRWAY PRESSURE RELEASE VENTILATION

Airway pressure release ventilation is a technique designed to achieve lung volume recruitment and relies on patient's spontaneous breathing to achieve the bulk of minute ventilation. The ventilator maintains a high inflation pressure for most of each ventilator cycle with periodic "release" of this pressure for brief periods.[135] This alternating pattern of low and high airway pressure is, in essence, a form of extreme inverse ratio ventilation. Similar to biphasic CPAP it relies on spontaneous breathing and aims to optimize lung volume recruitment, but in a more extreme way. Airway pressure release ventilation is usually used as a rescue technique and in contrast to biphasic CPAP, the upper pressure level "P high" is maintained for most of the cycle "T high." The pressure to which the lungs are released is called "P low" and the release time is called

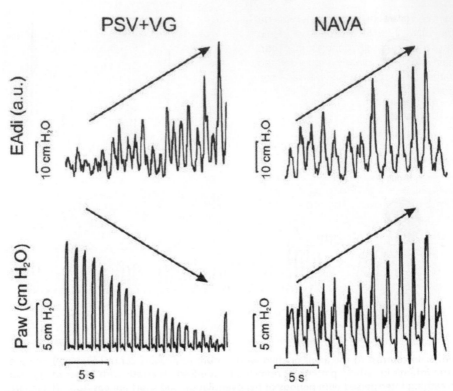

Fig. 6. The contrasting approaches to respiratory assist between VG ventilation (*left*) and NAVA (*right*). With VG, when the patient's respiratory effort, as indicated by the EAdi, is insufficient or absent, the ventilator generates a higher peak inflation pressure (PIP); when vigorous inspiratory effort generates excessive tidal volume, the ventilator pressure decreases to maintain a stable tidal volume. This is a negative feedback loop. With NAVA, mature respiratory control is assumed and the ventilator delivers PIP in direct proportion to the EAdi, a positive feedback mechanism. airway pressure (Paw); pressure support ventilation (PSV). (*From* Sinderby C, Beck J. Proportional assist ventilation and neurally adjusted ventilatory assist–better approaches to patient ventilator synchrony? Clin Chest Med. 2008;29(2):329-342, vii.)

"T low." The technique has primarily been used in adult patients with acute lung injury, where there is evidence for short-term benefits in terms of oxygenation but no demonstrable improvement in survival or reduction in complications.[135] There is insufficient evidence to assess the utility of this technique in newborn infants with only a handful of case reports available and no controlled trials, but it is concerning that a recent randomized trial in pediatric patients was terminated early because of increased mortality in the airway pressure release ventilation arm.[136]

MANDATORY MINUTE VENTILATION

Mandatory minute ventilation may be useful in preterm infants who have inconsistent respiratory effort. Mandatory minute ventilation is a modification of SIMV with PS that maintains a low baseline rate of mandatory inflations as long as the patient's spontaneous effort, augmented by PS, is adequate to meet the user-selected mandatory minute ventilation target. When the patient's respiratory rate falls, the device increases the SIMV rate in a proactive fashion if the projected minute ventilation is falling short.[137] Although conceptually attractive, the potential benefits of this approach have not been clearly demonstrated.[138] Other approaches, such as assist control with an appropriate backup rate combined with VG, can already achieve the same goal.

ADAPTIVE SUPPORT VENTILATION

Adaptive support ventilation is modality of ventilation used in pediatric and adult patients that uses automatic adjustments to respiratory rate and V_T.[139] The clinician determines the desired minute ventilation, and the adaptive support ventilation algorithm determines the optimal respiratory rate/V_T combination according to the patient's respiratory mechanics. The optimal respiratory rate and V_T are reassessed on a breath-to-breath basis based on continuous measurement of lung mechanics. In periods during which the spontaneous breathing rate decreases, mandatory inflations are provided to maintain the desired respiratory rate. The modality is unlikely to be adapted to neonatal ventilation, because of its complexity, need for accurate measurement of lung mechanics and V_T, and the erratic respiratory pattern of preterm infants.

AUTOMATED CONTROL OF FRACTION OF INSPIRED OXYGEN

Automated oxygen controllers reduce the percent of time infants spend outside target oxygen saturation as measured by pulse oximetry levels.[140,141] Both hyperoxemia and hypoxemia are reduced and thus this technology might reduce oxidative stress and proinflammatory stimuli in preterm infants at risk for BPD, a hypothesis being tested in a current multicenter trial.[142] Unfortunately, these devices have not yet received approval for clinical use by the Food and Drug Administration and are thus not available in the United States.

SUMMARY

Prevention of lung injury remains an elusive goal of neonatal respiratory support. Careful delivery room stabilization with early application of distending pressure to facilitate establishment of FRC and clearance of lung fluid is an essential first step. CPAP remains the mainstay of noninvasive respiratory support, but a variety of other approaches to noninvasive ventilation are being explored with NIV NAVA potentially the most promising strategy. Less invasive means of surfactant administration have shown promising results, but evidence is still accumulating as to which approach is best. If mechanical ventilation is needed, optimization of lung inflation, avoidance of volutrauma, and atelectrauma are essential. Of the novel techniques of mechanical ventilation NAVA has been more extensively studied, but larger clinical trials with important clinical outcomes are needed. Clinicians should exercise caution regarding adoption of novel therapeutic interventions until more evidence of safety and efficacy are available.

BEST PRACTICES

Current Practice: Large practice style variation persists in neonatal respiratory support, in part because of incomplete evidence to guide best practice. Lack of a consistent approach with frequent changes in support based on individual clinician preference is common. Uncertainty remains about optimal delivery room stabilization of preterm infants. Pressure-controlled synchronized intermittent mandatory ventilation remains the most prevalent approach in the United States, despite evidence that alternate approaches lead to better outcomes. The open lung strategy is not often practiced with conventional ventilation. Adoption of less invasive surfactant administration, non-invasive support and advanced modalities of support remains uneven.

Steps that would improve outcome: Adoption of an evidence-based consistent approach to respiratory support is an important step toward improving outcome. The adopted strategies should start with initial stabilization and address surfactant administration, non-invasive support, criteria for escalation of support to invasive ventilation and for progression to novel strategies.

Best Practice: Gentle application of continuous positive airway pressure (CPAP) is appropriate in all preterm infants to facilitate lung aeration and clearance of lung fluid. The pressure used may need to be titrated to effect. Sustained inflation should be avoided. Positive pressure ventilation should be delivered via a T-piece resuscitator with care to use minimal pressures needed to achieve a chest rise and improved heart rate. Intubation and invasive ventilation should be reserved for infants with inadequate respiratory effort who fail to respond to initial non-invasive positive pressure ventilation. Intubation solely for the purpose of prophylactic surfactant is not indicated. Less invasive surfactant administration via a thin catheter or laryngeal mask airway appears to be the best option for avoiding the need for mechanical ventilation.Most infants born at 26 weeks and beyond are able to be supported, at least initially with non-invasive support. CPAP remains the gold standard and there is some evidence that bubble CPAP via short binasal prongs is superior to ventilator CPAP.The RAM cannula has very high resistance resulting in delivery of less pharyngeal pressure than the set value. It functions more lake a high flow cannula and is not the preferred interface for small preterm infants.High-flow nasal cannula therapy is a reasonable alternative in larger preterm infants, but less effective than CPAP in very low birth weight infants.Observational data and early randomized trials suggest that prolongation of CPAP use until 32 weeks promotes lung growth and may reduce the incidence of bronchopulmonary dysplasia.Nasal intermittent positive pressure ventilation (NIPPV) appears to be more effective than CPAP, but non-synchronized NIPPV does not generate a measurable tidal volume - its apparent benefits stem from the use of higher mean airway pressure, compared to CPAP. Synchronized NIPPV, only available outside of the United States, appears to be more effective than CPAP. Non-invasive neurally adjusted ventilatory assist (NIV NAVA) is a form of synchronized NIPPV that is available in the United States appears to be superior to CPAP or non-synchronized NIPPV, but current evidence is weak.Nasal high-frequency ventilation is a promising novel approach that needs further study before widespread use can be advocated.Volume-targeted ventilation is the preferred mode of invasive respiratory support, based on several meta-analyses, resulting in a significant reduction in most complications of respiratory support. It is best combined with assist-control or pressure support ventilation.The use of adequate distending pressure to achieve an open lung strategy is a key element in avoiding ventilator associated lung injury with all forms of non-invasive and invasive ventilation.High frequency ventilation may not be superior to state of the art conventional ventilation, but it does facilitate lung volume recruitment. When combined with optimal lung volume strategy and volume-targeting, as currently available outside the United States, it may provide the best lung-protective ventilation approach.Invasive neurally adjusted ventilatory assist (NAVA) support of very preterm infants has been widely embraced but lacks a solid evidence base. There are potential risks of this approach that provides inflation pressure in proportion to infant's effort in preterm infants with immature respiratory control and frequent periodic breathing, apnea and brief bursts of strong inspiratory effort when disturbed. For this reason, it cannot currently be recommended as best practice.

DISCLOSURE

The author has received research support for a study of high-frequency oscillatory ventilation and lecture honoraria from Draeger Medical, Inc.

REFERENCES

1. Stoll BJ, Hansen NI, Bell EF, et al. Trends in care practices, morbidity, and mortality of extremely preterm neonates, 1993-2012. JAMA 2015;314(10):1039-51.
2. Horbar JD, Edwards EM, Greenberg LT, et al. Variation in performance of neonatal intensive care units in the United States. JAMA Pediatr 2017;171(3):e164396.
3. Vom Hove M, Prenzel F, Uhlig HH, et al. Pulmonary outcome in former preterm, very low birth weight children with bronchopulmonary dysplasia: a case-control follow-up at school age. J Pediatr 2014;164(1):40-5.e4.
4. Short EJ, Klein NK, Lewis BA, et al. Cognitive and academic consequences of bronchopulmonary dysplasia and very low birth weight: 8-year-old outcomes. Pediatrics 2003;112(5):e359.
5. Klinger G, Sokolover N, Boyko V, et al. Perinatal risk factors for bronchopulmonary dysplasia in a national cohort of very-low-birthweight infants. Am J Obstet Gynecol 2013;208(2):115.e1-9.
6. Lapcharoensap W, Bennett MV, Xu X, et al. Hospitalization costs associated with bronchopulmonary dysplasia in the first year of life. J Perinatol 2020;40(1):130-7.
7. Lapcharoensap W, Gage SC, Kan P, et al. Hospital variation and risk factors for bronchopulmonary dysplasia in a population-based cohort. JAMA Pediatr 2015; 169(2):e143676.
8. Ambalavanan N, Walsh M, Bobashev G, et al. Intercenter differences in bronchopulmonary dysplasia or death among very low birth weight infants. Pediatrics 2011;127(1):e106-16.
9. Clark RH, Gerstmann DR, Jobe AH, et al. Lung injury in neonates: causes, strategies for prevention, and long-term consequences. J Pediatr 2001;139(4):478-86.
10. Slutsky AS, Ranieri VM. Ventilator-induced lung injury. N Engl J Med 2013; 369(22):2126-36.
11. Keszler M, Sant'Anna G. Mechanical ventilation and bronchopulmonary dysplasia. Clin Perinatol 2015;42(4):781-96.
12. Dreyfuss D, Soler P, Basset G, et al. High inflation pressure pulmonary edema. Respective effects of high airway pressure, high tidal volume, and positive end-expiratory pressure. Am Rev Respir Dis 1988;137(5):1159-64.
13. Hernandez LA, Peevy KJ, Moise AA, et al. Chest wall restriction limits high airway pressure-induced lung injury in young rabbits. J Appl Physiol 1989; 66(5):2364-8.
14. Lachmann B. Open up the lung and keep the lung open. Intensive Care Med 1992;18(6):319-21.
15. Jobe AH. Effects of chorioamnionitis on the fetal lung. Clin Perinatol 2012;39(3): 441-57.
16. Jobe AH, Hillman N, Polglase G, et al. Injury and inflammation from resuscitation of the preterm infant. Neonatology 2008;94(3):190-6.
17. Bjorklund LJ, Ingimarsson J, Curstedt T, et al. Manual ventilation with a few large breaths at birth compromises the therapeutic effect of subsequent surfactant replacement in immature lambs. Pediatr Res 1997;42(3):348-55.
18. te Pas AB, Siew M, Wallace MJ, et al. Establishing functional residual capacity at birth: the effect of sustained inflation and positive end-expiratory pressure in a preterm rabbit model. Pediatr Res 2009;65(5):537-41.
19. te Pas AB, Walther FJ. A randomized, controlled trial of delivery-room respiratory management in very preterm infants. Pediatrics 2007;120(2):322-9.
20. Lista G, Boni L, Scopesi F, et al. Sustained lung inflation at birth for preterm infants: a randomized clinical trial. Pediatrics 2015;135(2):e457-64.

21. Kirpalani H, Ratcliffe SJ, Keszler M, et al. Effect of sustained inflations vs inter-mittent positive pressure ventilation on bronchopulmonary dysplasia or death among extremely preterm infants: the SAIL randomized clinical trial. JAMA 2019;321(12):1165–75.

22. Foglia EE, Te Pas AB, Kirpalani H, et al. Sustained inflation vs standard resuscitation for preterm infants: a systematic review and meta-analysis. JAMA Pediatr 2020;174(4):e195897.

23. Hussey SG, Ryan CA, Murphy BP. Comparison of three manual ventilation devices using an intubated mannequin. Arch Dis Child Fetal Neonatal Ed 2004; 89(6):F490–3.

24. Dawson JA, Gerber A, Kamlin CO, et al. Providing PEEP during neonatal resuscitation: which device is best? J Paediatr Child Health 2011;47(10):698–703.

25. Poulton DA, Schmolzer GM, Morley CJ, et al. Assessment of chest rise during mask ventilation of preterm infants in the delivery room. Resuscitation 2011; 82(2):175–9.

26. Solevag AL, Haemmerle E, van Os S, et al. A novel prototype neonatal resuscitator that controls tidal volume and ventilation rate: a comparative study of mask ventilation in a newborn manikin. Front Pediatr 2016;4:129.

27. Aziz K, Lee CHC, Escobedo MB, et al. Part 5: neonatal resuscitation 2020 American Heart Association guidelines for cardiopulmonary resuscitation and emergency cardiovascular care. Pediatrics 2021;147(Suppl 1). e2020038505E.

28. Welsford M, Nishiyama C, Shortt C, et al. Initial oxygen use for preterm newborn resuscitation: a systematic review with meta-analysis. Pediatrics 2019;143(1): e20181828.

29. Dawson JA, Kamlin CO, Vento M, et al. Defining the reference range for oxygen saturation for infants after birth. Pediatrics 2010;125(6):e1340–7.

30. Challis P, Nydert P, Hakansson S, et al. Association of adherence to surfactant best practice uses with clinical outcomes among neonates in Sweden. JAMA Netw Open 2021;4(5):e217269.

31. Ammari A, Suri M, Milisavljevic V, et al. Variables associated with the early failure of nasal CPAP in very low birth weight infants. J Pediatr 2005;147(3):341–7.

32. Schmolzer GM, Kumar M, Pichler G, et al. Non-invasive versus invasive respiratory support in preterm infants at birth: systematic review and meta-analysis. BMJ 2013;347:f5980.

33. Fischer HS, Buhrer C. Avoiding endotracheal ventilation to prevent bronchopulmonary dysplasia: a meta-analysis. Pediatrics 2013;132(5):e1351–60.

34. Vento M, Bohlin K, Herting E, et al. Surfactant administration via thin catheter: a practical guide. Neonatology 2019;116(3):211–26.

35. Roberts KD, Brown R, Lampland AL, et al. Laryngeal mask airway for surfactant administration in neonates: a randomized, controlled trial. J Pediatr 2018;193: 40–46 e41.

36. Reininger A, Khalak R, Kendig JW, et al. Surfactant administration by transient intubation in infants 29 to 35 weeks' gestation with respiratory distress syndrome decreases the likelihood of later mechanical ventilation: a randomized controlled trial. J Perinatol 2005;25(11):703–8.

37. Cummings JJ, Gerday E, Minton S, et al. Aerosolized calfactant for newborns with respiratory distress: a randomized trial. Pediatrics 2020;146(5):e20193967.

38. Minocchieri S, Berry CA, Pillow JJ, et al. Nebulised surfactant to reduce severity of respiratory distress: a blinded, parallel, randomised controlled trial. Arch Dis Child Fetal Neonatal Ed 2019;104(3):F313–9.

39. Pillow JJ, Hillman N, Moss TJ, et al. Bubble continuous positive airway pressure enhances lung volume and gas exchange in preterm lambs. Am J Respir Crit Care Med 2007;176(1):63–9.
40. Bharadwaj SK, Alonazi A, Banfield L, et al. Bubble versus other continuous positive airway pressure forms: a systematic review and meta-analysis. Arch Dis Child Fetal Neonatal Ed 2020;105(5):526–31.
41. Miedema M, van der Burg PS, Beuger S, et al. Effect of nasal continuous and biphasic positive airway pressure on lung volume in preterm infants. J Pediatr 2013;162(4):691–7.
42. Owen LS, Morley CJ, Davis PG. Effects of synchronisation during SiPAP-generated nasal intermittent positive pressure ventilation (NIPPV) in preterm infants. Arch Dis Child Fetal Neonatal Ed 2015;100(1):F24–30.
43. Lampland AL, Plumm B, Worwa C, et al. Bi-level CPAP does not improve gas exchange when compared with conventional CPAP for the treatment of neonates recovering from respiratory distress syndrome. Arch Dis Child Fetal Neonatal Ed 2015;100(1):F31–4.
44. Victor S, Roberts SA, Mitchell S, et al. Biphasic positive airway pressure or continuous positive airway pressure: a randomized trial. Pediatrics 2016; 138(2):e20154095.
45. Lemyre B, Davis PG, De Paoli AG, et al. Nasal intermittent positive pressure ventilation (NIPPV) versus nasal continuous positive airway pressure (NCPAP) for preterm neonates after extubation. Cochrane Database Syst Rev 2017;(2):CD003212.
46. Kirpalani H, Millar D, Lemyre B, et al. A trial comparing noninvasive ventilation strategies in preterm infants. N Engl J Med 2013;369(7):611–20.
47. Owen LS, Morley CJ, Dawson JA, et al. Effects of non-synchronised nasal intermittent positive pressure ventilation on spontaneous breathing in preterm infants. Arch Dis Child Fetal Neonatal Ed 2011;96(6):F422–8.
48. van Vonderen JJ, Hooper SB, Hummler HD, et al. Effects of a sustained inflation in preterm infants at birth. J Pediatr 2014;165(5):903–8.e1.
49. Buzzella B, Claure N, D'Ugard C, et al. A randomized controlled trial of two nasal continuous positive airway pressure levels after extubation in preterm infants. J Pediatr 2014;164(1):46–51.
50. Mukerji A, Belik J. Neonatal nasal intermittent positive pressure ventilation efficacy and lung pressure transmission. J Perinatol 2015;35(9):716–9.
51. Gerdes JS, Sivieri EM, Abbasi S. Factors influencing delivered mean airway pressure during nasal CPAP with the RAM cannula. Pediatr Pulmonol 2016; 51(1):60–9.
52. Singh N, McNally MJ, Darnall RA. Does the RAM cannula provide continuous positive airway pressure as effectively as the Hudson prongs in preterm neonates? Am J Perinatol 2019;36(8):849–54.
53. Iyer NP, Chatburn R. Evaluation of a nasal cannula in noninvasive ventilation using a lung simulator. Respir Care 2015;60(4):508–12.
54. Gokce IK, Kaya H, Ozdemir R. A randomized trial comparing the short binasal prong to the RAM cannula for noninvasive ventilation support of preterm infants with respiratory distress syndrome. J Matern Fetal Neonatal Med 2021;34(12): 1868–74.
55. Matlock DN, Bai S, Weisner MD, et al. Tidal volume transmission during non-synchronized nasal intermittent positive pressure ventilation via RAM((R)) cannula. J Perinatol 2019;39(5):723–9.

56. Gibu C, Cheng P, Ward RJ, et al. Feasibility and physiological effects of non-invasive neurally-adjusted ventilatory assist (NIV-NAVA) in preterm infants. Pediatr Res 2017;11(1):15778.

57. Colaizy TT, Kummet GJ, Kummet CM, et al. Noninvasive neurally adjusted ventilatory assist in premature infants Postextubation. Am J Perinatol 2017;34(6):593–8.

58. Lee BK, Shin SH, Jung YH, et al. Comparison of NIV-NAVA and NCPAP in facilitating extubation for very preterm infants. BMC Pediatr 2019;19(1):298.

59. Yagui AC, Meneses J, Zolio BA, et al. Nasal continuous positive airway pressure (NCPAP) or noninvasive neurally adjusted ventilatory assist (NIV-NAVA) for preterm infants with respiratory distress after birth: a randomized controlled trial. Pediatr Pulmonol 2019;54(11):1704–11.

60. Yagui AC, Goncalves PA, Murakami SH, et al. Is noninvasive neurally adjusted ventilatory assistance (NIV-NAVA) an alternative to NCPAP in preventing extubation failure in preterm infants? J Matern Fetal Neonatal Med 2021;34(22):3756–60.

61. Rochon ME, Lodygensky G, Tabone L, et al. Continuous neurally adjusted ventilation: a feasibility study in preterm infants. Arch Dis Child Fetal Neonatal Ed 2020;105(6):640–5.

62. van der Hoeven M, Brouwer E, Blanco CE. Nasal high frequency ventilation in neonates with moderate respiratory insufficiency. Arch Dis Child Fetal Neonatal Ed 1998;79(1):F61–3.

63. Mukerji A, Sarmiento K, Lee B, et al. Non-invasive high-frequency ventilation versus bi-phasic continuous positive airway pressure (BP-CPAP) following CPAP failure in infants <1250 g: a pilot randomized controlled trial. J Perinatol 2017;37(1):49–53.

64. Zhu XW, Zhao JN, Tang SF, et al. Noninvasive high-frequency oscillatory ventilation versus nasal continuous positive airway pressure in preterm infants with moderate-severe respiratory distress syndrome: a preliminary report. Pediatr Pulmonol 2017;52(8):1038–42.

65. Chen L, Wang L, Ma J, et al. Nasal high-frequency oscillatory ventilation in preterm infants with respiratory distress syndrome and ARDS after extubation: a randomized controlled trial. Chest 2019;155(4):740–8.

66. Iranpour R, Armanian AM, Abedi AR, et al. Nasal high-frequency oscillatory ventilation (nHFOV) versus nasal continuous positive airway pressure (NCPAP) as an initial therapy for respiratory distress syndrome (RDS) in preterm and near-term infants. BMJ Paediatr Open 2019;3(1):e000443.

67. Malakian A, Bashirnezhadkhabaz S, Aramesh MR, et al. Noninvasive high-frequency oscillatory ventilation versus nasal continuous positive airway pressure in preterm infants with respiratory distress syndrome: a randomized controlled trial. J Matern Fetal Neonatal Med 2020;33(15):2601–7.

68. Li J, Li X, Huang X, et al. Noninvasive high-frequency oscillatory ventilation as respiratory support in preterm infants: a meta-analysis of randomized controlled trials. Respir Res 2019;20(1):58.

69. Haidar Shehadeh AM. Non-invasive high flow oscillatory ventilation in comparison with nasal continuous positive pressure ventilation for respiratory distress syndrome, a literature review. J Matern Fetal Neonatal Med 2021;34(17):2900–9.

70. Zhu XW, Shi Y, Shi LP, et al. Non-invasive high-frequency oscillatory ventilation versus nasal continuous positive airway pressure in preterm infants with respiratory distress syndrome: study protocol for a multi-center prospective randomized controlled trial. Trials 2018;19(1):319.

71. Shi Y, De Luca D, group NAOp-Es. Continuous positive airway pressure (CPAP) vs noninvasive positive pressure ventilation (NIPPV) vs noninvasive high frequency oscillation ventilation (NHFOV) as post-extubation support in preterm neonates: protocol for an assessor-blinded, multicenter, randomized controlled trial. BMC Pediatr 2019;19(1):256.
72. De Luca D, Piastra M, Pietrini D, et al. Effect of amplitude and inspiratory time in a bench model of non-invasive HFOV through nasal prongs. Pediatr Pulmonol 2012;47(10):1012–8.
73. Colaizy TT, Younis UM, Bell EF, et al. Nasal high-frequency ventilation for premature infants. Acta Paediatr 2008;97(11):1518–22.
74. Czernik C, Schmalisch G, Buhrer C, et al. Weaning of neonates from mechanical ventilation by use of nasopharyngeal high-frequency oscillatory ventilation: a preliminary study. J Matern Fetal Neonatal Med 2012;25(4):374–8.
75. Mukerji A, Finelli M, Belik J. Nasal high-frequency oscillation for lung carbon dioxide clearance in the newborn. Neonatology 2013;103(3):161–5.
76. Yoder BA, Albertine KH, Null DM Jr. High-frequency ventilation for non-invasive respiratory support of neonates. Semin Fetal Neonatal Med 2016;21(3):162–73.
77. Dumas De La Roque E, Bertrand C, Tandonnet O, et al. Nasal high frequency percussive ventilation versus nasal continuous positive airway pressure in transient tachypnea of the newborn: a pilot randomized controlled trial (NCT00556738). Pediatr Pulmonol 2011;46(3):218–23.
78. Keel J, De Beritto T, Ramanathan R, et al. Nasal high-frequency jet ventilation (NHFJV) as a novel means of respiratory support in extremely low birth weight infants. J Perinatol 2021;41(7):1697–703.
79. Zhang S, Garbutt V, McBride JT. Strain-induced growth of the immature lung. J Appl Physiol 1996;81(4):1471–6.
80. Nobuhara KK, Fauza DO, DiFiore JW, et al. Continuous intrapulmonary distension with perfluorocarbon accelerates neonatal (but not adult) lung growth. J Pediatr Surg 1998;33(2):292–8.
81. Hedrick MH, Estes JM, Sullivan KM, et al. Plug the lung until it grows (PLUG): a new method to treat congenital diaphragmatic hernia in utero. J Pediatr Surg 1994;29(5):612–7.
82. Deprest JA, Nicolaides KH, Benachi A, et al. Randomized trial of fetal surgery for severe left diaphragmatic hernia. N Engl J Med 2021;385(2):107–18.
83. Polin RA, Sahni R. Newer experience with CPAP. Semin Neonatol 2002;7(5):379–89.
84. Lam R, Schilling D, Scottoline B, et al. The effect of extended continuous positive airway pressure on changes in lung volumes in stable premature infants: a randomized controlled trial. J Pediatr 2020;217:66–72.e1.
85. Abman SH, Collaco JM, Shepherd EG, et al. Interdisciplinary care of children with severe bronchopulmonary dysplasia. J Pediatr 2017;181:12–28.e1.
86. Muscedere JG, Mullen JB, Gan K, et al. Tidal ventilation at low airway pressures can augment lung injury. Am J Respir Crit Care Med 1994;149(5):1327–34.
87. Tremblay L, Valenza F, Ribeiro SP, et al. Injurious ventilatory strategies increase cytokines and c-fos m-RNA expression in an isolated rat lung model. J Clin Invest 1997;99(5):944–52.
88. van Kaam AH, de Jaegere A, Haitsma JJ, et al. Positive pressure ventilation with the open lung concept optimizes gas exchange and reduces ventilator-induced lung injury in newborn piglets. Pediatr Res 2003;53(2):245–53.
89. Tsuchida S, Engelberts D, Peltekova V, et al. Atelectasis causes alveolar injury in nonatelectatic lung regions. Am J Respir Crit Care Med 2006;174(3):279–89.

90. Morley CJ, Davis PG, Doyle LW, et al. Nasal CPAP or intubation at birth for very preterm infants. N Engl J Med 2008;358(7):700–8.

91. Mukerji A, Abdul Wahab MG, Razak A, et al. High CPAP vs. NIPPV in preterm neonates: a physiological cross-over study. J Perinatol 2021;41(7):1690–6.

92. van Kaam AH, Rimensberger PC. Lung-protective ventilation strategies in neonatology: what do we know–what do we need to know? Crit Care Med 2007;35(3):925–31.

93. De Jaegere A, van Veenendaal MB, Michiels A, et al. Lung recruitment using oxygenation during open lung high-frequency ventilation in preterm infants. Am J Respir Crit Care Med 2006;174(6):639–45.

94. Castoldi F, Daniele I, Fontana P, et al. Lung recruitment maneuver during volume guarantee ventilation of preterm infants with acute respiratory distress syndrome. Am J Perinatol 2011;28(7):521–8.

95. Halter JM, Steinberg JM, Schiller HJ, et al. Positive end-expiratory pressure after a recruitment maneuver prevents both alveolar collapse and recruitment/derecruitment. Am J Respir Care Med 2003;167(12):1620–6.

96. van der Burg PS, Miedema M, de Jongh FH, et al. Cross-sectional changes in lung volume measured by electrical impedance tomography are representative for the whole lung in ventilated preterm infants. Crit Care Med 2014;42(6): 1524–30.

97. Keszler M. What if you could see lung inflation in real time? J Pediatr 2013; 162(4):670–2.

98. Tingay DG, Mills JF, Morley CJ, et al. The deflation limb of the pressure-volume relationship in infants during high-frequency ventilation. Am J Respir Crit Care Med 2006;173(4):414–20.

99. Krause MF, Jakel C, Haberstroh J, et al. Alveolar recruitment promotes homogeneous surfactant distribution in a piglet model of lung injury. Pediatr Res 2001; 50(1):34–43.

100. Wheeler K, Klingenberg C, McCallion N, et al. Volume-targeted versus pressure-limited ventilation in the neonate. Cochrane Database Syst Rev 2010;(11):CD003666.

101. Peng W, Zhu H, Shi H, et al. Volume-targeted ventilation is more suitable than pressure-limited ventilation for preterm infants: a systematic review and meta-analysis. Arch Dis Child Fetal Neonatal Ed 2014;99(2):F158–65.

102. Gupta A, Keszler M. Survey of ventilation practices in the neonatal intensive care units of the United States and Canada: use of volume-targeted ventilation and Barriers to its use. Am J Perinatol 2019;36(5):484–9.

103. Singh J, Sinha SK, Clarke P, et al. Mechanical ventilation of very low birth weight infants: is volume or pressure a better target variable? J Pediatr 2006;149(3): 308–13.

104. Keszler M. Update on mechanical ventilatory strategies. Neoreviews 2013; 14(5):e237–51.

105. Nassabeh-Montazami S, Abubakar KM, Keszler M. The impact of instrumental dead-space in volume-targeted ventilation of the extremely low birth weight (ELBW) infant. Pediatr Pulmonol 2009;44(2):128–33.

106. Sharma S, Clark S, Abubakar K, et al. Tidal volume requirement in mechanically ventilated infants with meconium aspiration syndrome. Am J Perinatol 2015; 32(10):916–9.

107. Sharma S, Abubakar KM, Keszler M. Tidal volume in infants with congenital diaphragmatic hernia supported with conventional mechanical ventilation. Am J Perinatol 2015;32(6):577–82.

108. Keszler M, Nassabeh-Montazami S, Abubakar K. Evolution of tidal volume requirement during the first 3 weeks of life in infants <800 g ventilated with volume guarantee. Arch Dis Child Fetal Neonatal Ed 2009;94(4):F279–82.

109. Keszler M. Volume-targeted ventilation: one size does not fit all. Evidence-based recommendations for successful use. Arch Dis Child Fetal Neonatal Ed 2018; 104(1):F108–12.

110. Keszler M, Abubakar K. Volume-targeted ventilation. In: Keszler M, Suresh Gautham K, editors. Assisted ventilation of the neonate: an evidence-based approach to neonatal respiratory care. 7th edition. Philadelphia: Elsevier; 2022.

111. Cools F, Offringa M, Askie LM. Elective high frequency oscillatory ventilation versus conventional ventilation for acute pulmonary dysfunction in preterm infants. Cochrane Database Syst Rev 2015;(3):CD000104.

112. Keszler M, Donn SM, Bucciarelli RL, et al. Multicenter controlled trial comparing high-frequency jet ventilation and conventional mechanical ventilation in newborn infants with pulmonary interstitial emphysema. J Pediatr 1991;119(1 Pt 1):85–93.

113. Iscan B, Duman N, Tuzun F, et al. Impact of volume guarantee on high-frequency oscillatory ventilation in preterm infants: a randomized crossover clinical trial. Neonatology 2015;108(4):277–82.

114. Belteki G, Morley CJ. High-frequency oscillatory ventilation with volume guarantee: a single-centre experience. Arch Dis Child Fetal Neonatal Ed 2019; 104(4):F384–9.

115. Enomoto M, Keszler M, Sakuma M, et al. Effect of volume guarantee in preterm infants on high-frequency oscillatory ventilation: a pilot study. Am J Perinatol 2017;34(1):26–30.

116. Sindelar R, McKinney RL, Wallstrom L, et al. Proportional assist and neurally adjusted ventilation: clinical knowledge and future trials in newborn infants. Pediatr Pulmonol 2021;56(7):1841–9.

117. Schulze A, Rich W, Schellenberg L, et al. Effects of different gain settings during assisted mechanical ventilation using respiratory unloading in rabbits. Pediatr Res 1998;44(1):132–8.

118. Schulze A, Gerhardt T, Musante G, et al. Proportional assist ventilation in low birth weight infants with acute respiratory disease: a comparison to assist/control and conventional mechanical ventilation. J Pediatr 1999;135(3):339–44.

119. Schulze A, Rieger-Fackeldey E, Gerhardt T, et al. Randomized crossover comparison of proportional assist ventilation and patient-triggered ventilation in extremely low birth weight infants with evolving chronic lung disease. Neonatology 2007;92(1):1–7.

120. Shetty S, Bhat P, Hickey A, et al. Proportional assist versus assist control ventilation in premature infants. Eur J Pediatr 2016;175(1):57–61.

121. Hunt KA, Dassios T, Greenough A. Proportional assist ventilation (PAV) versus neurally adjusted ventilator assist (NAVA): effect on oxygenation in infants with evolving or established bronchopulmonary dysplasia. Eur J Pediatr 2020; 179(6):901–8.

122. Firestone KS, Fisher S, Reddy S, et al. Effect of changing NAVA levels on peak inspiratory pressures and electrical activity of the diaphragm in premature neonates. J Perinatol 2015;35(8):612–6.

123. Nam SK, Lee J, Jun YH. Neural feedback is insufficient in preterm infants during neurally adjusted ventilatory assist. Pediatr Pulmonol 2019;54(8):1277–83.

124. Beck J, Reilly M, Grasselli G, et al. Patient-ventilator interaction during neurally adjusted ventilatory assist in low birth weight infants. Pediatr Res 2009;65(6): 663–8.
125. Stein H, Howard D. Neurally adjusted ventilatory assist in neonates weighing <1500 grams: a retrospective analysis. J Pediatr 2012;160(5):786–9.e1.
126. Lee J, Kim HS, Sohn JA, et al. Randomized crossover study of neurally adjusted ventilatory assist in preterm infants. J Pediatr 2012;161(5):808–13.
127. Longhini F, Ferrero F, De Luca D, et al. Neurally adjusted ventilatory assist in preterm neonates with acute respiratory failure. Neonatology 2015;107(1):60–7.
128. Shetty S, Hunt K, Peacock J, et al. Crossover study of assist control ventilation and neurally adjusted ventilatory assist. Eur J Pediatr 2017;176(4):509–13.
129. Stein H, Alosh H, Ethington P, et al. Prospective crossover comparison between NAVA and pressure control ventilation in premature neonates less than 1500 grams. J Perinatol 2013;33(6):452–6.
130. Kallio M, Koskela U, Peltoniemi O, et al. Neurally adjusted ventilatory assist (NAVA) in preterm newborn infants with respiratory distress syndrome-a randomized controlled trial. Eur J Pediatr 2016;175(9):1175–83.
131. Jung YH, Kim HS, Lee J, et al. Neurally adjusted ventilatory assist in preterm infants with established or evolving bronchopulmonary dysplasia on high-intensity mechanical ventilatory support: a single-center experience. Pediatr Crit Care Med 2016;17(12):1142–6.
132. Lee J, Kim HS, Jung YH, et al. Neurally adjusted ventilatory assist for infants under prolonged ventilation. Pediatr Int 2017;59(5):540–4.
133. Rong X, Liang F, Li YJ, et al. Application of neurally adjusted ventilatory assist in premature neonates less than 1,500 grams with established or evolving bronchopulmonary dysplasia. Front Pediatr 2020;8:110.
134. McKinney RL, Keszler M, Truog WE, et al. Multicenter experience with neurally adjusted ventilatory assist in infants with severe bronchopulmonary dysplasia. Am J Perinatol 2021;38(S 01):e162–6.
135. Daoud EG, Farag HL, Chatburn RL. Airway pressure release ventilation: what do we know? Respir Care 2012;57(2):282–92.
136. Lalgudi Ganesan S, Jayashree M, Chandra Singhi S, et al. Airway pressure release ventilation in pediatric acute respiratory distress syndrome. A randomized controlled trial. Am J Respir Crit Care Med 2018;198(9):1199–207.
137. Claure N, Gerhardt T, Hummler H, et al. Computer-controlled minute ventilation in preterm infants undergoing mechanical ventilation. J Pediatr 1997;131(6): 910–3.
138. Guthrie SO, Lynn C, Lafleur BJ, et al. A crossover analysis of mandatory minute ventilation compared to synchronized intermittent mandatory ventilation in neonates. J Perinatol 2005;25(10):643–6.
139. Burns KE, Lellouche F, Lessard MR. Automating the weaning process with advanced closed-loop systems. Intensive Care Med 2008;34(10):1757–65.
140. Sturrock S, Williams E, Dassios T, et al. Closed loop automated oxygen control in neonates: a review. Acta Paediatr 2019;109(5):914–22.
141. Dani C. Automated control of inspired oxygen (FiO2) in preterm infants: literature review. Pediatr Pulmonol 2019;54(3):358–63.
142. Maiwald CA, Niemarkt HJ, Poets CF, et al. Effects of closed-loop automatic control of the inspiratory fraction of oxygen (FiO2-C) on outcome of extremely preterm infants: study protocol of a randomized controlled parallel group multicenter trial for safety and efficacy. BMC Pediatr 2019;19(1):363.

Pharmacologic Analgesia and Sedation in Neonates

Christopher McPherson, PharmD[a,b,*], Ruth E. Grunau, PhD[c,d]

KEYWORDS

- Dexmedetomidine • Fentanyl • Morphine • Neonate • Pain • Stress • Sucrose

KEY POINTS

- Nonpharmacologic interventions form the foundation of analgesia and sedation to mitigate neonatal pain and agitation; oral sweet-tasting solutions should be treated as a pharmacologic intervention and used judiciously for mild painful procedures preferably more than 27-weeks postmenstrual age.
- Moderately painful procedures, including endotracheal intubations, require utilization of a rapidly acting opioid (eg, fentanyl or remifentanil); adjunctive pharmacologic agents should be tailored to the patient and specific clinical situation.
- Preterm neonates experiencing stress from mechanical ventilation and term neonates experiencing stress from therapeutic hypothermia may benefit from appropriately dosed continuous pharmacologic sedation; optimal agents with a clearly favorable benefit:risk ratio have not been clearly defined.

INTRODUCTION

The past 4 decades have witnessed enormous leaps in understanding of the acute and long-term impacts of neonatal pain and stress. Healthy infants experience roughly 12 skin-breaking procedures in the first year of life. Hospitalized neonates born very prematurely encounter 1 to 3 skin breaks in concert with 4 to 12 invasive stressful or painful procedures *daily* during hospitalization.[1] Initially, in 1987, a landmark study documented the unique susceptibility of the most immature preterm neonates to dramatically increased morbidity including brain injury from insufficiently treated acute surgical pain.[2] While severe brain injury has the potential to impact survival, brain dysmaturation is a more reliable predictor of neurodevelopmental impairments in

[a] Department of Pharmacy, St. Louis Children's Hospital, 1 Children's Place, St. Louis, MO 63110, USA; [b] Department of Pediatrics, Washington University School of Medicine, 660 South Euclid Avenue, St. Louis, MO 63110, USA; [c] Department of Pediatrics, University of British Columbia, F605B, 4480 Oak Street, Vancouver, BC V6H 3V4, Canada; [d] BC Children's Hospital Research Institute, 938 West 28th Avenue, Vancouver BC V5Z 4H4, Canada
* Corresponding author. Department of Pharmacy, St. Louis Children's Hospital, 1 Children's Place, St. Louis, MO 63110, USA.
E-mail address: mcphersonc@wustl.edu

Clin Perinatol 49 (2022) 243–265
https://doi.org/10.1016/j.clp.2021.11.014
0095-5108/22/© 2021 Elsevier Inc. All rights reserved.
perinatology.theclinics.com

neonates with severe illness in early life.[3] Extensive subsequent investigation has associated a greater burden of procedural pain and stress with microstructural changes in white matter and subcortical gray matter, decreased frontal and parietal brain width, and smaller thalamic and cortical volumes near discharge from intensive care, altered neuromagnetic activity, and poorer functional outcomes up to age 8 years (**Fig. 1**).[4–6] Despite increased understanding of the profound impacts of neonatal pain and stress on short-term and long-term outcomes, an evidence-based, standardized approach has not been achieved for the most common clinical situations encountered during intensive care. As with all therapies in neonatology, *le bon Dieu est dans le détail* (the good Lord is in the detail). Multidisciplinary research is urgently needed to define the optimal dose and long-term impact of all pain and stress mitigating interventions used in neonates. Nonpharmacologic comfort measures have been widely studied for minor procedural pain, but limited standardization of specific procedures and duration (ie, "dose") and lacking longitudinal studies have hindered universal adoption. Often misclassified as nonpharmacologic, oral sweet-tasting solutions have been widely adopted to limit the behavioral response to minor acute pain due to their simplicity. However, studies have very limited inclusion of extremely preterm, unstable, and/or ventilated neonates and lack long-term follow-up regarding the impact of daily repetitive sweet-tasting solutions on the vulnerable developing extremely preterm brain. Hence, administration of sweet-tasting solutions for infants less than 27-weeks postmenstrual age is questionable and ongoing investigations are warranted.[7] Opioids represent the long-standing standard of care for moderately or severely painful procedures, ranging from endotracheal intubation to bedside

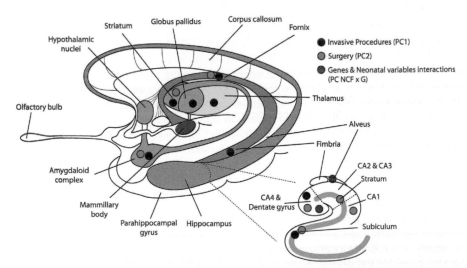

Fig. 1. Reduced regional volumes in limbic system, basal ganglia, and thalamus at 8 years of age in children born preterm exposed to pain, surgical interventions, and neonatal intensive care. The results of a constrained principal component analysis document the association of regional brain growth with a number of invasive procedures (principal component 1 [PC1], blue dots), number of surgeries (principal component 2 [PC2], green dots), and neonatal clinical factors and genotype (principal component of the interaction term [PC NCFxG], red dots). (*From* Chau CMY, Ranger M, Bichin M, et al. Hippocampus, Amygdala, and Thalamus Volumes in Very Preterm Children at 8 Years: Neonatal Pain and Genetic Variation. *Front Behav Neurosci.* 2019;13:51;with permission.)

surgery. Clear guidelines exist to inform the selection of the optimal agents to use before nonemergent endotracheal intubation; however, the data underpinning these guidelines are incomplete and significant variability still exists in clinical practice. Finally, recent focus on the longitudinal developmental impact of chronic pain and stress underscores the void of evidence that pharmacologic intervention improves outcomes in preterm and term neonates. Extensive research has investigated pharmacotherapy to limit stress from mechanical ventilation in preterm neonates, uncovering numerous dose-limiting adverse effects. The utilization of pharmacologic sedatives to limit stress during therapeutic hypothermia in term neonates is controversial, with clinical practice preceding careful study to the potential detriment of many neonates. This review summarizes data informing the current standards of care for mild, moderate, and chronic neonatal pain and stress in hospitalized preterm and term neonates. Given the incomplete nature of these data, we also highlight novel research efforts in this field and potential opportunities to improve interventions that may optimize efficacy, safety, and long-term outcomes.

MILD PAINFUL PROCEDURES

Critically ill neonates undergo a high burden of invasive painful and noninvasive stressful procedures. A robust body of literature documents clear associations between this burden and long-term developmental impacts on childhood. These findings highlight the vital nature of judicious utilization of tests and procedures and thoughtful construction of bundles to mitigate pain including the consideration of both nonpharmacologic and pharmacologic interventions.

Judicious Utilization

Painful procedures such as heel lance or venipuncture for laboratory monitoring may be essential to care but may also be protocoled or habitual. Every laboratory test in neonatal care must be undertaken thoughtfully and have a potential impact on care or outcome.[8] Protocols for laboratory monitoring should consider both the risks associated with insufficient testing and the harm associated with acute pain and stress on the immature brain. When possible, laboratory-based assays like blood gas analysis should be replaced, or limited in number, with noninvasive measurements like transcutaneous carbon dioxide monitoring. In many cases, invasive procedures are unavoidable; these situations must be approached with a standardized bundle of nonpharmacologic interventions with or without additional pharmacologic analgesia or sedation.

Nonpharmacologic Interventions

Nonpharmacologic interventions form the foundation of the multimodal approach to manage neonatal pain and stress. These interventions vary in both effect size and feasibility. In a recent Cochrane review, nonnutritive sucking and swaddling/facilitated tucking provided the largest standardized mean difference for treatment improvement over control conditions on pain reactivity in neonates.[9] Swaddling/facilitated tucking, nonnutritive sucking, and skin-to-skin care all effectively reduce physiologic and behavioral pain responses to mildly painful invasive procedures such as needle sticks, and promote self-regulation and attenuate stress from acute pain[9,10]; however, efficacy varies depending on neonatal maturity.

Skin-to-skin care may be the most studied nonpharmacologic intervention for mild pain, consistently producing reduced pain scale scores and improved regulation. This intervention also benefits parents through involvement and empowerment. However, skin-to-skin care requires careful staff education and involvement, with a host of pragmatic safety challenges.[11] When nonpharmacologic interventions offer incomplete comfort or are not feasible, clinicians must consider the benefits and risks of pharmacotherapy.

Oral Sweet-Tasting Solutions

Sweet-tasting solutions, most commonly oral sucrose, have been studied in at least 200 trials including well more than 5000 neonates over the course of 30 years.[12,13] Before heel lance, venipuncture, and intramuscular injection, sweet-tasting solutions consistently reduce crying, facial grimacing, and motor activity. Although often classified as nonpharmacologic, sweet-tasting solutions in this context clearly meet the Oxford definition of a drug as "a medicine or other substance which has a physiologic effect when ingested or otherwise introduced into the body." Despite consistent impact on behavioral responses at a variety of doses across a spectrum of mildly painful stimuli, administration of sweet-tasting solutions has not been documented to positively impact oxygen saturation, cerebral blood flow or tissue oxygenation, salivary or plasma cortisol concentrations, or neural activity of nociception-evoked circuits in the spinal cord or brain.[7] Sweet-tasting solutions also do not prevent the development of remote hyperalgesia in neonates when given consistently before repeated skin-breaking procedures, despite a clear impact on pain scale scores during each procedure.[14]

The mechanism of oral sweet-tasting solutions may be as simplistic as the encouragement of nonnutritive sucking, or involve the stimulation of endogenous opioid, dopaminergic, and/or cholinergic pathways. The latter possibility highlights the importance of considering the long-term impact of repetitive and/or high-dose oral sucrose, considering the clear role of these pathways on the development of motor function and attention.[15] Preclinical studies support concern. Repeated exposure to sucrose (10 times daily) as compared with placebo in mice before handling or superficial needle-prick during the first week of life produced smaller white and gray matter volumes (corpus callosum, stria terminalis, fimbria, hippocampus, cerebellum) in adulthood.[16] These structural changes may have functional impacts. Oral sucrose compared with placebo before handling in mice compromised spatial memory in adulthood, while the combination of sucrose and needle-prick did not protect against impairments in spatial memory associated with repetitive pain.[17] The lack of efficacy of sucrose on physiologic parameters has potential for adverse consequences, especially repeated use in fragile preterm infants and/or at high cumulative doses.

An historic randomized, controlled trial exposed a population of preterm neonates (N = 107) to sucrose or placebo for all painful procedures during the first week of life. Assessment at term equivalent age revealed delayed motor development and decreased vigor when greater than 10 doses per day of oral sucrose were administered in the first week of life.[18] However, these findings were not reproduced by a subsequent study randomizing preterm neonates (N = 66) to 28 days of sucrose or exclusively nonpharmacologic interventions before all painful procedures.[19]

Importantly, in a longitudinal cohort study of brain development in very preterm neonates, oral glucose before painful procedures provided no protective effect for adverse effects of pain on brain growth, functional connectivity between the thalamus and sensorimotor cortices, and neurodevelopmental outcomes at 18 months of age.[20] These data highlight the need for judicious utilization of sweet-tasting solutions in clinical practice, especially in extremely preterm, unstable, and/or ventilated infants, and liberal ongoing study.

Research Directions

Outstanding research questions abound regarding nonpharmacologic interventions. The duration of nonnutritive sucking and skin-to-skin care before painful stimuli varies dramatically between studies. Additionally, research efforts of nonpharmacologic interventions have focused on single events, rather than efficacy over a prolonged period including multiple painful events. Therefore, the optimal "dose" and long-term impact of nonpharmacologic intervention(s) remain urgent outstanding research questions.

Emerging data highlight a potential path forward for oral sweet-tasting solutions with a focus on dose-finding, efficacy, safety, and long-term impact. A recent Canadian study focused on the pharmacodynamics of oral sucrose in 245 neonates, performing a dose-finding study comparing the impact of varying doses (0.1 mL, 0.5 mL, and 1 mL of 24% solution) 2 minutes before heel lance on Premature Infant Pain Profile (PIPP-R) scores.[21] All doses in the study were effective, leading to the identification of 0.1 mL as a minimal effective dose. The study of even smaller doses (by volume or concentration) would be fascinating, but this represents a reasonable solution in clinical practice leading to the lowest accurately measurable dose of the most used sucrose concentration.

In term neonates undergoing a heel stick, oral glucose with or without maternal holding blunted cortical activation in parietal, temporal, and frontal cortices on multichannel near-infrared spectroscopy.[22] The lowest pain expression was associated with oral glucose with maternal holding or breastfeeding. These findings reveal a complex interplay between interventions to mitigate mild pain, cortical processing, and apparent analgesic effects. Somatic sensations processed by the cortex seem to interact with the potentially subcortical activity of sweet-tasting solutions. The authors of the above study make 2 astute conclusions—(1) maternal relationship seems superior to independent administration of oral solutions (breastmilk or glucose) and (2) a multidimensional approach including behavioral, physiologic, neurophysiological, and hormonal markers of pain seems a requirement for future studies of the analgesic efficacy of sweet-tasting solutions.

There is urgent need for studies of sweet-tasting solutions in the preterm neonatal population that focus on the impact of repetitive exposures and long-term outcomes. A recent large randomized controlled trial comparing maternal skin-to-skin contact alone or in combination with oral sucrose throughout neonatal intensive care documented no difference in pain scores between treatment groups or over time.[23] Robust follow-up of such a cohort would likely provide valuable data to inform clinical practice. A multidimensional approach for long-term follow-up including brain structure and function, as well as neurodevelopmental assessments of outcomes at school age, seems prudent.

MODERATELY PAINFUL PROCEDURES

Moderately painful procedures in neonates require providers to leverage analgesics to appropriately blunt the nociceptive response. Although recent efforts in neonatology have focused on increased utilization of continuous positive airway pressure in very preterm neonates, endotracheal intubation for surfactant administration and/or mechanical ventilation remains a common moderately painful procedure in neonatal intensive care units (NICUs). Endotracheal intubation occurs with high risk of adverse effects, including physiologic disruptions such as hypoxemia, bradycardia *via* vagal stimulation, and systemic, pulmonary, and intracranial hypertension.[24] Although procedural skill is highly variable between providers of different experience levels and at different medical centers, tertiary care centers report success rates of less than half for endotracheal intubation attempts.[25] The confluence of frequent physiologic adverse effects and repeated attempts results in increased morbidity, with both intraventricular hemorrhage and severe cognitive impairment, cerebral palsy, hearing impairment, visual impairment, or death at 18 to 22-month follow-up associated with multiple intubation attempts.[26,27] Premedication with a foundation of safe and effective analgesic administration minimizes the risk of airway trauma and reduces physiologic instability.[28] Vitally, appropriate premedication also reduces procedure time and the number of attempts required to intubate, regardless of the experience of the provider.[29] Despite consensus on the value of premedication, survey data document frequent utilization of drug cocktails with negative or absent supporting data.[30]

Optimal Analgesics for Procedural Pain

The ideal analgesic for procedural pain must have a rapid onset and short duration of action with minimal impact on respiratory mechanics. Opioids have traditionally formed the foundation of procedural analgesia. These agents provide analgesia through agonism of G-protein coupled μ-opioid receptors; however, dramatic differences in pharmacokinetic profiles result in clinically meaningful differences in efficacy. Intravenous fentanyl at a dose of 2 mcg/kg rapidly achieves peak concentrations with roughly 2-fold variability in very preterm neonates.[31] Elimination is even more dramatically variable, with half-life ranging from 4 to 33 hours in a small pharmacokinetic study (N = 20). The prolonged effective half-life of fentanyl in preterm neonates has an impact on clinical practice in scenarios whereby the INSURE (INtubation, SURfactant therapy, Extubation) approach is used, and immediate extubation may not be feasible.[32] Despite this limitation, fentanyl does blunt the physiologic adverse effects of endotracheal intubation as the analgesic component of a premedication cocktail.[33] Of equal importance, fentanyl is stable in a formulation that allows accurate measurement of doses appropriate for neonates.[34] For these reasons, fentanyl is listed as the preferred analgesic in the American Academy of Pediatrics (AAP) premedication guideline.[28]

This profile contrasts sharply with the frequently used, "acceptable analgesic agent" morphine.[28] Morphine fails to blunt the physiologic adverse effects of endotracheal intubation, in contrast *increasing* the duration of hypoxia when used as premedication.[35] When compared with a rapid-acting opioid, morphine is less likely to produce favorable intubation conditions and improve first-attempt success.[36] These clinical results likely arise from the pharmacokinetic profile of morphine, with delayed onset (5–10 minutes) and prolonged and highly variable elimination in preterm neonates (mean half-life of 2–12 hours in available studies; 12 studies including 166 preterm neonates).[37] In fairness to the AAP guideline, "acceptable analgesic agent" is immediately followed by the caveat "use only if other opioids are not available; if selected, must wait at least 5 min for onset of action," suggesting morphine should not be included as the standard analgesic in premedication cocktails used in neonates in the vast majority of modern NICUs.

Anesthetic Doses of Hypnotic Agents for Procedural Pain

The AAP guideline includes an important decision point when determining the foundation of premedication for endotracheal intubation, allowing "analgesic agents or anesthetic doses of a hypnotic drug." The desire for a single agent solution to premedication has led to intense interest in the sedative/hypnotic propofol, a potent rapidly acting γ-aminobutyric acid$_A$ (GABA$_A$) receptor agonist and N-methyl-D-aspartate (NMDA) receptor antagonist. In a small randomized trial (N = 63), propofol facilitated successful intubation, reduced desaturation events, and had a shorter recovery time compared with a multi-agent approach.[38] Of prime importance, the comparator cocktail used morphine for analgesia, raising questions regarding the efficacy of propofol compared with an optimal analgesic agent. A recent *double-blind* randomized controlled trial has shed significant light on the potential and pitfalls of propofol compared with more traditional agents used for premedication. Neonates premedicated with propofol-atropine were more likely to preserve oxygenation and recovered more rapidly (as assessed by both limb movement and spontaneous respiration) compared with a cocktail including a rapidly acting opioid, atropine, and a muscle relaxant. However, propofol produced a lower quality of sedation as judged by the operator, negatively impacted mean arterial blood pressure, and prolonged procedural time.[39] These results highlight currently unresolved issues regarding the potential for effective and safe dosing of propofol in preterm neonates. The pharmacokinetics of propofol in this population are variable and relatively unpredictable, with rapid initial redistribution half-life (5–20 minutes) but slow overall clearance, especially in preterm neonates and/or neonates in the first week of life.[40] Dose-finding studies to determine the minimum effective dose of propofol have produced widely disparate results, with a relatively large study (N = 50) suggesting 0.7 to 1.4 mg/kg for efficacy in 50% of neonates contrasted by efficacy in only 37% of neonates given 2 mg/kg (N = 60).[41,42] The former study with much more conservative dosing noted a 28.5% to 39.1% reduction in mean arterial blood pressure with a brief impact on cerebral oxygen saturation. In the latter study, 39% of neonates required an intravenous fluid bolus after propofol. This line of investigation recently culminated with the NEOPROP-2 study, the largest prospective multicenter stratified dose-finding study to date in neonates.[43] The study was halted after the inclusion of 91 patients with effective sedation without side effects achieved in 13% of the study population. The median cumulative dose of propofol was 3 mg/kg (range 1–6 mg/kg). Fifty-nine percent of study patients had hypotension as defined by mean arterial pressure less than gestational age. Hypotension was prolonged (beyond 60 min after infusion) and dose-dependent.[44] These results cast significant doubt on the role of propofol as a viable premedication before endotracheal intubation in neonates.

Research Directions

Controversies in this field have led to poor adoption of premedication before endotracheal intubation as a standard of care.[45] Several future research directions seem warranted. It must be noted that historic as well as recent data highlight the role of muscle relaxants in the objective efficacy of opioid-based premedication regimens.[46,47] Short-acting opioids have demonstrated superiority to slower acting agents in a blinded trial as monotherapy (N = 20), but with a single, experienced anesthesiologist as the operator.[36] Two potential pathways arise from this observation. First, clinician-scientists may continue to pursue alternative single agents. Ketamine, an NMDA antagonist with sedative and analgesic effects, has limited data, producing lower pain scores and less vagal bradycardia compared with no treatment in one study, but inferior sedation than intranasal midazolam in another.[48,49] Ketamine has become a popular premedication before less invasive surfactant administration (LISA) and would benefit from rigorous investigation including pharmacokinetic/pharmacodynamic, safety, and efficacy studies.[50] Alternatively, researchers may consider further exploration of the optimal premedication cocktail, comprised of a rapid-acting opioid with or without a sedative and with or without muscle relaxation. The opioid remifentanil seems to be a strong candidate for a series of pharmacokinetic, safety, and efficacy studies. This series should also include the definition of a stable formulation allowing for accurate measurement of small dose volumes required in neonates (in other words, more dilute than the current commercially available 50 mcg/mL or rigorously tested 20 mcg/mL dilution). Importantly, blinded randomized controlled trials with clinicians reflective of real-world NICUs are complex, but feasible and necessary for optimal scientific rigor.[39,51]

A one-size-fits-all approach may never be achieved, and randomized trials should recruit neonates accordingly. In this area, personalized medicine will likely dictate utilization in different regimens in different neonates. It is clear that muscle relaxants should be avoided in patients with airway anomalies and for LISA procedures. Potent GABA agonists (including midazolam and propofol) do not seem to have a role in extremely preterm neonates. Defining safe and effective regimens for all neonatal subpopulations, potentially comprised of different drug and/or dosing approaches, remains a vital and outstanding question currently impairing optimal and compassionate care.

PROLONGED STRESS IN PRETERM NEONATES

After successful intubation, clinicians must consider the role of pharmacologic sedation in the care of neonates requiring persistent mechanical ventilation. The indication for any pharmacologic sedation in preterm infants receiving stable invasive ventilation remains an area of active debate, despite more than 25 years of research on this topic.[52,53] Clear distress from invasive mechanical ventilation in older patients along with frequent elevations in stress hormones and ventilator asynchrony in neonates make a strong case for routine sedation.[54–56] Controversy centers on the lack of effective sedatives with short-term and long-term safety data supporting use in preterm neonates.

Sedatives for Prolonged Stress – Misadventures with Benzodiazepines

Benzodiazepines represent the historic foundation of pharmacologic sedation in older patients requiring mechanical ventilation, providing sedation via the $GABA_A$ receptor complex. Continuous infusion of midazolam produces significantly lower sedation scores during mechanical ventilation of preterm neonates than placebo.[57] Both short-term and long-term safety concerns prohibit widespread utilization. Pharmacokinetic studies undertaken to inform randomized controlled trials in preterm neonates document a high risk of transient hypotension and decreased mean cerebral blood flow velocity from bolus doses of midazolam.[58] The clinical importance of these adverse effects was emphasized by results of a pilot randomized controlled trial (NOPAIN) documenting an unacceptable risk of severe intraventricular hemorrhage, periventricular leukomalacia, or death in preterm neonates who received midazolam infusion during invasive mechanical ventilation.[59] Given the pilot nature of this trial, long-term follow-up studies are limited to retrospective cohorts. Significant concern exists in the setting of preclinical studies consistently documenting neuroapoptosis and long-term functional deficits following early benzodiazepine exposure.[60] Clinical cohort studies in humans support this concern, demonstrating decreased hippocampal growth and development at term equivalent age associated with lower cognitive scores at 18 months corrected age associated with higher midazolam exposure.[61] These data highlight the importance of avoiding benzodiazepines for the sedation of preterm neonates, even outside of the window of highest vulnerability to acute neurologic injury.

Analgesics for Prolonged Stress—Relatively Safe and Relatively Mismatched to the Problem

Morphine, predominantly used as an analgesic, has sedative properties in most patients before pain relief.[62] Continuous morphine infusion increases ventilator synchrony and decreases noradrenaline concentrations in mechanically ventilated preterm neonates.[63,64] Morphine rose to prominence for the relief of prolonged stress in preterm neonates based on the NOPAIN trial, documenting a high rate of early neurologic injury with continuous midazolam infusion contrasted by a very low rate with continuous morphine infusion.[59] Unfortunately, large randomized controlled trials (NEOPAIN [N = 898] and the European morphine trial [N = 150]) of morphine for sedation of mechanically ventilated preterm neonates subsequently found no impact on the composite incidence of intraventricular hemorrhage, periventricular leukomalacia, or death (in the absence of preexisting hypotension).[65,66] These trials consistently document clear short-term adverse effects from morphine infusion, including prolonged duration of mechanical ventilation and time to tolerate enteral feedings.[67,68]

Continuous fentanyl has been used in clinical practice as an alternative to morphine in the hopes that the synthetic opioid will produce fewer cardiovascular and gastrointestinal adverse effects.[69,70] Continuous infusion fentanyl also decreases the neuroendocrine stress response in mechanically ventilated preterm neonates.[71] However, a randomized controlled trial in mechanically ventilated preterm neonates documented no impact on open-label boluses of opioid with an increased duration of mechanical ventilation and a trend toward a longer time to full enteral feedings.[72] In the setting of unclear benefit and clear short-term adverse effects, the AAP and Canadian Pediatric Society agree that continuous opioid infusions should not be routinely used in mechanically ventilated preterm neonates, although utilization in clinical practice remains common.

The tenuous, acute benefit:risk profile of continuous opioid infusions highlights the importance of considering long-term outcomes.[60] Randomized controlled trials of low-dose continuous morphine (100 mcg/kg bolus followed by 10 mcg/kg/h continuous infusion for 7 days or less) have been reassuring.[66,73,74] However, cohort data highlight the potential associations between high-level morphine exposure and adverse brain development and long-term outcomes, even after accounting for confounding clinical factors.[6,75–78] Historic gaps in knowledge regarding the pharmacokinetics of continuous fentanyl in preterm neonates have led to high-level opioid exposure in clinical trials and clinical practice. Continuous infusion of fentanyl at "standard doses" (1 mcg/kg bolus followed by 1 mcg/kg/h continuous infusion) results in significant accumulation of drug in preterm neonates.[79] Exposure to this regimen for 1 week was associated with neurodevelopmental impairment at 24 months corrected age in randomized controlled trial.[72,80] A retrospective cohort study with even more dramatic fentanyl exposure demonstrated that cerebellar growth decreases as cumulative fentanyl exposure increases on term equivalent magnetic resonance imaging.[81] These findings characterizing real-world opioid exposure in preterm neonates emphasize the importance of limiting or eliminating exposure and carefully evaluating potential alternative agents.

Sedative for Prolonged Stress – Alpha-2 Agonists Have Promise or in Practice?

Dexmedetomidine, a highly selective alpha-2-adrenergic receptor agonist, provides analgesia, anxiolysis, and sedation. This agent has the potential to solve the riddle of providing comfort during chronic mechanical ventilation in preterm neonates. Clinical data comparing dexmedetomidine to current standards are limited to a retrospective case series, but suggests superior efficacy compared with fentanyl infusion.[82] Dexmedetomidine does not cause respiratory depression or gastrointestinal dysmotility, dramatically shifting the short-term benefit:risk calculation. Preclinical data suggest the possibility of neuroprotection of the immature brain[83]; long-term follow-up of preterm neonates treated with dexmedetomidine has not occurred. It is clearly preliminary to suggest the utilization of dexmedetomidine infusion in all mechanically ventilated preterm neonates. However, incorporation of dexmedetomidine into sedation protocols before escalation from a low-dose morphine infusion in a clinically symptomatic neonate would be reasonable in the setting of current knowledge regarding the benefits and risks of available sedative agents.

Research Directions

Recent studies refine the observation that level of exposure to opioids impacts long-term outcome. Morphine has complex pharmacokinetics, undergoing hepatic metabolism by UDP-glucuronosyltransferases to an opioid agonist (morphine-6-glucuronide) and an opioid antagonist (morphine-3-glucuronide), both of which are eliminated renally. Pharmacokinetic studies informed the design of the NEOPAIN and European morphine trials.[84,85] Although these studies provided data on the relationship between morphine infusion rate and serum concentrations of parent drug and metabolites, they do not account for interindividual variation in morphine biotransformation or pharmacodynamics.[86] Given the disparate actions of morphine's metabolites and known variability in patient-specific dose–response, these differences have the potential to impact exposure and/or long-term outcome. In fact, a recent study suggests genetic variability impacting the metabolism of morphine in neonates modulates the association between exposure and behavioral problems at 18 months of age (**Fig. 2**).[77] Variations in UDP-glucuronosyltransferase activity influence the relationship between morphine exposure and internalizing (anxiety/depression) behavior at 18 months of age, with more rapid metabolizers exhibiting long-term impact possibly via excess accumulation of morphine's active and competing metabolites. Combined variations in the OPRM1 gene, responsible for encoding the μ-opioid receptor, and catechol-O-methyltransferase (COMT) activity, a protein that regulates μ-opioid receptor expression, influence the need for rescue bolus doses of morphine in mechanically ventilated neonates in a randomized trial.[87] Additionally, COMT activity mediated the relationship between morphine exposure and externalizing behavior at 18 months, with neonates more susceptible to morphine's effects driving associations between exposure and outcome.[77] Although these findings require careful validation in animal models and additional human cohorts, they raise the prospect of personalized morphine dosing in neonates through genotyping.

Pharmacokinetic data regarding continuous infusion fentanyl in preterm neonates have lagged behind clinical practice and trials. Fentanyl undergoes hepatic metabolism by CYP3A4 enzymes to inactive metabolites preceding renal elimination. Recently, the Drug dosage Improvement in Neonates (DINO) study prospectively collected 442 opportunistic plasma samples from 98 neonates born at less than 32 weeks gestation receiving fentanyl. The resulting robust population pharmacokinetic model documented the dramatic influence of gestational age and postnatal age on fentanyl clearance, suggesting alternative dosing to the current standard of care in most units (0.5 mcg/kg/h for the first 4 days of life and 0.75 mcg/kg/h from day of life 5–9).[88] The efficacy and safety of this approach must be validated in clinical trials, offering an evidence-based alternative to the standard bodyweight-based dosing used historically. Consideration of pharmacogenetic variation should be prioritized in future pharmacokinetic and clinical studies of fentanyl in neonates.

A major challenge encountered by all prospective trials of analgesics and sedatives in preterm neonates remains the evaluation of short-term efficacy. Pain behaviors are typically used to measure efficacy in research studies and indicate the need for dose titration in clinical practice, but these responses are known to be less robust in more premature neonates.[89] For example, a recent study of continuous fentanyl in preterm

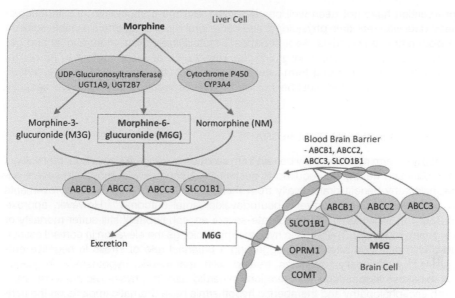

Fig. 2. Genetic influences of morphine activity and clearance in neonates. UGT1A9 and UGT2B7 glucuronidate morphine to morphine-3-glucuronide and morphine-6-glucuronide; cytochrome P450 3A4 biotransforms morphine to normorphine; greater activity in these pathways increases the concentrations of morphine metabolites. ABCB1, ABCC2, ABCC3, and SLCO1B1 influence the excretion of morphine and its metabolites, and also facilitate efflux across the blood–brain barrier; greater density of these enzymes is associated with less analgesic effect from morphine. Inside the brain, genes encode enzymes involved in morphine pharmacokinetics/pharmacodynamics (eg, COMT which regulates endogenous opioid level and OPRM1 which encodes the μ-opioid receptor); greater density of OPRM1 is associated with greater analgesia from morphine. (*From* Chau CMY, Ross CJD, Chau V, et al. Morphine biotransformation genes and neonatal clinical factors predicted behavior problems in very preterm children at 18months. *EBioMedicine*. Feb 2019;40:655-662; with permission)

neonates failed to document any impact on pain scores after the initial 3 days of therapy.[72] Additional measures like the magnitude of noxious-evoked brain activity on electroencephalogram have the potential to augment scoring tools.[90] Regardless of the specific components of a multidimensional approach to pain assessment, clinical trials and clinical practice must collate all available patient data to inform decision making. This approach was recently described for morphine, with pharmacokinetic model-informed dosing guidance provided directly in the electronic health record based on patient-specific drug concentrations in concert with physiologic data and bedside assessment (NeoRelief).[91] Large scale combination of data regarding both exposure and effect allows the refinement of pharmacokinetic targets based on patient-specific pharmacodynamic data. Incorporation of genotyping has the potential to further improve functionality; this line of research should be prioritized.

The combination of pharmacokinetics, pharmacodynamics, genetics, and outcomes research represents the only path forward for novel interventions like dexmedetomidine. Dexmedetomidine is also hepatically metabolized, to inactive metabolites by CPY2A6 and UDP-glucuronosyltransferases, before renal elimination. Pharmacokinetic studies of dexmedetomidine exist, but include relatively low numbers and do not describe dosing in extremely preterm neonates.[92] The pharmacodynamic goals of this intervention have not been well characterized, but the combination of pharmacokinetic data with real-time physiologic and behavioral monitoring offers a viable solution in both practice and trials. As a hepatically-metabolized drug, maturational and genetic variance is certain, highlighting the importance of these factors in modeling. Finally, short-term and long-term safety data represent the lynchpin of any intervention in preterm neonates and must be included in all prospective studies of novel sedative agents.

PROLONGED STRESS IN TERM NEONATES

Critically ill, term neonates may benefit from sedation to mitigate stress from physiologic instability and treatments required to sustain life. Neonates with moderate-severe encephalopathy benefit dramatically from therapeutic hypothermia, with improvements in both mortality and long-term neurodevelopmental outcome.[93] However, approximately 1 in 3 neonates with moderate-severe encephalopathy still suffer mortality or long-term morbidity. Therapeutic hypothermia prolongs the elevation in cortisol associated with asphyxia after birth, suggesting a potential role of stress in negative outcomes.[94] Additionally, neonates treated with therapeutic hypothermia frequently exhibit stress associated with alterations in cardiovascular physiologic homeostasis.[95] Both encephalopathy and therapeutic hypothermia have dramatic impacts on the benefit:risk profile of available agents for pharmacologic sedation.

Analgesics for Prolonged Stress – Relatively Safe and Relatively Mismatched to the Problem

Morphine is the most widely used sedative during therapeutic hypothermia, in spite of limited data supporting clinical benefit.[96] Sedation or analgesia from morphine may have a role in reducing cerebral metabolic demand in the absence of therapeutic hypothermia, with a retrospective study identifying less brain injury and better scores on the Pediatric Cerebral Performance Category Scale at discharge in morphine-treated neonates than untreated controls, despite greater severity of illness.[97] Standing sedation or analgesia was not standard of care in randomized controlled trials documenting the profound benefits of therapeutic hypothermia, with the sole exception of the neo.n-EURO study (morphine 0.1 mg/kg every 4 hours or an equivalent dose of fentanyl).[93,98] This trial identified a larger effect size (32% absolute risk reduction [ARR] of death or severe disability) compared with previous trials (ARR = 15%); however, the relatively high incidence of death or severe disability in the control group may have contributed.

Recent retrospective studies examining morphine infusion in neonates with moderate-severe encephalopathy treated with therapeutic hypothermia have produced mixed results. The observational Magnetic Resonance Biomarkers in Neonatal Encephalopathy (MARBLE) study evaluated outcomes in 169 neonates and documented no difference in magnetic resonance imaging at 1 week of age or neurodevelopmental testing at 22 months of age in infants who received open-label morphine infusion (N = 141) compared with those who did not (N = 28).[99] These results are bolstered by a recent report from the Bristol cooling program (N = 229) documenting no significant association between cumulative morphine dose in the first week of life and Bayley-3 scores at 18 to 24 months of age in infants treated with therapeutic hypothermia for encephalopathy.[100] However, in the MARBLE study, neonates who received open-label morphine infusion, dosed typically at 10 to 20 mcg/kg/h, were more likely to be hypotensive (49% vs 25%, P = .02) and had a longer hospital stay (12 days vs 9 days, P = .009). Lack of benefit in the setting of potential adverse effects encourages the consideration of alternative agents.

Sedative for Prolonged Stress – Alpha-2 Agonists Have Promise or in Practice?

Brain recovery during the latent phase of neonatal encephalopathy relies on reduced brain blood flow and metabolism via norepinephrine-mediated stimulation of the alpha-2 receptor.[101] Inhibition of alpha-2 receptor stimulation exacerbates neuronal loss; infusion of an alpha-2 receptor agonist is neuroprotective.[102] Dexmedetomidine specifically increases the expression of hippocampal phosphorylated extracellular signal-regulated protein kinase 1 and 2 (mediators of neuronal survival and synaptic plasticity) and suppresses cytokine-mediated brain injury, reducing brain tissue loss and improving neurologic function in preclinical models of perinatal hypoxia-ischemia.[103,104]

Dexmedetomidine provides adequate sedation and reduces shivering threshold in adults exposed to mild hypothermia without producing respiratory depression.[105] Emerging use of dexmedetomidine in neonatal clinical practice has resulted in the publication of a retrospective case series (N = 19) and a retrospective cohort study (N = 70) with standing morphine as the comparator (0.1 mg/kg/dose every 4 hours).[106,107] In these experiences, dexmedetomidine successfully eliminates the need for open-label boluses or infusion of opioid for pain/agitation perceived by the bedside clinician, shivering, or tachycardia.[106] Sedation is accomplished without impacting respiratory drive, allowing sustained noninvasive ventilation or facilitating reduction in invasive respiratory support. Trophic feedings are well tolerated during dexmedetomidine infusion. Cardiovascular complications seem to be rare and transient. Based on these outcomes, future use in clinical practice and accompanying retrospective studies are inevitable, but do not eliminate the need for careful pharmacokinetic studies and randomized trials evaluating efficacy, safety, and long-term outcomes.

Research Directions

Consistent with the pitfalls encountered in the optimal sedation of preterm neonates, clinical practice has preceded robust pharmacokinetic studies of both morphine and dexmedetomidine in term neonates with encephalopathy treated with therapeutic hypothermia. Neonatal encephalopathy often coincides with multi-organ injury, with acute liver and kidney injury reported in up to 60% and 40% of cases, respectively.[108] Additionally, therapeutic hypothermia independently reduces drug clearance through the alteration of temperature-dependent metabolic processes and/or organ blood flow.[109] The impacts of these alterations in drug distribution, metabolism, and elimination must be evaluated carefully to ensure appropriate dosing of all pharmacologic agents used during therapeutic hypothermia.

Morphine disposition is altered during therapeutic hypothermia due to reduced volume of distribution from peripheral vasoconstriction, decreased activity of cytochrome P450 enzymes, and reduced glucuronidation.[110] Two recent pharmacokinetic studies have documented the impact of neonatal encephalopathy and therapeutic hypothermia on the dosing approach required to achieve therapeutic serum concentrations for analgesia (10–40 ng/mL) and avoid excessive drug accumulation. The studies agree on a more conservative dosing approach than previously described in clinical reports, with a loading dose of morphine 50 mcg/kg followed by 5 mcg/kg/h or 40 to 50 mcg/kg every 6 hours (Fig. 3).[110,111] The impact of this dose modification on efficacy, safety, and long-term outcomes requires careful prospective evaluation. Additionally, the impact of genetic variability on the interindividual difference in pharmacokinetics in term and postterm neonates would benefit from additional exploration.[112]

The pharmacokinetics of dexmedetomidine, a hepatically metabolized and renally eliminated drug, are also altered by both hypoxia–ischemia and therapeutic

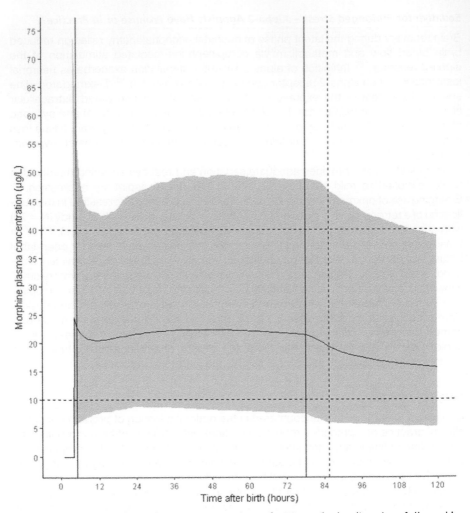

Fig. 3. Simulated morphine plasma concentrations of a 50 mcg/kg loading dose followed by 5 mcg/kg/h. Solid line indicates the mean plasma morphine concentration; gray area indicates the 95% confidence interval. Dotted horizontal lines indicate the proposed therapeutic window of 10 to 40 mcg/L. Solid vertical lines indicate the period of therapeutic hypothermia; dashed vertical line indicates the end of rewarming. (*From* Favie LMA, Groenendaal F, van den Broek MPH, et al. Pharmacokinetics of morphine in encephalopathic neonates treated with therapeutic hypothermia. *PLoS One.* 2019;14(2):e0211910; with permission.)

hypothermia. In animal models, clearance is reduced by 56% following experimental hypoxia–ischemia and an additional 33% during therapeutic hypothermia.[113] Retrospective clinical data have defined the effective dose of dexmedetomidine as a median of 0.3 mcg/kg/h (range 0.1–0.5 mcg/kg/h).[106,107] However, pharmacokinetic studies to verify the appropriateness of this approach as well as evaluate the impact of degree of encephalopathy on clearance are extremely limited. The pharmacokinetics of dexmedetomidine have been evaluated in only 7 human neonates with moderate–severe encephalopathy treated with therapeutic hypothermia.[114] The maximum dexmedetomidine dose evaluated was 0.4 mcg/kg/h and no firm conclusions regarding safe and effective dosing are possible based on this limited report. Focus in this area is required as the prevalence of dexmedetomidine increases in clinical practice.

SUMMARY

Hospitalized preterm and term neonates are exposed to a high burden of pain and stress with clear negative impact on the quality of care and long-term outcome. Mildly painful procedures must be minimized and approached with a standardized bundle of nonpharmacologic interventions optimized for the maturation of specific neonatal subpopulations. Sweet-tasting solution may be used judiciously at the lowest effective dose, but also require further evaluation including longitudinal exposures and assessment of long-term outcomes. Moderately painful procedures require pharmacotherapy, including a rapidly acting opioid as the backbone of a cocktail potentially including muscle relaxation for nonemergent endotracheal intubation. Prolonged mechanical ventilation is likely a source of stress in preterm neonates, but only low-dose morphine infusions have palatable short-term adverse effects and long-term safety data in symptomatic neonates; clinicians should strongly consider continuous dexmedetomidine as an alternative or adjunct. Similarly, term neonates receiving therapeutic hypothermia may experience stress, but the role of continuous pharmacologic sedation has not yet been clarified. Low-dose morphine is widely used in the setting of strong pharmacokinetic data, but limited clinical data suggest concerning adverse effects; dexmedetomidine requires additional evaluation but may be a more effective and safer alternative agent. Carefully designed and executed clinical research remains essential to define an optimal approach to neonatal pain in various clinical situations, and should consider efficacy, safety, pharmacokinetics, and long-term outcomes.

DISCLOSURE

The authors have nothing to disclose.

CLINICS CARE POINTS

- Develop protocols for feasible, evidence-based nonpharmacologic care, and train staff to ensure safety and optimize efficacy
- Use nonnutritive sucking and swaddling/facilitated tucking as standard care for mildly painful procedures. Addition of sucrose 0.1 mL 2 minutes before the procedure may be appropriate for physiologically stable neonates. Avoid sweet-tasting solutions for other indications and consider alternatives when a neonate requires more than 10 mildly painful procedures daily.
- A rapidly acting opioid (generally fentanyl or remifentanil) should be given before all nonemergent endotracheal intubations in neonates; muscle relaxation should be strongly considered.
- Preterm neonates exhibiting signs of agitation during stable mechanical ventilation should receive a low-dose morphine infusion. Dexmedetomidine may be considered as alternative or adjunctive therapy with careful monitoring for acute adverse effects.
- Term neonates exhibiting signs of agitation during therapeutic hypothermia should receive low-dose morphine infusion or dexmedetomidine infusion; regardless of the agent used, careful monitoring for adverse effects is required.

Best practices

What is the current practice for managing pain and stress in neonates?

- Despite frequent mild and moderate pain and prolonged stress in critically ill neonates, pharmacologic interventions to mitigate acute and long-term adverse effects have not been standardized.
- Clinicians must consider available evidence and implement standardized interventions with the most favorable safety and efficacy profile, carefully monitoring outcomes in their own population of neonates and evaluating emerging evidence.

What changes in current practice are likely to improve outcomes?

- Robust research is required regarding the pharmacokinetics, pharmacogenomics, safety, efficacy, and long-term impact of pharmacologic agents used in clinical practice to mitigate neonatal pain and stress.

Major recommendations

- Nonpharmacologic interventions form the foundation of neonatal pain and stress relief; rapidly acting, safe, and effective pharmacologic analgesia should be provided before all moderately painful procedures.
- Continuous analgesia or sedation should be considered in the setting of prolonged stress; however, safe and effective therapies have not been adequately studied to support standardization and universal utilization.

Summary

Pain and stress have a profound impact on the long-term outcomes of neonates who require intensive care. Clinicians and clinician-scientists must provide interventions supported by available evidence and perform research to close gaps in knowledge to ensure compassionate developmental care for these vulnerable patients.

Data from Refs.[1,4,28,30]

REFERENCES

1. McNair C, Campbell-Yeo M, Johnston C, et al. Nonpharmacologic management of pain during common needle puncture procedures in infants: current research evidence and practical considerations: an update. Clin Perinatol 2019;46(4): 709–30. https://doi.org/10.1016/j.clp.2019.08.006.
2. Anand KJS. Discovering pain in newborn infants. Anesthesiology 2019;131(2): 392–5. https://doi.org/10.1097/ALN.0000000000002810.
3. Volpe JJ. Dysmaturation of premature brain: importance, cellular mechanisms, and potential interventions. Pediatr Neurol 2019;95:42–66. https://doi.org/10.1016/j.pediatrneurol.2019.02.016.
4. McPherson C, Miller SP, El-Dib M, et al. The influence of pain, agitation, and their management on the immature brain. Pediatr Res 2020. https://doi.org/10.1038/s41390-019-0744-6.
5. Chau CMY, Ranger M, Bichin M, et al. Hippocampus, amygdala, and thalamus volumes in very preterm children at 8 years: neonatal pain and genetic variation. Front Behav Neurosci 2019;13:51. https://doi.org/10.3389/fnbeh.2019.00051.
6. Nunes AS, Kozhemiako N, Hutcheon E, et al. Atypical neuromagnetic resting activity associated with thalamic volume and cognitive outcome in very preterm children. Neuroimage Clin 2020;27:102275. https://doi.org/10.1016/j.nicl.2020.102275.

7. Stevens B, Yamada J, Ohlsson A, et al. Sucrose for analgesia in newborn infants undergoing painful procedures. Cochrane Database Syst Rev 2016;(1):CD001069. https://doi.org/10.1002/14651858.CD001069.pub5.
8. Lin JC, Strauss RG, Kulhavy JC, et al. Phlebotomy overdraw in the neonatal intensive care nursery. Pediatrics 2000;106(2):E19. https://doi.org/10.1542/peds.106.2.e19.
9. Pillai Riddell RR, Racine NM, Gennis HG, et al. Non-pharmacological management of infant and young child procedural pain. Cochrane Database Syst Rev 2015;(12):CD006275. https://doi.org/10.1002/14651858.CD006275.pub3.
10. Hatfield LA, Murphy N, Karp K, et al. A systematic review of behavioral and environmental interventions for procedural pain management in preterm infants. J Pediatr Nurs 2019;44:22–30. https://doi.org/10.1016/j.pedn.2018.10.004.
11. Benoit B, Campbell-Yeo M, Johnston C, et al. Staff nurse utilization of kangaroo care as an intervention for procedural pain in preterm infants. Adv Neonatal Care 2016;16(3):229–38. https://doi.org/10.1097/ANC.0000000000000262.
12. Harrison D, Larocque C, Bueno M, et al. Sweet solutions to reduce procedural pain in neonates: a meta-analysis. Pediatrics 2017;139(1):e20160955. https://doi.org/10.1542/peds.2016-0955.
13. Huang RR, Xie RH, Wen SW, et al. Sweet solutions for analgesia in neonates in China: a systematic review and meta-analysis. Can J Nurs Res 2019;51(2): 116–27. https://doi.org/10.1177/0844562118803756.
14. Taddio A, Shah V, Atenafu E, et al. Influence of repeated painful procedures and sucrose analgesia on the development of hyperalgesia in newborn infants. Pain 2009;144(1–2):43–8. https://doi.org/10.1016/j.pain.2009.02.012.
15. McPherson C, Grunau RE. Neonatal pain control and neurologic effects of anesthetics and sedatives in preterm infants. Clin Perinatol 2014;41(1):209–27. https://doi.org/10.1016/j.clp.2013.10.002.
16. Tremblay S, Ranger M, Chau CMY, et al. Repeated exposure to sucrose for procedural pain in mouse pups leads to long-term widespread brain alterations. Pain 2017;158(8):1586–98. https://doi.org/10.1097/j.pain.0000000000000961.
17. Ranger M, Tremblay S, Chau CMY, et al. Adverse behavioral changes in adult mice following neonatal repeated exposure to pain and sucrose. Front Psychol 2018;9:2394. https://doi.org/10.3389/fpsyg.2018.02394.
18. Johnston CC, Filion F, Snider L, et al. Routine sucrose analgesia during the first week of life in neonates younger than 31 weeks' postconceptional age. Pediatrics 2002;110(3):523–8.
19. Stevens B, Yamada J, Beyene J, et al. Consistent management of repeated procedural pain with sucrose in preterm neonates: is it effective and safe for repeated use over time? Clin J Pain 2005;21(6):543–8. https://doi.org/10.1097/01.ajp.0000149802.46864.e2.
20. Schneider J, Duerden EG, Guo T, et al. Procedural pain and oral glucose in preterm neonates: brain development and sex-specific effects. Pain 2018;159(3): 515–25. https://doi.org/10.1097/j.pain.0000000000001123.
21. Stevens B, Yamada J, Campbell-Yeo M, et al. The minimally effective dose of sucrose for procedural pain relief in neonates: a randomized controlled trial. BMC Pediatr 2018;18(1):85. https://doi.org/10.1186/s12887-018-1026-x.
22. Bembich S, Cont G, Causin E, et al. Infant analgesia with a combination of breast milk, glucose, or maternal holding. Pediatrics 2018;142(3):e20173416. https://doi.org/10.1542/peds.2017-3416.
23. Campbell-Yeo M, Johnston CC, Benoit B, et al. Sustained efficacy of kangaroo care for repeated painful procedures over neonatal intensive care unit

hospitalization: a single-blind randomized controlled trial. Pain 2019;160(11): 2580–8. https://doi.org/10.1097/j.pain.0000000000001646.

24. Kelly MA, Finer NN. Nasotracheal intubation in the neonate: physiologic responses and effects of atropine and pancuronium. J Pediatr 1984;105(2):303–9.

25. Haubner LY, Barry JS, Johnston LC, et al. Neonatal intubation performance: room for improvement in tertiary neonatal intensive care units. Resuscitation 2013;84(10):1359–64. https://doi.org/10.1016/j.resuscitation.2013.03.014.

26. Sauer CW, Kong JY, Vaucher YE, et al. Intubation attempts increase the risk for severe intraventricular hemorrhage in preterm infants-A retrospective cohort study. J Pediatr 2016;177:108–13. https://doi.org/10.1016/j.jpeds.2016.06.051.

27. Wallenstein MB, Birnie KL, Arain YH, et al. Failed endotracheal intubation and adverse outcomes among extremely low birth weight infants. J Perinatol 2016; 36(2):112–5. https://doi.org/10.1038/jp.2015.158.

28. Kumar P, Denson SE, Mancuso TJ. Committee on fetus and newborn section on anesthesiology and pain medicine. Premedication for nonemergency endotracheal intubation in the neonate. Pediatrics 2010;125(3):608–15. https://doi.org/10.1542/peds.2009-2863.

29. Le CN, Garey DM, Leone TA, et al. Impact of premedication on neonatal intubations by pediatric and neonatal trainees. J Perinatol 2014;34(6):458–60. https://doi.org/10.1038/jp.2014.32.

30. Mari J, Franczia P, Margas W, et al. International consensus is neededon premedication for non-emergency neonatal intubation after survey found wide-ranging policies and practices in 70 countries. Acta Paediatr 2020;109(7): 1369–75. https://doi.org/10.1111/apa.15119.

31. Norman E, Kindblom JM, Rane A, et al. Individual variations in fentanyl pharmacokinetics and pharmacodynamics in preterm infants. Acta Paediatr 2019; 108(8):1441–6. https://doi.org/10.1111/apa.14744.

32. Elmekkawi A, Abdelgadir D, Van Dyk J, et al. Use of naloxone to minimize extubation failure after premedication for INSURE procedure in preterm neonates. J Neonatal Perinatal Med 2016;9(4):363–70. https://doi.org/10.3233/NPM-915141.

33. Choong K, AlFaleh K, Doucette J, et al. Remifentanil for endotracheal intubation in neonates: a randomised controlled trial. Arch Dis Child Fetal Neonatal Ed 2010;95(2):F80–4. https://doi.org/10.1136/adc.2009.167338.

34. McCluskey SV, Graner KK, Kemp J, et al. Stability of fentanyl 5 microg/mL diluted with 0.9% sodium chloride injection and stored in polypropylene syringes. Am J Health Syst Pharm 2009;66(9):860–3. https://doi.org/10.2146/ajhp080255.

35. Lemyre B, Doucette J, Kalyn A, et al. Morphine for elective endotracheal intubation in neonates: a randomized trial [ISRCTN43546373]. BMC Pediatr 2004;4:20. https://doi.org/10.1186/1471-2431-4-20.

36. Pereira e Silva Y, Gomez RS, Marcatto Jde O, et al. Morphine versus remifentanil for intubating preterm neonates. Arch Dis Child Fetal Neonatal Ed 2007;92(4): F293–4. https://doi.org/10.1136/adc.2006.105262.

37. Altamimi MI, Choonara I, Sammons H. Inter-individual variation in morphine clearance in children. Eur J Clin Pharmacol 2015;71(6):649–55. https://doi.org/10.1007/s00228-015-1843-x.

38. Ghanta S, Abdel-Latif ME, Lui K, et al. Propofol compared with the morphine, atropine, and suxamethonium regimen as induction agents for neonatal endotracheal intubation: a randomized, controlled trial. Comparative study

randomized controlled trial. Pediatrics 2007;119(6):e1248–55. https://doi.org/10.1542/peds.2006-2708.

39. Durrmeyer X, Breinig S, Claris O, et al. Effect of atropine with propofol vs atropine with atracurium and sufentanil on oxygen desaturation in neonates requiring nonemergency intubation: a randomized clinical trial. JAMA 2018; 319(17):1790–801. https://doi.org/10.1001/jama.2018.3708.

40. Allegaert K, Peeters MY, Verbesselt R, et al. Inter-individual variability in propofol pharmacokinetics in preterm and term neonates. Br J Anaesth 2007;99(6): 864–70. https://doi.org/10.1093/bja/aem294.

41. Smits A, Thewissen L, Caicedo A, et al. Propofol dose-finding to reach optimal effect for (Semi-)Elective intubation in neonates. J Pediatr 2016;179:54–60.e9. https://doi.org/10.1016/j.jpeds.2016.07.049.

42. Simons SH, van der Lee R, Reiss IK, et al. Clinical evaluation of propofol as sedative for endotracheal intubation in neonates. Acta Paediatr 2013;102(11): e487–92. https://doi.org/10.1111/apa.12367.

43. de Kort EHM, Prins SA, Reiss IKM, et al. Propofol for endotracheal intubation in neonates: a dose-finding trial. Arch Dis Child Fetal Neonatal Ed 2020;105(5): 489–95. https://doi.org/10.1136/archdischild-2019-318474.

44. de Kort EHM, Twisk JWR, van t Verlaat EPG, et al. Propofol in neonates causes a dose-dependent profound and protracted decrease in blood pressure. Acta Paediatr 2020;109(12):2539–46. https://doi.org/10.1111/apa.15282.

45. Muniraman HK, Yaari J, Hand I. Premedication use before nonemergent intubation in the newborn infant. Am J Perinatol 2015;32(9):821–4. https://doi.org/10.1055/s-0034-1543987.

46. Roberts KD, Leone TA, Edwards WH, et al. Premedication for nonemergent neonatal intubations: a randomized, controlled trial comparing atropine and fentanyl to atropine, fentanyl, and mivacurium. Pediatrics 2006;118(4):1583–91. https://doi.org/10.1542/peds.2006-0590.

47. Ozawa Y, Ades A, Foglia EE, et al. Premedication with neuromuscular blockade and sedation during neonatal intubation is associated with fewer adverse events. J Perinatol 2019;39(6):848–56. https://doi.org/10.1038/s41372-019-0367-0.

48. Barois J, Tourneux P. Ketamine and atropine decrease pain for preterm newborn tracheal intubation in the delivery room: an observational pilot study. Acta Paediatr 2013;102(12):e534–8. https://doi.org/10.1111/apa.12413.

49. Milesi C, Baleine J, Mura T, et al. Nasal midazolam vs ketamine for neonatal intubation in the delivery room: a randomised trial. Arch Dis Child Fetal Neonatal Ed 2018;103(3):F221–6. https://doi.org/10.1136/archdischild-2017-312808.

50. Krajewski P, Szpecht D, Hozejowski R. Premedication practices for less invasive surfactant administration - results from a nationwide cohort study. J Matern Fetal Neonatal Med 2020;1–5. https://doi.org/10.1080/14767058.2020.1863365.

51. Tauzin M, Marchand-Martin L, Lebeaux C, et al. Neurodevelopmental outcomes after premedication with atropine/propofol vs atropine/atracurium/sufentanil for neonatal intubation: 2-year follow-up of a randomized clinical trial. J Pediatr 2020. https://doi.org/10.1016/j.jpeds.2020.12.001.

52. American Academy of Pediatrics Committee on Fetus and Newborn, American Academy of Pediatrics Section on Surgery, Canadian Paediatric Society Fetus and Newborn Committee, Batton DG, Barrington KJ, Wallman C. Prevention and management of pain in the neonate: an update. Practice guideline. Pediatrics 2006;118(5):2231–41. https://doi.org/10.1542/peds.2006-2277.

53. Ancora G, Lago P, Garetti E, et al. Evidence-based clinical guidelines on analgesia and sedation in newborn infants undergoing assisted ventilation and endotracheal intubation. Acta Paediatr 2019;108(2):208–17. https://doi.org/10.1111/apa.14606.

54. Gelinas C, Fortier M, Viens C, et al. Pain assessment and management in critically ill intubated patients: a retrospective study. Am J Crit Care 2004;13(2):126–35.

55. Quinn MW, de Boer RC, Ansari N, et al. Stress response and mode of ventilation in preterm infants. Arch Dis Child Fetal Neonatal Ed 1998;78(3):F195–8.

56. Longhini F, Ferrero F, De Luca D, et al. Neurally adjusted ventilatory assist in preterm neonates with acute respiratory failure. Neonatology 2015;107(1):60–7. https://doi.org/10.1159/000367886.

57. Jacqz-Aigrain E, Daoud P, Burtin P, et al. Placebo-controlled trial of midazolam sedation in mechanically ventilated newborn babies. Lancet 1994;344(8923):646–50.

58. van Straaten HL, Rademaker CM, de Vries LS. Comparison of the effect of midazolam or vecuronium on blood pressure and cerebral blood flow velocity in the premature newborn. Dev Pharmacol Ther 1992;19(4):191–5.

59. Anand KJ, Barton BA, McIntosh N, et al. Analgesia and sedation in preterm neonates who require ventilatory support: results from the NOPAIN trial. Neonatal outcome and prolonged analgesia in neonates. Arch Pediatr Adolesc Med 1999;153(4):331–8.

60. Durrmeyer X, Vutskits L, Anand KJ, et al. Use of analgesic and sedative drugs in the NICU: integrating clinical trials and laboratory data. Review. Pediatr Res 2010;67(2):117–27.

61. Duerden EG, Guo T, Dodbiba L, et al. Midazolam dose correlates with abnormal hippocampal growth and neurodevelopmental outcome in preterm infants. Ann Neurol 2016;79(4):548–59. https://doi.org/10.1002/ana.24601.

62. Paqueron X, Lumbroso A, Mergoni P, et al. Is morphine-induced sedation synonymous with analgesia during intravenous morphine titration? Br J Anaesth 2002;89(5):697–701.

63. Dyke MP, Kohan R, Evans S. Morphine increases synchronous ventilation in preterm infants. J Paediatr Child Health 1995;31(3):176–9.

64. Simons SH, van Dijk M, van Lingen RA, et al. Randomised controlled trial evaluating effects of morphine on plasma adrenaline/noradrenaline concentrations in newborns. Arch Dis Child Fetal Neonatal Ed 2005;90(1):F36–40. https://doi.org/10.1136/adc.2003.046425.

65. Anand KJ, Hall RW, Desai N, et al. Effects of morphine analgesia in ventilated preterm neonates: primary outcomes from the NEOPAIN randomised trial. Lancet 2004;363(9422):1673–82. https://doi.org/10.1016/S0140-6736(04)16251-X.

66. Simons SH, van Dijk M, van Lingen RA, et al. Routine morphine infusion in preterm newborns who received ventilatory support: a randomized controlled trial. JAMA 2003;290(18):2419–27. https://doi.org/10.1001/jama.290.18.2419.

67. Bhandari V, Bergqvist LL, Kronsberg SS, et al. Morphine administration and short-term pulmonary outcomes among ventilated preterm infants. Pediatrics 2005;116(2):352–9. https://doi.org/10.1542/peds.2004-2123.

68. Menon G, Boyle EM, Bergqvist LL, et al. Morphine analgesia and gastrointestinal morbidity in preterm infants: secondary results from the NEOPAIN trial. Multicenter Study Randomized Controlled Trial. Arch Dis Child Fetal Neonatal Ed 2008;93(5):F362–7. https://doi.org/10.1136/adc.2007.119297.

69. Saarenmaa E, Huttunen P, Leppaluoto J, et al. Advantages of fentanyl over morphine in analgesia for ventilated newborn infants after birth: a randomized trial. J Pediatr 1999;134(2):144–50.

70. Hamon I, Hascoet JM, Debbiche A, et al. Effects of fentanyl administration on general and cerebral haemodynamics in sick newborn infants. Acta Paediatr 1996;85(3):361–5.

71. Lago P, Benini F, Agosto C, et al. Randomised controlled trial of low dose fentanyl infusion in preterm infants with hyaline membrane disease. Arch Dis Child Fetal Neonatal Ed 1998;79(3):F194–7.

72. Ancora G, Lago P, Garetti E, et al. Efficacy and safety of continuous infusion of fentanyl for pain control in preterm newborns on mechanical ventilation. J Pediatr 2013;163(3):645–51.e1. https://doi.org/10.1016/j.jpeds.2013.02.039.

73.. de Graaf J, van Lingen RA, Simons SH, et al. Long-term effects of routine morphine infusion in mechanically ventilated neonates on children's functioning: five-year follow-up of a randomized controlled trial. Pain 2011;152(6): 1391–7. https://doi.org/10.1016/j.pain.2011.02.017.

74. de Graaf J, van Lingen RA, Valkenburg AJ, et al. Does neonatal morphine use affect neuropsychological outcomes at 8 to 9 years of age? Pain 2013;154(3): 449–58. https://doi.org/10.1016/j.pain.2012.12.006.

75. Steinhorn R, McPherson C, Anderson PJ, et al. Neonatal morphine exposure in very preterm infants-cerebral development and outcomes. J Pediatr 2015; 166(5):1200–7.e4. https://doi.org/10.1016/j.jpeds.2015.02.012.

76. Zwicker JG, Miller SP, Grunau RE, et al. Smaller cerebellar growth and poorer neurodevelopmental outcomes in very preterm infants exposed to neonatal morphine. J Pediatr 2016;172:81–7.e2. https://doi.org/10.1016/j.jpeds.2015. 12.024.

77. Chau CMY, Ross CJD, Chau V, et al. Morphine biotransformation genes and neonatal clinical factors predicted behaviour problems in very preterm children at 18months. EBioMedicine 2019;40:655–62. https://doi.org/10.1016/j.ebiom. 2019.01.042.

78. Ranger M, Zwicker JG, Chau CM, et al. Neonatal pain and infection relate to smaller cerebellum in very preterm children at school age. J Pediatr 2015; 167(2):292–8.e1. https://doi.org/10.1016/j.jpeds.2015.04.055.

79. Saarenmaa E, Neuvonen PJ, Fellman V. Gestational age and birth weight effects on plasma clearance of fentanyl in newborn infants. J Pediatr 2000;136(6): 767–70.

80. Ancora G, Lago P, Garetti E, et al. Follow-up at the corrected age of 24 months of preterm newborns receiving continuous infusion of fentanyl for pain control during mechanical ventilation. Pain 2017;158(5):840–5. https://doi.org/10. 1097/j.pain.0000000000000839.

81. McPherson C, Haslam M, Pineda R, et al. Brain injury and development in preterm infants exposed to fentanyl. Ann Pharmacother 2015;49(12):1291–7. https://doi.org/10.1177/1060028015606732.

82. O'Mara K, Gal P, Wimmer J, et al. Dexmedetomidine versus standard therapy with fentanyl for sedation in mechanically ventilated premature neonates. J Pediatr Pharmacol Ther 2012;17(3):252–62. https://doi.org/10.5863/1551-6776-17.3.252.

83.. Laudenbach V, Mantz J, Lagercrantz H, et al. Effects of alpha(2)-adrenoceptor agonists on perinatal excitotoxic brain injury: comparison of clonidine and dexmedetomidine. Anesthesiology 2002;96(1):134–41.

84. Chay PC, Duffy BJ, Walker JS. Pharmacokinetic-pharmacodynamic relationships of morphine in neonates. Clin Pharmacol Ther 1992;51(3):334–42.
85. Hartley R, Green M, Quinn M, et al. Pharmacokinetics of morphine infusion in premature neonates. Arch Dis Child 1993;69(1 Spec No):55–8.
86. Allegaert K, Simons SHP, Tibboel D, et al. Non-maturational covariates for dynamic systems pharmacology models in neonates, infants, and children: filling the gaps beyond developmental pharmacology. Eur J Pharm Sci 2017;109S: S27–31. https://doi.org/10.1016/j.ejps.2017.05.023.
87. Matic M, Simons SH, van Lingen RA, et al. Rescue morphine in mechanically ventilated newborns associated with combined OPRM1 and COMT genotype. Pharmacogenomics 2014;15(10):1287–95. https://doi.org/10.2217/pgs.14.100.
88. Völler S, Flint RB, Andriessen P, et al. Rapidly maturing fentanyl clearance in preterm neonates. Arch Dis Child Fetal Neonatal Ed 2019;104(6):F598–603. https://doi.org/10.1136/archdischild-2018-315920.
89. Johnston CC, Stevens BJ, Franck LS, et al. Factors explaining lack of response to heel stick in preterm newborns. J Obstet Gynecol Neonatal Nurs 1999;28(6): 587–94. https://doi.org/10.1111/j.1552-6909.1999.tb02167.x.
90. Hartley C, Moultrie F, Hoskin A, et al. Analgesic efficacy and safety of morphine in the Procedural Pain in Premature Infants (Poppi) study: randomised placebo-controlled trial. Lancet 2018;392(10164):2595–605. https://doi.org/10.1016/S0140-6736(18)31813-0.
91. Vinks AA, Punt NC, Menke F, et al. Electronic health record-embedded decision support platform for morphine precision dosing in neonates. Clin Pharmacol Ther 2020;107(1):186–94. https://doi.org/10.1002/cpt.1684.
92. Chrysostomou C, Schulman SR, Herrera Castellanos M, et al. A phase II/III, multicenter, safety, efficacy, and pharmacokinetic study of dexmedetomidine in preterm and term neonates. J Pediatr 2014;164(2):276–82. https://doi.org/10.1016/j.jpeds.2013.10.002, e1–3.
93. Jacobs SE, Berg M, Hunt R, et al. Cooling for newborns with hypoxic ischaemic encephalopathy. Cochrane Database Syst Rev 2013;(1):CD003311. https://doi.org/10.1002/14651858.CD003311.pub3.
94. Davidson JO, Fraser M, Naylor AS, et al. Effect of cerebral hypothermia on cortisol and adrenocorticotropic hormone responses after umbilical cord occlusion in preterm fetal sheep. Pediatr Res 2008;63(1):51–5. https://doi.org/10.1203/PDR.0b013e31815b8eb4.
95. Hoffman K, Bromster T, Hakansson S, et al. Monitoring of pain and stress in an infant with asphyxia during induced hypothermia: a case report. Adv Neonatal Care 2013;13(4):252–61. https://doi.org/10.1097/ANC.0b013e31829d8baf.
96. Montaldo P, Vakharia A, Ivain P, et al. Pre-emptive opioid sedation during therapeutic hypothermia. Arch Dis Child Fetal Neonatal Ed 2020;105(1):108–9. https://doi.org/10.1136/archdischild-2019-317050.
97. Angeles DM, Wycliffe N, Michelson D, et al. Use of opioids in asphyxiated term neonates: effects on neuroimaging and clinical outcome. Pediatr Res 2005; 57(6):873–8. https://doi.org/10.1203/01.PDR.0000157676.45088.8C.
98. Simbruner G, Mittal RA, Rohlmann F, et al. neo.nEURO.network trial participants. Systemic hypothermia after neonatal encephalopathy: outcomes of neo.nEURO.network RCT. Pediatrics 2010;126(4):e771–8. https://doi.org/10.1542/peds.2009-2441.
99. Liow N, Montaldo P, Lally PJ, et al. Preemptive morphine during therapeutic hypothermia after neonatal encephalopathy: a secondary analysis. Ther Hypothermia Temp Manag 2020;10(1):45–52. https://doi.org/10.1089/ther.2018.0052.

100. Gundersen JK, Chakkarapani E, Jary S, et al. Morphine and fentanyl exposure during therapeutic hypothermia does not impair neurodevelopment. EClinical-Medicine 2021.

101. Wassink G, Lear CA, Gunn KC, et al. Analgesics, sedatives, anticonvulsant drugs, and the cooled brain. Semin Fetal Neonatal Med 2015;20(2):109–14. https://doi.org/10.1016/j.siny.2014.10.003.

102. Dean JM, George S, Naylor AS, et al. Partial neuroprotection with low-dose infusion of the alpha2-adrenergic receptor agonist clonidine after severe hypoxia in preterm fetal sheep. Neuropharmacology 2008;55(2):166–74. https://doi.org/10.1016/j.neuropharm.2008.05.009.

103. Dahmani S, Paris A, Jannier V, et al. Dexmedetomidine increases hippocampal phosphorylated extracellular signal-regulated protein kinase 1 and 2 content by an alpha 2-adrenoceptor-independent mechanism: evidence for the involvement of imidazoline I1 receptors. Anesthesiology 2008;108(3):457–66. https://doi.org/10.1097/ALN.0b013e318164ca81.

104. Ma D, Hossain M, Rajakumaraswamy N, et al. Dexmedetomidine produces its neuroprotective effect via the alpha 2A-adrenoceptor subtype. Eur J Pharmacol 2004;502(1–2):87–97. https://doi.org/10.1016/j.ejphar.2004.08.044.

105. Callaway CW, Elmer J, Guyette FX, et al. Dexmedetomidine reduces shivering during mild hypothermia in waking subjects. PLoS One 2015;10(8):e0129709. https://doi.org/10.1371/journal.pone.0129709.

106. O'Mara K, Weiss MD. Dexmedetomidine for sedation of neonates with HIE undergoing therapeutic hypothermia: a single-center experience. AJP Rep 2018; 8(3):e168–73. https://doi.org/10.1055/s-0038-1669938.

107. Cosnahan AS, Angert RM, Jano E, et al. Dexmedetomidine versus intermittent morphine for sedation of neonates with encephalopathy undergoing therapeutic hypothermia. J Perinatol 2021. https://doi.org/10.1038/s41372-021-00998-8.

108. O'Dea M, Sweetman D, Bonifacio SL, et al. Management of multi organ dysfunction in neonatal encephalopathy. Front Pediatr 2020;8:239. https://doi.org/10.3389/fped.2020.00239.

109. Smits A, Annaert P, Van Cruchten S, et al. A physiology-based pharmacokinetic framework to support drug development and dose precision during therapeutic hypothermia in neonates. Front Pharmacol 2020;11:587. https://doi.org/10.3389/fphar.2020.00587.

110. Favie LMA, Groenendaal F, van den Broek MPH, et al. Pharmacokinetics of morphine in encephalopathic neonates treated with therapeutic hypothermia. PLoS One 2019;14(2):e0211910. https://doi.org/10.1371/journal.pone.0211910.

111. Frymoyer A, Bonifacio SL, Drover DR, et al. Decreased morphine clearance in neonates with hypoxic ischemic encephalopathy receiving hypothermia. J Clin Pharmacol 2017;57(1):64–76. https://doi.org/10.1002/jcph.775.

112. Hahn D, Emoto C, Euteneuer JC, et al. Influence of OCT1 ontogeny and genetic variation on morphine disposition in critically ill neonates: lessons from PBPK modeling and clinical study. Clin Pharmacol Ther 2019;105(3):761–8. https://doi.org/10.1002/cpt.1249.

113. Ezzati M, Broad K, Kawano G, et al. Pharmacokinetics of dexmedetomidine combined with therapeutic hypothermia in a piglet asphyxia model. Acta Anaesthesiol Scand 2014;58(6):733–42. https://doi.org/10.1111/aas.12318.

114. McAdams RM, Pak D, Lalovic B, et al. Dexmedetomidine pharmacokinetics in neonates with hypoxic-ischemic encephalopathy receiving hypothermia. Anesthesiol Res Pract 2020;2020:2582965.

Controversies in Fetal Surgery

Prenatal Repair of Myelomeningocele in the Modern Era

John P. Marquart, MD[a], Andrew B. Foy, MD[b],
Amy J. Wagner, MD[c],*

KEYWORDS

- Fetal surgery • Myelomeningocele • Spina bifida • Fetoscopy • Prenatal • Preterm
- Accessibility

KEY POINTS

- Fetal surgery has evolved significantly over the years with advancement in animal models, imaging, and collaborative trials.
- Prenatal surgical intervention for myelomeningocele, a nonlethal congenital anomaly, has proven to be effective; however there remain controversies over patient selection, technique, obstetric outcomes, and accessibility.
- Inclusion and exclusion criteria are slowly being evaluated and adjusted at certain centers for consideration of repair.
- There are a variety of technical approaches for repair with similar results regarding shunting and mortality, but differences in obstetric outcomes.
- The personal and financial burden on families undergoing therapy is significantly relegating care to a group of patients with higher socioeconomic status.

INTRODUCTION

Fetal surgery began to show clinical potential in the 1980s, and since then has evolved into a complex and diverse field.[1,2] Over four decades of progress, the field has shown that the course of congenital diseases can be altered by intervening in the prenatal time period. Today, a variety of procedures exist for treatment of prenatal defects

Disclosure Statement: None.
[a] Children's Wisconsin, 999 North 92nd Street, Suite C320, Milwaukee, WI 53226, USA;
[b] Department of Pediatric Neurosurgery, Children's Wisconsin, 8915 W. Connell Court, Milwaukee, WI 53226, USA; [c] Division of Pediatric Surgery, Children's Wisconsin, 999 North 92nd Street, Suite C320, Milwaukee, WI 53226, USA
* Corresponding author.
E-mail address: awagner@chw.org

Clin Perinatol 49 (2022) 267–277
https://doi.org/10.1016/j.clp.2021.11.015
0095-5108/22/© 2021 Elsevier Inc. All rights reserved.

including genitourinary obstruction, diaphragmatic hernia, sacrococcygeal teratoma, congenital lung lesions, and myelomeningocele (MMC), among others. Although these interventions can greatly improve outcomes, they require careful patient selection and carry significant risk.[3–8]

One of the most common indications for fetal surgery is MMC. MMC is a relatively frequent congenital defect that has shown improvement of postnatal quality-of-life outcomes with fetal surgical intervention.[4] MMC is a severe form of spina bifida with exposed neural tissue that leads to significant neurologic and physical disability. MMC historically was treated with postnatal repair and further management of downstream issues such as hydrocephalus with ventricular shunting. Prenatal surgical repair was established by the Management of Myelomeningocele Study (MOMS) from 2011, which was a large, multicenter, randomized, controlled trial that showed significant improvement for multiple fetal outcomes when compared with postnatal intervention.[5] This improvement in quality of life was an important adjustment in the considerations of maternal–fetal therapy, because previously prenatal interventions were generally reserved for lethal disease processes due to the ethical challenges and trade offs.[9]

Although the current evidence for fetal surgery in MMC favors prenatal surgical care to mitigate life-long morbidity, there continue to be controversies largely in patient selection, obstetric outcomes, technique, and accessibility.[10] This article discusses the history, current management, and controversies surrounding surgical intervention for MMC.

HISTORY OF FETAL SURGERY

Fetal surgery should be considered when multiple specific criteria are met. These criteria include an accurate prenatal diagnosis, a known natural history with severe consequences including the possibility of fetal demise or severe morbidity without intervention, a defect amenable to surgical correction, no other significant fetal defects, and a reasonable risk to benefit ratio for both patients involved.[11] To achieve these requirements with positive results has taken significant effort, time, and innovation.

The development of fetal surgery relied on the advancement of imaging techniques, notably ultrasound assessments, to allow for the accurate prenatal diagnosis of congenital defects. Being able to visualize these malformations has not only allowed for early diagnosis, but also the ability to observe their formation, natural history, and then develop treatment.[1,2,12] Initially starting in the 1920s, plain radiography was used in obstetrics to evaluate osseous structures and gross anomalies, but this was soon found to be harmful to the developing fetus.[13] Although other imaging modalities such as computed tomography scans and MRI have been used, the most important tool has been ultrasound technology. Ultrasound imaging was developed in the 1940s and 1950s into a diagnostic tool, with the first publication presented by Goldberg in the 1960s to measure fetal dimensions.[14] This development progressed through the 1980s to the point of real time continuous imaging, allowing for the further delineation of fetal structures and internal organs. Currently, ultrasound examination has become a routine evaluation for the majority of pregnant women in developed countries, it now has the ability to create 3-dimensional images of a fetal face with surface rendering.[15] All of this advancement in imaging technology has significantly improved the ability to accurately visualize, diagnose, and treat congenital anomalies.

Another critical feature for the advancement of the field has been the creation of animal models of congenital disease and their surgical repair. This process began in the late 1800s with observation of fetal guinea pigs, and progressed through the 1940s with the creation of the lamb fetal model, which Barcroft used to perform surgical experiments.[1] A key step followed in the 1950s through the 1970s when researchers created fetal defects in animals to mimic human disease. Although these studies would eventually lead to surgical interventions, one of the earliest fetal therapies was actually initiated in 1962 when Liley treated hydrops fetalis with fetal blood transfusions.[12,16] This procedure changed the field and showed that prenatal procedures could alter the course of a fatal disease. This procedure initially involved accessing fetal circulation through open uterine incisions.[1] Although this was not largely successful at the time, it paved the way for future work. In the late 1970s at University of California San Francisco (UCSF), there was notable advancement using the fetal lamb model to evaluate various anomalies such as congenital diaphragmatic hernia.[17] One major drawback, however, is that the human uterus is significantly more prone to premature contraction and labor with surgical incisions when compared with sheep animal models. This necessitated the use of the rhesus monkey at both UCSF and University of California Davis to better imitate human fetal surgery. Although extensive animal testing was completed and laboratory studies showed that prenatal intervention could change the course of disease, it was still a leap forward to begin operating on human patients.

The exact beginning of human fetal surgery is difficult to identify, but many consider it to be around 1981 at UCSF when Dr Michael Harrison created a vesicostomy for urinary obstruction with ultrasound guidance.[12] Further work was completed at other centers, and as the field began to grow this prompted collaboration and the creation of the International Fetal Medicine and Surgery Society. Since then, as fetal surgical care has consistently improved, the effectiveness of these interventions and their possible associated adverse effects must be evaluated continually. One important example was congenital diaphragmatic hernia that, despite having a rational anatomic basis for fetal repair, did not initially show benefit from open surgery after rigorous study.[17–19] More recently, benefit has been shown with a fetoscopic tracheal occlusion approach for the most severely affected patients with diaphragmatic hernia.[20] Eventually, the field evolved to fetal intervention for the first-ever indication of improvement of quality of life instead of to improve survival with MMC. The first open repair of MMC was performed in 1997 with promising results.[4]

BACKGROUND OF FETAL SURGERY FOR MYELOMENINGOCELE

MMC, a form of spina bifida, involves failure of the complete closure of the caudal neuropore, leaving exposed neural tissue.[21] It is the most common neural tube defect with an estimated incidence of 3.6 in 10,000 live births in the United States.[21–23] This defect occurs during the fourth week of gestation and can be associated with inadequate maternal folic acid intake. Additional folate supplementation and fortified foods have helped to decrease the incidence, but there continue to be a significant number of cases in the United States. The open spinal defect causes a loss of cerebrospinal fluid and is often associated with hindbrain herniation, the Arnold–Chiari II malformation, and the development of hydrocephalus[10] (Fig. 1). In addition, the already malformed tissue undergoes further damage by open trauma and exposure to amniotic fluid. Although the majority of patients survive to adulthood, they do so with significant impairments requiring ongoing medical treatment at extensive financial costs.[24] These effects commonly includes cognitive defects and bowel and bladder dysfunction, as well as sensorimotor deficits that depend on the level of the lesion.[21]

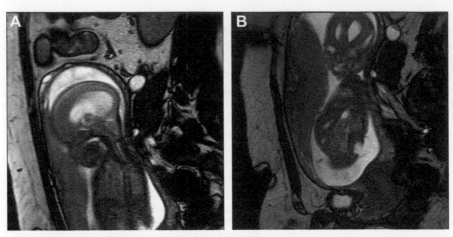

Fig. 1. Hindbrain herniation and fetal ventriculomegaly (*A*). Lumbosacral MMC with sac (*B*).

MMC was originally treated surgically with early repair after birth, largely to mitigate infection.[25,26] Despite this intervention, evidence showed damage had already been done to the exposed neural tissue. Patients were still at high risk of developing hydrocephalus, neurogenic bowel and bladder, and impaired ambulation.[7,21,27] The vast majority of patients also required management of hydrocephalus using a ventriculoperitoneal shunt. The use of shunting brings about its own difficulties, with the need for lifelong monitoring and additional procedures.[26,28] These complications, and the theory regarding progressive in utero damage from the open defect, became the impetus for pursuing prenatal repair. Thus, in the early 1980s Michejda[29] created a primate model of spina bifida by opening the vertebral column and moving the spinal cord in the uterus. Using an animal model, Meuli and colleagues[30] showed that exposure of the normal spinal cord to the intrauterine environment during the latter portion of gestation results in a similar phenotype to that of MMC. There was additional evidence to support prenatal intervention, including ultrasound studies of fetal leg movement decreasing throughout pregnancy, and reports of those patients born before a period of labor having improved neurologic outcomes.[27,31] Progress continued with multiple animal model experiments displaying improved neurologic outcomes with prenatal repair.[32,33] This work was expanded on in the 1990s, attempting human in utero intervention first using the fetoscopic technique.[34] Improved outcomes were noted with adjustment to open fetal repair, which was first completed at the end of the 1990s by groups at Vanderbilt and the Children's Hospital of Philadelphia (CHOP).[2,4,35]

These results and ongoing discussion of the possible benefits of fetal surgery led to the MOMS in the United States.[5] This multicenter randomized controlled trial compared prenatal and postnatal repair at UCSF, CHOP, and Vanderbilt and started in 2003. It had strict inclusion and exclusion criteria notable for no patients with a body mass index (BMI) of greater than 35, no additional anomalies, and all families in the prenatal intervention arm were required to remain nearby the fetal surgery center with a support person. Patients randomized to fetal surgery underwent in utero repair between 19.0 and 25.9 weeks of gestation, and then scheduled for planned cesarean section at 37 weeks if they did not have preterm labor prior. One notable feature of the study design was there was no back door opportunity for patients to undergo fetal surgery for MMC during the study period. All patients in the United States who were interested in fetal surgery for MMC had to do so through the trial at 1 of the 3 centers in the country.

The study extended over the majority of a decade to enroll enough patients. This commitment paid off; in utero intervention showed such success that the data safety monitoring board halted the trial in 2010 owing to the mounting evidence. The most notable differences were the decreased need for shunt placement at 40% in the pre-natal group versus 82% for postnatal, decreased hindbrain herniation from 96% to 64%, along with improved motor function and independent ambulation among the fetal surgery cohort (**Fig. 2**). Additional data obtained during long-term follow-up shows continued improvement in neurologic outcomes, with a large portion of patients able to ambulate and perform daily activities at a median age of 10 years.[36] There is ongoing research and some preliminary data on other important measures such as bowel and bladder function.

Despite the success that the MOMS trial showed with prenatal intervention, one must consider the fact that fetal surgery involves 2 patients with inherent risks to both the mother and child. Additionally, although MMC causes significant disability, it is not considered a lethal anomaly. Many of these risks increased significantly in the prenatal repair group including placental abruption, preterm birth (38% prenatal vs 14% post), premature rupture of membranes (46% vs 8%), oligohydramnios (21% vs 4%), chorioamniotic membrane separation (26% vs 0), and dehiscence of the hysterotomy closure (9%).[6,24] These potential risks must be clearly explained, and then weighed by both the patient and clinicians when proceeding with fetal intervention.

MODERN TREATMENT CONTROVERSIES

Because the MOMS trial displayed a clear improvement in outcomes with prenatal surgical intervention, this treatment has become standard, available to many patients with MMC diagnosed prenatally.[37] One controversy involves patient selection; the original MOMS trial had strict inclusion and exclusion criteria that excluded many pa-tients. Elucidating whether safe expansion of these parameters is possible is an impor-tant aspect to appropriate care of all patients with MMC.

One of the most common reasons for not meeting inclusion criteria for fetal interven-tion for MMC is maternal obesity. Obesity is known to complicate a normal pregnancy and adds risk to many adult operations, not to mention its challenges to prenatal

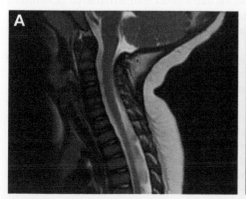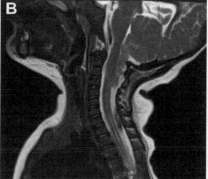

Fig. 2. Reversal of hindbrain herniation in fetal surgery patient (*A*) versus postnatal surgery patient (*B*).

surgical intervention. As obesity rates continue to increase, a recent study—the MOMS Plus trial—specifically evaluated prenatal surgery in patients with a higher BMI.[38] This retrospective review included patients treated from 2013 to 2016 at the University of Colorado with prenatal surgery. Complete data were obtained for 47 patients, including 11 with a BMI between 36 and 40, with follow-up at 1 year. In the higher BMI group, they found similar rates of shunting, but noted an earlier average delivery date by approximately 2 weeks when compared with the prenatal MOMS cohort. Overall, it is difficult to draw major conclusions from such a small patient population, but there were no obvious serious complications from expanded BMI criteria. Other exclusion criteria now being reconsidered include additional maternal comorbidities such as type 1 diabetes, prior preterm delivery, and chronic viral infections such as HIV or hepatitis C. Only a limited number of centers reportedly offer prenatal treatment in these conditions.[39]

An additional important consideration is the exclusion of patients with other fetal anomalies not related to MMC. Modern technology for noninvasive prenatal testing has shown continued promise and expansion of use.[40] Previously, karyotyping was the gold standard to diagnose chromosomal abnormalities, but recently this practice has shifted to chromosomal microarray analysis. Currently, these techniques are consistent for the major trisomies, but an ongoing question remains the clinical importance of various other abnormalities found in sequencing. These include copy number variants, which may be pathogenic, as well as variants of unknown significance. Santirocco and colleagues[41] specifically studied this testing in fetuses with central nervous system anomalies. Their rate of pathogenic copy number variants was 6.7%, but they also had 7.6% for variants of unknown significance. This information has not yet been investigated thoroughly to know if it changes the risk or outcome after fetal intervention. Additionally, this process requires careful interpretation and explanation, because abnormal results can cause serious psychological distress for families.[42] In a 2016 survey of 17 principle investigators from the Fetal Myelomeningocele consortium, 8 of the 11 responders require DNA microarray during diagnostic testing.[39] The implications of these unclear results in array testing warrant further study.

Another controversy has been the best technical approach in fetal MMC repair, namely, open versus fetoscopic. As mentioned elsewhere in this article, the MOMS trial was exclusively performed with open repair (**Fig. 3**). Despite this factor, multiple centers have recently moved to offering a minimally invasive version. This practice theoretically may decrease the complications associated with a maternal laparotomy and hysterotomy.[43–45] However, this approach can also make it difficult to achieve an adequate repair of the fetal defect and some studies have shown additional complications.[46,47]

It has been challenging to assess these 2 techniques; there are no randomized controlled trials directly comparing them. Additionally, there is a variability of technique within each method.[43,47–50] For example, how the uterus is accessed fetoscopically differs between surgeons and centers, with some using a completely percutaneous approach, whereas others perform a maternal laparotomy and then place uterine ports. Additionally, some fetoscopic repairs use a patch closure of varying materials, and others do primary closure (**Fig. 4**).

A recent meta-analysis by Kabagambe and colleagues[47] attempted to compare the modern versions of the 2 techniques by reviewing literature since the publication of the MOMS trial. They evaluated 11 studies looking at a variety of outcomes and notably found that percutaneous fetoscopic repair was associated with higher rates of premature rupture of membranes and preterm birth when compared with open repair. They

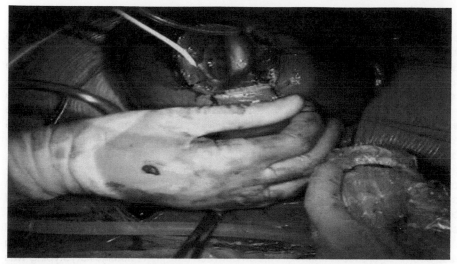

Fig. 3. Open fetal surgery for MMC.

did note that fetoscopic repair by way of maternal laparotomy decreased preterm birth compared with open repair. However, both fetoscopic procedures had increased rates of dehiscence and cerebrospinal fluid leaking from the surgical site, often requiring postnatal revision. Open repair had a significantly higher number of uterine dehiscences. The authors pointed out that some of the selected studies were lacking complete data and that long-term results are not available for many of the fetoscopic studies. Overall, both methods have similar results in terms of mortality and need for shunting. The fetoscopic technique seems to be in evolution still. Additionally, the specific method of closure can vary further, as Belfort and associates[51] showed by comparing single versus 3 layer repair. They found that a 3-layer closure decreased he rates of cerebrospinal fluid leakage and improved hindbrain herniation compared with a single-layer repair. This decision did not impact the larger concerns of shunt placement or mortality. The broad array of techniques in prenatal repair are still under investigation, and the variety makes it difficult to compare results between institutions with different approaches.

An important point of consideration with all of the controversies regarding prenatal surgery is who benefits from the operation and how accessible is the intervention to the general population? When looking at large tertiary care settings, only about one-third of annual cases are eligible for surgery, with an even smaller number following through with intervention.[52] The original MOMS study required patients and their families to move and stay near the hospital. Although this is not a specific requirement for

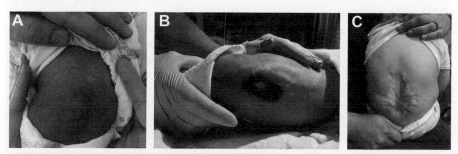

Fig. 4. Primary repair (*A*) versus AlloDerm patch closure (*B,C*).

ongoing centers, families often still have to travel far from home for treatment. For instance, after fetal therapy for MMC patients treated at CHOP may continue to receive care and deliver with their original referring providers. However, 90% of those families chose to deliver at CHOP, incurring any additional expense or travel that was required.[53]

As Alrefai and colleagues[52] noted at the University of Toronto, there was a clear differential in whether patients who were eligible for surgery actually followed through based on referral location. For those who were local, those eligible chose surgery 75% of the time, but this number drastically decreased to 18% if it was a cross-border patient. The limitations of access to fetal care cause an unintended consequence of relegating the possibility of fetal care to only those who either happen to live in urban locations with a fetal center, or those with significant resources (both financial and personal) to have the option of relocating temporarily. This situation creates a cohort of patients that tend to be Caucasian, well-educated, and of significant financial means.[52]

In addition to the challenges in accessibility of fetal surgery to patients, there has also been a difference in financial burden between fetal intervention and postnatal surgery. Riddle and colleagues[54] performed a retrospective study to evaluate the difference in morbidity and cost associated with prenatal versus postnatal repair. They noted significant increases in the rates of morbidity associated with prematurity for the fetal surgery group, which was also correlated with higher financial costs in the first year of life. Although the overall costs may tip in favor of fetal surgery when considering the long-term disability of MMC repaired after birth, these data are important because they present additional evidence of the burden families undertake when pursuing fetal surgical intervention.

There is limited direct evidence of socioeconomic disparities in regard to prenatal surgical care for MMC, but a noticeable difference is seen when comparing the demographics of patients who participated in the major studies relative to historical data for children born with spina bifida. The MOMS trial, for instance, had more than 90% of maternal race categorized as White, whereas Radcliff and coworkers[55] previously found closer to 50% for mothers of infants born with spina bifida in Florida reported as White. There may be geographic differences, but they additionally showed that one-half of those infants born had a public payer source. One can imagine how difficult this would be for families likely on public insurance to undertake the required travel, additional testing, and hospital visits associated with fetal surgery.

There is little doubt as to the obvious benefits derived from prenatal surgical intervention for MMC, and fetal surgery has become an accepted treatment for a disease to improve quality of life instead of survival. There remain areas of controversy that require ongoing investigation and efforts to improve care for all patients.

CLINICS CARE POINTS

- For patients who qualify, prenatal surgery for MMC has proven to be effective.
- The inclusion and exclusion criteria based on the MOMS trial is being slowly evaluated and expanded as able.
- There is no clear consensus yet on the best technical approach for prenatal surgery for MMC; each method seems to have trade-offs regarding outcomes from the current data.
- Evidence shows that prenatal repair tends to be for patients of higher socioeconomic backgrounds, likely based on the personal and financial requirements for treatment.

REFERENCES

1. Jancelewicz T, Harrison MR. A history of fetal surgery. Clin Perinatol 2009;36(2): 227–36, vii. (In eng).
2. Kitagawa H, Pringle KC. Fetal surgery: a critical review. Pediatr Surg Int 2017; 33(4):421–33.
3. Baumgarten HD, Flake AW. Fetal surgery. Pediatr Clin North Am 2019;66(2): 295–308 (In eng).
4. Adzick NS, Sutton LN, Crombleholme TM, et al. Successful fetal surgery for spina bifida. Lancet 1998;352(9141):1675–6.
5. Adzick NS, Thom EA, Spong CY, et al. A randomized trial of prenatal versus post-natal repair of myelomeningocele. N Engl J Med 2011;364(11):993–1004.
6. Winder FM, Vonzun L, Meuli M, et al. Maternal complications following open fetal myelomeningocele repair at the Zurich center for fetal diagnosis and therapy. Fetal Diagn Ther 2019;46(3):153–8 (In eng).
7. Licci M, Guzman R, Soleman J. Maternal and obstetric complications in fetal sur-gery for prenatal myelomeningocele repair: a systematic review. Neurosurg Focus 2019;47(4):E11 (In eng).
8. Kahr MK, Winder FM, Vonzun L, et al. Open intrauterine fetal myelomeningocele repair: changes in the surgical procedure and perinatal complications during the first 8 years of experience at a single center. Fetal Diagn Ther 2020;47(6):485–90 (In eng).
9. Flake AW. Prenatal intervention: ethical considerations for life-threatening and non-life-threatening anomalies. Semin Pediatr Surg 2001;10(4):212–21.
10. Elbabaa SK, Gildehaus AM, Pierson MJ, et al. First 60 fetal in-utero myelomenin-gocele repairs at Saint Louis Fetal Care Institute in the post-MOMS trial era: hy-drocephalus treatment outcomes (endoscopic third ventriculostomy versus ventriculo-peritoneal shunt). Childs Nerv Syst 2017;33(7):1157–68 (In eng).
11. Partridge EA, Flake AW. Maternal–fetal surgery for structural malformations. Best Pract Res Clin Obstet Gynaecol 2012;26:669–82.
12. Moise KJ Jr. The history of fetal therapy. Am J Perinatol 2014;31(7):557–66 (In eng).
13. Benson CB, Doubilet PM. The history of imaging in obstetrics. Radiology 2014; 273(2 Suppl):S92–110 (In eng).
14. Goldberg BB. Obstetric US imaging: the past 40 years. Radiology 2000;215(3): 622–9.
15. Newman PG, Rozycki GS. The history of ultrasound. Surg Clin North Am 1998; 78(2):179–95 (In eng).
16. Liley AW. Diagnosis and treatment of erythroblastosis in the fetus. Adv Pediatr 1968;15:29–63 (In eng).
17. Pringle KC, Turner JW, Schofield JC, et al. Creation and repair of diaphragmatic hernia in the fetal lamb: lung development and morphology. J Pediatr Surg 1984; 19(2):131–40 (In eng).
18. Harrison MR, Adzick NS, Bullard KM, et al. Correction of congenital diaphrag-matic hernia in utero VII: a prospective trial. J Pediatr Surg 1997;32(11): 1637–42 (In eng).
19. Grivell RM, Andersen C, Dodd JM. Prenatal interventions for congenital diaphrag-matic hernia for improving outcomes. Cochrane Database Syst Rev 2015;11: Cd008925 (In eng).
20. Cole FS. Fetal tracheal occlusion for congenital diaphragmatic hernia. N Engl J Med 2021. https://doi.org/10.1056/nejme2107446.

21. Copp AJ, Adzick NS, Chitty LS, et al. Spina bifida. Nat Rev Dis Primers 2015;1(1): 15007.
22. Mai CT, Isenburg JL, Canfield MA, et al. National population-based estimates for major birth defects, 2010-2014. Birth Defects Res 2019;111(18):1420–35 (In eng).
23. Parker SE, Mai CT, Canfield MA, et al. Updated National Birth Prevalence estimates for selected birth defects in the United States, 2004-2006. Birth Defects Res A Clin Mol Teratol 2010;88(12):1008–16 (In eng).
24. Moldenhauer JS, Flake AW. Open fetal surgery for neural tube defects. Best Pract Res Clin Obstet Gynaecol 2019;58:121–32.
25. Attenello FJ, Tuchman A, Christian EA, et al. Infection rate correlated with time to repair of open neural tube defects (myelomeningoceles): an institutional and national study. Child's Nervous Syst 2016;32(9):1675–81.
26. Cherian J, Staggers KA, Pan IW, et al. Thirty-day outcomes after postnatal myelomeningocele repair: a National Surgical Quality Improvement Program Pediatric database analysis. J Neurosurg Pediatr 2016;18(4):416–22.
27. Adzick NS. Fetal surgery for spina bifida: past, present, future. Semin Pediatr Surg 2013;22(1):10–7 (In eng).
28. Radmanesh F, Nejat F, Khashab ME, et al. Shunt complications in children with myelomeningocele: effect of timing of shunt placement. J Neurosurg Pediatr 2009;3(6):516–20.
29. Michejda M. Intrauterine treatment of spina bifida: primate model. Z Kinderchir 1984;39(4):259–61 (In eng).
30. Meuli M, Meuli-Simmen C, Yingling CD, et al. Creation of myelomeningocele in utero: a model of functional damage from spinal cord exposure in fetal sheep. J Pediatr Surg 1995;30(7):1028–32 ; discussion 1032-3. (In eng).
31. Yamashiro KJ, Galganski LA, Hirose S. Fetal myelomeningocele repair. Semin Pediatr Surg 2019;28(4):150823 (In eng).
32. Meuli M, Meuli-Simmen C, Yingling CD, et al. In utero repair of experimental myelomeningocele saves neurological function at birth. J Pediatr Surg 1996;31(3): 397–402 (In eng).
33. Bouchard S, Davey MG, Rintoul NE, et al. Correction of hindbrain herniation and anatomy of the vermis after in utero repair of myelomeningocele in sheep. J Pediatr Surg 2003;38(3):451–8, discussion 451-8. (In eng).
34. Bruner JP, Tulipan NE, Richards WO. Endoscopic coverage of fetal open myelomeningocele in utero. Am J Obstet Gynecol 1997;176(1 Pt 1):256–7 (In eng).
35. Tulipan N, Bruner JP. Myelomeningocele repair in utero: a report of three cases. Pediatr Neurosurg 1998;28(4):177–80.
36. Danzer E, Thomas NH, Thomas A, et al. Long-term neurofunctional outcome, executive functioning, and behavioral adaptive skills following fetal myelomeningocele surgery. Am J Obstet Gynecol 2016;214(2):269.e1–8.
37. Mazzola CA, Assassi N, Baird LC, et al. Congress of neurological surgeons systematic review and evidence-based guidelines for pediatric myelomeningocele: executive summary. Neurosurgery 2019;85(3):299–301.
38. Hilton SA, Hodges MM, Dewberry LC, et al. MOMS Plus: single-institution review of outcomes for extended BMI criteria for open fetal repair of myelomeningocele. Fetal Diagn Ther 2019;46(6):411–4 (In eng).
39. Moise KJ Jr, Moldenhauer JS, Bennett KA, et al. Current selection criteria and perioperative therapy used for fetal myelomeningocele surgery. Obstet Gynecol 2016;127(3):593–7 (In eng).

40. Sabbagh R, Van den Veyver IB. The current and future impact of genome-wide sequencing on fetal precision medicine. Hum Genet 2020;139(9):1121–30 (In eng).
41. Santirocco M, Plaja A, Rodó C, et al. Chromosomal microarray analysis in fetuses with central nervous system anomalies: an 8-year long observational study from a tertiary care university hospital. Prenatal Diagn 2021;41(1):123–35.
42. Bernhardt BA, Soucier D, Hanson K, et al. Women's experiences receiving abnormal prenatal chromosomal microarray testing results. Genet Med 2013; 15(2):139–45.
43. Kohl T. Percutaneous minimally invasive fetoscopic surgery for spina bifida aperta. Part I: surgical technique and perioperative outcome. Ultrasound Obstet Gynecol 2014;44(5):515–24 (In eng).
44. Kohl T. Impact of partial amniotic carbon dioxide insufflation (PACI) on middle cerebral artery blood flow in mid-gestation human fetuses undergoing fetoscopic surgery for spina bifida aperta. Ultrasound Obstet Gynecol 2016;47(4):521–2 (In eng).
45. Kohl T. Minimally invasive fetoscopic surgery for spina bifida aperta: learning and doing. Ultrasound Obstet Gynecol 2020;56(4):633 (In eng).
46. Sanz Cortes M, Chmait RH, Lapa DA, et al. Experience of 300 cases of prenatal fetoscopic open spina bifida repair: report of the International Fetoscopic Neural Tube Defect Repair Consortium. Am J Obstet Gynecol 2021. https://doi.org/10.1016/j.ajog.2021.05.044 (In eng).
47. Kabagambe SK, Jensen GW, Chen YJ, et al. Fetal surgery for myelomeningocele: a systematic review and meta-analysis of outcomes in fetoscopic versus open repair. Fetal Diagn Ther 2018;43(3):161–74 (In eng).
48. Degenhardt J, Schürg R, Winarno A, et al. Percutaneous minimal-access fetoscopic surgery for spina bifida aperta. Part II: maternal management and outcome. Ultrasound Obstet Gynecol 2014;44(5):525–31 (In eng).
49. Belfort MA, Whitehead WE, Shamshirsaz AA, et al. Fetoscopic repair of meningomyelocele. Obstet Gynecol 2015;126(4):881–4 (In eng).
50. Sanz Cortes M, Lapa DA, Acacio GL, et al. Proceedings of the first annual meeting of the International Fetoscopic Myelomeningocele Repair Consortium. Ultrasound Obstet Gynecol 2019;53(6):855–63.
51. Belfort MA, Whitehead WE, Shamshirsaz AA, et al. Comparison of two fetoscopic open neural tube defect repair techniques: single- vs three-layer closure. Ultrasound Obstet Gynecol 2020;56(4):532–40 (In eng).
52. Alrefai A, Drake J, Kulkarni AV, et al. Fetal myelomeningocele surgery: only treating the tip of the iceberg. Prenatal Diagn 2018. https://doi.org/10.1002/pd.5390.
53. Moldenhauer JS, Adzick NS. Fetal surgery for myelomeningocele: after the Management of Myelomeningocele Study (MOMS). Semin Fetal Neonatal Med 2017; 22(6):360–6 (In eng).
54. Riddle S, Huddle R, Lim F-Y, et al. Morbidity and cost burden of prenatal myelomeningocele repair. J Maternal-Fetal Neonatal Med 2021;34(10):1651–7.
55. Radcliff E, Cassell CH, Tanner JP, et al. Hospital use, associated costs, and payer status for infants born with spina bifida. Birth Defects Res A Clin Mol Teratol 2012; 94(12):1044–53 (In eng).

New Horizons in Mild Hypoxic-ischemic Encephalopathy: A Standardized Algorithm to Move past Conundrum of Care

Lina Chalak, MD, MSCS

KEYWORDS

- Mild HIE • Bayley • Therapeutic hypothermia

KEY POINTS

- Preclinical and observational data suggest that therapeutic hypothermia improves outcomes in mild HIE, though these infants were not studied in RCT trials.
- There is a loss of clinical equipoise regarding treatment in mild HIE despite insufficient risk–benefit information on vulnerable subgroups to benefit from treatment.
- Reasons for the loss of equipoise regarding treatment include overlapping definitions in the first 6 hours, the narrow therapeutic window for hypothermia, fear of litigations, and misclassifications due to the dynamic nature of the neonatal encephalopathy.
- It is important to standardize the definition and etiology of encephalopathy to confirm mild HIE and exclude other etiologies. We provide a detailed algorithm of care perform that includes serial examinations, Sarnat scoring, and a trajectory of outcomes.

INTRODUCTION AND SCOPE OF THE PROBLEM

Worldwide, hypoxic-ischemic encephalopathy (HIE) affects 2 million infants annually[1]; it presents clinically as neonatal encephalopathy(NE) is difficult to classify immediately after birth[2] leading to a global burden of 50.2 million disability-adjusted life years.[2] Although over half of infants with HIE present within a mild spectrum, past clinical trials have focused exclusively on moderately and severely affected infants.[3–7] This was understandable initially at that time when the safety profile of interventions was largely unknown.[8,9]

The establishment of hypothermia for moderate and severe HIE leads to a decrease of death and disability at 2 years from 45% to 29% as recently demonstrated in contemporary studies.[10,11] In contrast to such improvements, recent data in untreated

Funding: Dr Lina Chalak is funded by NIH Grant 5R01NS102617.
Neonatal-Perinatal Medicine, University of Texas Southwestern Medical School, 5323 Harry Hines Boulevard, Dallas, TX 75390-9063, USA
E-mail address: Lina.Chalak@utsouthwestern.edu

Clin Perinatol 49 (2022) 279–294
https://doi.org/10.1016/j.clp.2021.11.016
0095-5108/22/© 2021 Elsevier Inc. All rights reserved.

infants with "mild" HIE show a higher range of abnormal neurologic outcomes at 12 to 24 months through school age.[12–16] There is now compelling evidence that untreated neonates with mild HIE are at significant risk for adverse outcomes.[16–18] This resulted in a therapeutic drift such that presently, half of all US hospitals offer TH for mild HIE, with the remainder providing normothermia. This assumption of benefit has reduced equipoise for enrollment in randomized trials despite the lack of evidence to support the effectiveness or safety of TH in this unstudied, vulnerable patient population. Still, there are several risks to TH and these collectively may offset the potential benefits for mild HIE. These can include potential severe adverse events (bradycardia, thrombocytopenia, coagulopathy), as well as stress, pain, disrupted maternal-infant bonding, decreased breastfeeding, and prolonged length of stay.[10,19] Most concerning, preclinical studies have shown that TH is harmful to uninjured animals (sham controls), leading to neuronal injury/loss suggesting that caution is warranted when this is applied to infants with no brain injury.[20]

The conundrum of so-called "mild HIE" is rooted in the need to define severity within the therapeutic window of 6 hours, despite the evolving nature of neonatal encephalopathy in the first week after birth and heterogeneity in the timing of the insult

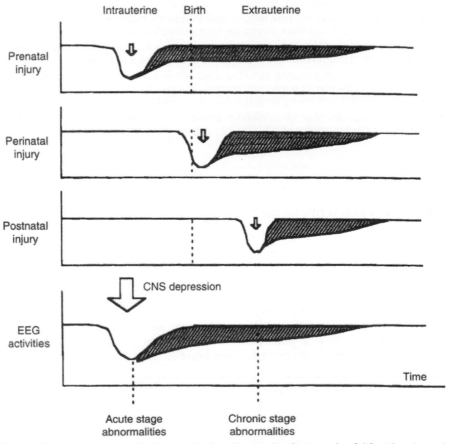

Fig. 1. Clinical evolution of the encephalopathy in the first week of life. The dynamic evolving nature of neonatal encephalopathy is illustrated, showing how the timing of the insult affects the initial presentation after birth. Examples of pre, peri, and postnatal insults, as well as the associated EEG manifestations, are highlighted.

(Fig. 1).[21] The research gap in mild HIE is compounded by both the dynamic evolution and overlap between mild and moderate asphyxia in the first hours of life, as well as a lack of a clear and consistent definition for what constitutes mild NE in the first 6 hours of life whereby decisions regarding therapies are made.[18] Notably, the modified Sarnat Exam—the gold standard for staging HIE—did not distinguish between mild and normal status on the examination form for decades.[22,23]

The PRIME (Prospective Research in Mild HIE), an international multicenter observational cohort (NCT01747863) at 6 academic centers[24] provided the first empirically validated definition of mild HIE within 6 hours using 2 steps, as in prior cooling trials: first step screening for fetal acidosis and acute perinatal events per NICHD criteria; the second step is a certified examiner performing a modified Sarnat scoring which was expanded to include mild in addition to the moderate and severe abnormalities (Figs. 2 and 3). PRIME showed that a substantial proportion of infants with this definition of mild HIE have abnormal outcomes when not treated with hypothermia. Specifically, 41% had abnormal neurologic findings at discharge, while 16% were diagnosed with disability using established NICHD criteria and 40% had delays in cognitive and language development (<85 Bayley Scales of Infant Development [Bayley]-3at 18 to 22 months).

There is strong biological plausibility and preclinical evidence supporting the efficacy of hypothermia but there is a lack of comparative clinical data for mild HIE to establish the risk–benefit of therapeutic hypothermia (TH) in mild HIE. Now that the PRIME definition has been established and validated in multiple studies,[15,25,26] the first part of the conundrum related to definitions is resolved. This review will summarize (1) evidence that neonates with mild HIE are at risk for adverse outcomes, (2) controversies regarding management, and (3) provide an algorithm of clinical care after birth to close the knowledge gaps regarding the management of mild HIE (as formulated for the COOL PRIME comparative effectiveness trial).

CUMULATIVE EVIDENCE SUGGESTS THAT MILD HIE IS NOT SO "MILD"
There is compelling evidence that neonates with mild HIE are at significant risk for adverse outcomes supporting a strong rationale for neuroprotective therapies for this population

Preclinical data support an association of TH with improved neuroprotection after a mild HIE insult.[27] New clinical studies demonstrate clearly abnormal neurologic

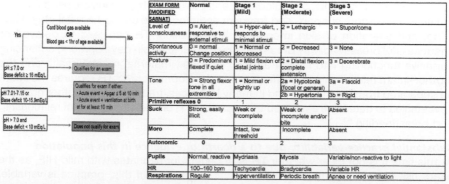

Fig. 2. The examination form for neonatal encephalopathy. PRIME definition of mild HIE requires ≥ 2 abnormal categories in mild but NOT greater than 3 moderate or severe findings.

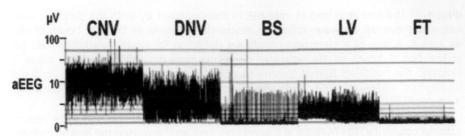

Fig. 3. Amplitude EEG patterns. Patterns are highlighted with pattern classification (CNV: continuous normal voltage, DNV: discontinuous normal voltage, BS: burst suppression, LV: low voltage, FT: flat tracings). Any tracing showing BS, LV, or FT represents exclusion criteria for the definition of mild HIE.

outcomes in mild HIE.[16–18,28–31] Recent systematic reviews report disabilities during infancy or childhood in 25% of infants with mild HIE.[12,16] However, the only clinical comparative data available are derived from a meta-analysis of mild HIE infants who were inadvertently enrolled in prior RCTs and included in the intent to treat analyses. These pooled data (n = 91) albeit not powered and lacking a definition for mild HIE, trended toward a reduction in the rate of disability among infants who received TH (29%) compared with normothermia (NT) (37%; OR: 0.67; 95% CI: 0.28–1.61, P = .59).[12,16] The NICHD NRN late hypothermia study[32,33] established that cooling could be initiated between 6 to 24 hours but that late TH initiation after 6 hours postnatal was less effective with a small benefit effect of only 2% (Bayesian analysis showed a 76% probability of reduction in death/disability). Encouragingly, recent data from the MARBLE (magnetic resonance biomarkers in neonatal encephalopathy) study suggests that infants with mild HIE who received TH within 6 hours have less white matter injury and improved MR Spectroscopy (MRS), compared with untreated.[34]

CURRENT MANAGEMENT OF MILD HYPOXIC-ISCHEMIC ENCEPHALOPATHY PARADIGMS AND LIMITATIONS
Although TH is relatively safe it is not without risks

TH safety has been well studied in moderate and severe HIE.[4–11] Pooled data from all RCTs also show that risks associated with TH include bradycardia, decreased cardiac output, thrombocytopenia, coagulopathy, and pulmonary hypertension, need for central lines, respiratory support, and frequent sedation[19] prolonged hospital stay, shivering, and alteration of skin integrity.[10,19] In addition, TH can lead to delayed or unsuccessful breastfeeding.[5] Breast milk is optimal for brain development, enhancing cognitive functioning into school age.[35–37] Further, maternal mental health and the mother–infant relationship also affects infant development.[38–40] TH requires the infant be separated from the mother, and in many instances, transferred to another hospital. Few studies to date have assessed the impact of TH on the mother–infant relationship and breastfeeding.[41]

Substantial practice variability due to a dearth of evidence in this population
At this time it is not clear whether TH is of benefit for neonates with mild HIE, as the exact risk–benefit ratio is not known.[20,30,42] In the face of this, practice is variable, with some opting for hypothermia, and others normothermia. There is a widespread therapeutic drift in 50% of US institutions toward using TH in Mild HIE despite the

absence of clinical effectiveness studies.[43] A drift toward cooling in mild HIE is also internationally rampant as reported in 61% of UK institutions.[44]

Limitations of existing registries

Current data, including clinical registries, summarize the rampant use of early TH for mild HIE but do not describe outcomes past hospital discharge in TH treated infants.[31] Data from the Vermont Oxford Network (VON) Neonatal Encephalopathy Registry from 99 centers reveals that 40% of infants receiving TH have mild HIE.[45] The state of California reported the use of TH in 50% of mild HIE using the California Perinatal Quality Care Collaborative datasets.[46] The Children's Hospital Neonatal Consortium registry from 27 NICUs in the United States reports abnormal short-term outcomes in mild HIE with TH but provides no comparison to noncooled infants.[47] A single site retrospective small study reported that infants with mild HIE who underwent TH had similar outcomes to case-matched normal controls.[48] Overall there are no prior data comparing longitudinal outcomes in a large, multicenter cohort with mild HIE with/without TH.

TIME TO SEEK NONTRADITIONAL DESIGNS TO END THIS CONUNDRUM

The fundamental question of how to optimally manage mild HIE after birth remains unanswered. In 2018, the Neonatal Neurocritical Care Special Interest Group first summarized the critical knowledge gaps in evidence to support TH in mild HIE.[30] There is definitive agreement among experts that studies assessing the efficacy of TH in mild HIE are necessary. Yet dismantling of equipoise through the implementation of TH without scientific evidence Is worsening each year.[1,11,30,43,49,50] While this has been a topic of yearly panels,[11] commentaries and opinions,[30,49,50] no new RCT data have emerged to support or refute treatment. The therapeutic drift is rendering a multicenter neonatal RCT for mild HIE challenging to perform but traditionalists are struggling to accept the loss of equipoise in real life. Camps are divided into those who have persisted in the traditional approach of aiming for an ideal RCT[50] and those that adapted into the necessity of a pragmatic approach to find the best evidence in the real-world setting.[51]

We recently conducted a large international Physicians survey (n = 487) involving 50 countries that used 2 cases descriptions demonstrating that 57% of participants cool mild HIE in their site practice.[52]

We also conducted an interactive poll with cases of mild HIE on a forum of Newborn Brain Society (NBS, March 2021) with 400 participating members whereby 70% of responders confirmed the TH practice for mild HIE.

We also recently conducted a parental focus survey that recruited parents of children with mild HIE via Hope for HIE Foundation (**Fig. 4**). Results showed that 87% of parents preferred a nonrandomized real-world study design whereby neonatologists choose treatment of mild HIE. Further, because the definitions overlap between mild and moderate asphyxia in the first hours of life whereby decisions regarding therapies are made, it might not be ethically acceptable to withhold a treatment if this is offered as a site standard practice.

In neonatal RCTs, lack of equipoise for randomization of fragile newborns has resulted in nonparticipation, enrollment bias, and has threatened the external validity of findings, leading to higher budgets, early terminations, and squandering of resources.[26,53–58] Prior attempts to randomize in neonatal studies as for example, Prophylactic Phenobarbital Neonatal Seizures (PROPHENO) RCT have been met with challenges related to equipoise that lead to termination after failure to enroll. A recent large CER study[58] was subsequently completed to establish the safety of early

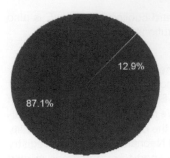

● Comparative effectiveness study
(Consent is required at time of injury,
there is no double-blind/placebo. All who
opt-in receive treatment).

● Randomized trial (Consent is required,
but your child may or may not receive
the therapeutic intervention).

Fig. 4. Standardized algorithm for Mild HIE. Screening, testing, and trajectory of outcomes are highlighted to provide a correct classification and facilitate early referrals.

discontinuation of antiseizure medications before hospital discharge in neonates with acute symptomatic seizures.

Collectively, the data presented suggest that at present, an RCT design in the United States to study TH for mild HIE is likely not feasible, due to increasing drift in practice, loss of equipoise, ethical concerns, physician bias, and a low rate of parental consent.[59] A newly proposed Comparative Effectiveness Study for Mild HIE (COOL-PRIME)- ClinicalTrials.gov Identifier: NCT04621279 is being proposed that promises to systematically address the knowledge gap and resolve the disjunction between the evolving clinical practice and the limited scientific basis for TH in mild HIE, by leveraging practice variation across sites to provide an accurate estimate treatment effects and associated risk. Below is the proposed algorithm of care for COOL PRIME.

ALGORITHM OF CARE

A Standardized algorithm (**Fig. 5**) is suggested to mitigate the current heterogeneity of care (see **Fig. 3**). This is recommended irrespective of the decisions to provide normothermia or hypothermia to infants with mild HIE.[30,34,43,52,60–88]

Examination

The dynamic evolution in neurologic examination findings coupled with the need to initiate therapeutic hypothermia within the first 6 hours of life presents challenges in using clinical examination to identify newborns with mild HIE for clinical trials. Thus, the PRIME examination form is recommended with serial examinations using the Total Sarnat Score (TSS)

- **Epic automated entry to trigger completion of the enhanced infant neurologic exam**. Any patient with a base deficit greater than 10 on blood gas EPIC system prompts the Pediatrician to do an enhanced neuro examination and contact cooling center.
- **Certification of examiners on Sarnat and mild HIE diagnosis with PRIME criteria**. To maintain skills, annual teaching and testing should be done and include video filming for surveillance.
- **Serial examinations are recommended with a threshold effect for decision making**. For example, if an infant has at any point in time 3 abnormalities in the moderate or severe categories or has seizures then the infant need to be reclassified as moderate or severe and treatment initiated accordingly, even if a subsequent examination shows improvements.

Mild HIE Algorithm

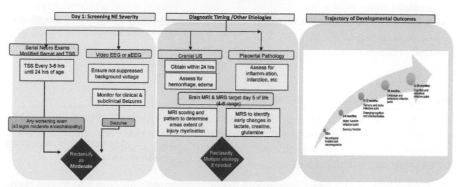

Fig. 5. Survey of parental mild HIE focus group. Parents of infants with mild HIE (n = 31) were queried via Hope for HIE Foundation regarding preferences for study designs.

- **Total Sarnat Score (TSS)** as in **Fig. 2** is recommended to allow the representation of the encephalopathy burden, by accounting for the number and the severity in each function and has been associated with disability at 2 years.[89]

Neurophysiology studies (EEG/aEEG)

Infants with mild HIE can have mild aEEG/EEG discontinuity/asymmetry or poor sleep–wake cycling[90–92] which can be associated with abnormal outcomes.[28] Infants with mild HIE also show discreet abnormalities consisting of incomplete SWC, intermittent discontinuity, diffuse slow wave activity, or excessive sharp/transient waves.[93] Further, besides the subtle qualitative EEG abnormalities, we and others identified other noninvasive quantification of EEG metrics that are distinctive in mild HIE.[94–96]

- *EEG:* Even in the absence of obvious seizures, a 24 hour EEG recording is recommended and in cooled infants 72 hours is optimal to cover the duration of hypothermia.
- *Amplitude EEG:* this is a good option if EEG is not available. A cerebral function monitor via a single channel EEG (aEEG) records activity from biparietal electrodes. The signal is smoothed and the amplitude integrated and shows the baseline background electrical activity. Visual analysis can exclude suppressed patterns[97] and seizures that point to moderate/severe encephalopathy (**Fig. 5**).

Neuroimaging

MRI and MRS biomarkers provide a quantitative measurement of brain injury and treatment response and are validated predictors of death and/or neurodevelopmental impairment.[25,98–105] MRI studies in infants with mild HIE have demonstrated a range of abnormalities in 20% to 60% of infants. Each MRI scoring system has a variable ability to label or detect these subtle abnormalities, and many MRI scoring systems are being used in infants with mild HIE.[26,31] The pattern of injury in mild HIE can be subtle and more likely to involve white matter rather than the deep central gray matter.

- Cranial ultrasound with Doppler: Ultrasound is cheap, noninvasive, and portable. It can reveal intracranial hemorrhages, cerebral edema but is not ideal for detailed mapping or to provide information about intracellular energy failure.

Recommended to obtain on day 1 of life before decisions about cooling and to exclude other etiologies.

- MRI/MRS Brain: This is the recommended gold standard for any HIE evaluation optimal timing is around day 5 of life with an acceptable 48 hours window and before discharge.

Trajectory of neurocognitive outcomes

A comprehensive and sensitive profile is needed to reflect the impact of even mild HIE, which has a more subtle outcome than moderate to severe HIE. Neurodevelopment is a complex continuum and trajectories can change with experience and environmental factors, whereby infants can develop new functionality.[106,107]

- Bayley testing at 2 years represents the gold standard outcome and allows comparison with prior hypothermia trials.[108,109]
- The Hammersmith Neurologic Examinations (HNNE/HINE): These examinations are standardized reliable and reproducible[110] with measures of tone, motor patterns, observation of movements, reflexes, and visual and auditory attention.[111,112] The examinations have well-studied optimality scores allowing for assessment from birth to 2 years.[113,114]
- The Child Behavior Checklist-parent report (CBCL) provides a profile of child's behavior and social functioning in relation to child's age and gender and in particular internalizing and externalizing tendencies associated with major psychological diagnoses into adolescence.[107]
- **Laboratory testing** Monitor *glucose* levels closely, every 4 to 6 hours, especially in the first 24 hours after birth. Actively manage to maintain serum levels 50 to 150 mg/dL as both hypoglycemia and hyperglycemia could be associated with secondary brain injury. *BUN, Creatinine, AST, and ALT* within 24 hours of age. Repeat at age 2–3 days, and continue testing until normal. *CBC with platelets* within the first 24 hours to assess for infection and thrombocytopenia. *PT, PTT, INR* Coagulation studies as needed within the first 24 hours based on the clinical assessment.
- **CO2 goal-** Avoid hypocapnia in ventilated neonates. Attempt to maintain $Paco_2$ 45 to 55 mm Hg after correction for temperature **(factor 0.83 at 33.5 C).**
- **Blood pressure** - Avoid hypotension, which may cause additional brain injury. Maintain blood pressure in the normal range (via invasive or cuff monitoring), using inotropic medications as needed. Continuous monitoring via intravascular catheter is preferred if inotropes are needed.
- **Infections-** Obtain blood culture before antibiotic administration. Treat with antibiotics if concerns for chorioamnionitis or infections. Consider LP if there is a concern for meningitis.
- **Sedation:** Provide sedation only if clinically indicated based on shiver/pain scores
    Avoid drips as the first line due to new data showing accumulation so sites will first intermittent morphine, fentanyl, or intermittent benzodiazepines to avoid cold stress.
    - Morphine boluses, 0.05 mg/kg IV q 6 hrs (repeat 0.05 mg/kg/dose PRN discomfort or shivering). If need Load dose 0.05–0.1 mg/kg IV. Start continuous infusion, and titrate for discomfort: 10 to 20 mcg/kg/h IV drip watch for accumulation. If ongoing sedation is required, continue infusion at lowest dose tolerated.

- Benzodiazepine avoids continuous infusions unless clinically indicated (eg, severe persistent pulmonary hypertension of the newborn).
- **Seizures.** Suggested algorithm for treatment if seizures are noted:
  - Will treat prolonged (>1 minute) or recurrent (≥2) clinical or electrographic seizures: *Phenobarbital* 20 mg/kg IV load.
  - For ongoing electrographic seizures, *Repeat phenobarbital* 20 mg/kg IV, for a total load of 40 mg/kg, followed by *Fosphenytoin* 20 mg/kg x IV; can repeat 10 mg/kg if needed; then *Levetiracetam* 40 to 60 mg/kg × IV, then *midazolam* drip
  - For brief, suspected clinical seizures in a neonate a benzodiazepine is a reasonable alternative. *Lorazepam* 0.05 to 0.1 mg/kg IV
  - Medication should be administered within 15 minutes of the identification of seizure(s).
  - Discontinuing antiseizure medications once the patient has been free from electrographic seizures for 24 to 72 hours and before discharge.

SUMMARY

1. Each normothermia and therapeutic hypothermia for mild HIE is accepted practices in standardized tertiary care settings able to provide intensive and follow-up care per AAP guidelines. However hypothermia is clearly not advised in low-resource settings whereby inappropriate cooling can result in poor outcomes
2. Avoidance of hyperthermia is strongly recommended. A core central temperature must be measured. As axillary temperature is on average 0.5°, lower sites will need to correct by 0.5 to avoid dangers associated with hyperthermia.
   a. If site provides hypothermia for mild HIE, consider limiting to those with TSS greater than 4: Whole body hypothermia will begin before 6 hours of age (ideal goal is within 3 hours).
      i. Target core temperature = 33.5°C (+/− 0.5°C)
      ii. Maintain core target temperature for 72 hours.
      iii. Rewarm patient slowly.
   b. Warm no faster than 0.5°C Increments every hour.
   c. Goal core temperature 36.5°- 37.0°C, or adjust if skin/axillary temperature as above.
   d. If site provides normothermia for mild HIE
      Maintain Goal core temperature 36.0–37.0°C
      Avoid temperature greater than 37°Core as hyperthermia can be associated with adverse outcomes
3. A standardized protocol that includes neuroimaging and neurodevelopmental follow-up is essential when providing care for any infant with HIE irrespective of its initial severity and decisions of cooling.
4. There is heterogeneity in outcomes with mild HIE. As such Total Sarnat score could be used to guide therapeutic decisions to target those at higher risk (TSS> 4 within 6 hours is significantly associated with disability at 2 years of age.
5. Hypothermia for mild HIE needs to be supported by systematic evidence that establishes the risk–benefit ratio with treatment and identifies subgroups at highest risk. Ongoing pragmatic effectiveness study COOL PRIME (NCT04621279) in planned along with pilot feasibility COMET study (NCT03409770) and TIME Study (NCT04176471) to help improve our knowledge of care in infants with mild HIE.

DISCLOSURE

The authors have nothing to disclose.

REFERENCES

1. Shipley L, Gale C, Sharkey D. Trends in the incidence and management of hypoxic-ischaemic encephalopathy in the therapeutic hypothermia era: a national population study. Arch Dis Child Fetal Neonatal Ed 2021.
2. Bryce J, Boschi-Pinto C, Shibuya K, et al. WHO estimates of the causes of death in children. Lancet 2005;365(9465):1147–52.
3. Azzopardi D, Brocklehurst P, Edwards D, et al. The TOBY Study. Whole body hypothermia for the treatment of perinatal asphyxial encephalopathy: a randomised controlled trial. BMC Pediatr 2008;8:17.
4. Shankaran S, Laptook AR, Ehrenkranz RA, et al. Whole-body hypothermia for neonates with hypoxic-ischemic encephalopathy. N Engl J Med 2005;353(15): 1574–84.
5. Jacobs SE, Morley CJ, Inder TE, et al. Whole-body hypothermia for term and near-term newborns with hypoxic-ischemic encephalopathy: a randomized controlled trial. Arch Pediatr Adolesc Med 2011;165(8):692–700.
6. Gluckman PD, Wyatt JS, Azzopardi D, et al. Selective head cooling with mild systemic hypothermia after neonatal encephalopathy: multicentre randomised trial. Lancet 2005;365(9460):663–70.
7. Gunn AJ, Laptook AR, Robertson NJ, et al. Therapeutic hypothermia translates from ancient history in to practice. Pediatr Res 2017;81(1–2):202–9.
8. Higgins RD, Raju T, Edwards AD, et al. Hypothermia and other treatment options for neonatal encephalopathy: an executive summary of the Eunice Kennedy Shriver NICHD workshop. J Pediatr 2011.
9. Higgins RD, Raju TN, Perlman J, et al. Hypothermia and perinatal asphyxia: executive summary of the national institute of child health and human development workshop. J Pediatr 2006;148(2):170–5.
10. Shankaran S, Laptook AR, Pappas A, et al. Effect of depth and duration of cooling on deaths in the NICU among neonates with hypoxic ischemic encephalopathy: a randomized clinical trial. JAMA 2014;312(24):2629–39.
11. Sabir H, Bonifacio SL, Gunn AJ, et al. Unanswered questions regarding therapeutic hypothermia for neonates with neonatal encephalopathy. Semin Fetal Neonatal Med 2021;101257.
12. Kariholu U, Montaldo P, Markati T, et al. Therapeutic hypothermia for mild neonatal encephalopathy: a systematic review and meta-analysis. Arch Dis Child Fetal Neonatal Ed 2020;105(2):225–8.
13. van Handel M, Swaab H, de Vries LS, et al. Behavioral outcome in children with a history of neonatal encephalopathy following perinatal asphyxia. J Pediatr Psychol 2010;35(3):286–95.
14. van Kooij BJ, van Handel M, Nievelstein RA, et al. Serial MRI and neurodevelopmental outcome in 9- to 10-year-old children with neonatal encephalopathy. J Pediatr 2010;157(2):221–227 e222.
15. Finder M, Boylan GB, Twomey D, et al. Two-year neurodevelopmental outcomes after mild hypoxic ischemic encephalopathy in the era of therapeutic hypothermia. JAMA Pediatr 2019.
16. Conway JM, Walsh BH, Boylan GB, et al. Mild hypoxic ischaemic encephalopathy and long term neurodevelopmental outcome - a systematic review. Early Hum Dev 2018;120:80–7.

17. Chalak L, Ferriero DM, Gressens P, et al. A 20 years conundrum of neonatal encephalopathy and hypoxic ischemic encephalopathy: are we closer to a consensus guideline? Pediatr Res 2019;86(5):548–9.
18. Chalak L, Latremouille S, Mir I, et al. A review of the conundrum of mild hypoxic-ischemic encephalopathy: current challenges and moving forward. Early Hum Dev 2018;120:88–94.
19. Jacobs SE, Berg M, Hunt R, et al. Cooling for newborns with hypoxic ischaemic encephalopathy. Cochrane Database Syst Rev 2013;(1):CD003311.
20. Wang B, Armstrong JS, Reyes M, et al. White matter apoptosis is increased by delayed hypothermia and rewarming in a neonatal piglet model of hypoxic ischemic encephalopathy. Neuroscience 2016;316:296–310.
21. Ferriero DM. Neonatal brain injury. N Engl J Med 2004;351(19):1985–95.
22. Sarnat HB, Sarnat MS. Neonatal encephalopathy following fetal distress. A clinical and electroencephalographic study. Arch Neurol 1976;33(10):696–705.
23. Shalak LF, Laptook AR, Velaphi SC, et al. Amplitude-integrated electroencephalography coupled with an early neurologic examination enhances prediction of term infants at risk for persistent encephalopathy. Pediatrics 2003;111(2):351–7.
24. Chalak LF, Nguyen KA, Prempunpong C, et al. Prospective research in infants with mild encephalopathy identified in the first six hours of life: neurodevelopmental outcomes at 18-22 months. Pediatr Res 2018;84(6):861–8.
25. Lally PJ, Pauliah S, Montaldo P, et al. Magnetic resonance biomarkers in neonatal encephalopathy (MARBLE): a prospective multicountry study. BMJ Open 2015;5(9):e008912.
26. Montaldo P, Lally PJ, Oliveira V, et al. Therapeutic hypothermia initiated within 6 hours of birth is associated with reduced brain injury on MR biomarkers in mild hypoxic-ischaemic encephalopathy: a non-randomised cohort study. Arch Dis Child Fetal Neonatal Ed 2019;104(5):F515–20.
27. Lodygensky GA, Battin MR, Gunn AJ. Mild neonatal encephalopathy-how, when, and how much to treat? JAMA Pediatr 2018;172(1):3–4.
28. Murray DM, O'Connor CM, Ryan CA, et al. Early EEG grade and outcome at 5 years after mild neonatal hypoxic ischemic encephalopathy. Pediatrics 2016.
29. Chalak LF, Pavageau L, Huet B, et al. Statistical rigor and kappa considerations: which, when and clinical context matters. Pediatr Res 2020.
30. El-Dib M, Inder TE, Chalak LF, et al. Should therapeutic hypothermia be offered to babies with mild neonatal encephalopathy in the first 6hafter birth? Pediatr Res 2019;85(4):442–8.
31. Prempunpong C, Chalak LF, Garfinkle J, et al. Prospective research on infants with mild encephalopathy: the PRIME study. J Perinatol 2018;38(1):80–5.
32. Laptook A, Tyson JE, Pedroza C, et al. Response to a different view concerning the NICHD neonatal research network late hypothermia trial. Acta Paediatr 2019;108(4):772–3.
33. Laptook AR, Shankaran S, Tyson JE, et al. Effect of therapeutic hypothermia initiated after 6 hours of age on death or disability among newborns with hypoxic-ischemic encephalopathy: a randomized clinical trial (vol 318, pg 1550, 2017). JAMA 2018;319(10):1051.
34. Montaldo P, Ivain P, Lally P, et al. White matter injury after neonatal encephalopathy is associated with thalamic metabolite perturbations. EBioMedicine 2020; 52:102663.
35. Deoni SCL. Neuroimaging of the developing brain and impact of nutrition. Nestle Nutr Inst Workshop Ser 2018;89:155–74.

36. Deoni S, Dean D 3rd, Joelson S, et al. Early nutrition influences developmental myelination and cognition in infants and young children. Neuroimage 2018;178: 649–59.

37. Remer J, Croteau-Chonka E, Dean DC 3rd, et al. Quantifying cortical development in typically developing toddlers and young children, 1-6 years of age. Neuroimage 2017;153:246–61.

38. McCrory C, Murray A. The effect of breastfeeding on neuro-development in infancy. Matern Child Health J 2013;17(9):1680–8.

39. Koutra K, Chatzi L, Bagkeris M, et al. Antenatal and postnatal maternal mental health as determinants of infant neurodevelopment at 18 months of age in a mother-child cohort (Rhea Study) in Crete, Greece. Soc Psychiatry Psychiatr Epidemiol 2013;48(8):1335–45.

40. Simcock G, Kildea S, Elgbeili G, et al. Age-related changes in the effects of stress in pregnancy on infant motor development by maternal report: the Queensland Flood Study. Dev Psychobiol 2016;58(5):640–59.

41. Deoni SC, Dean DC 3rd, Piryatinsky I, et al. Breastfeeding and early white matter development: a cross-sectional study. Neuroimage 2013;82:77–86.

42. Koo E, Sheldon RA, Lee BS, et al. Effects of therapeutic hypothermia on white matter injury from murine neonatal hypoxia-ischemia. Pediatr Res 2017;82(3): 518–26.

43. Chalak LF. Best practice guidelines on management of mild neonatal encephalopathy: is it really mild? Early Hum Dev 2018;120:74.

44. Oliveira V, Singhvi DP, Montaldo P, et al. Therapeutic hypothermia in mild neonatal encephalopathy: a national survey of practice in the UK. Arch Dis Child Fetal Neonatal Ed 2018;103(4):F388–90.

45. Soll RF. Cooling for newborns with hypoxic ischemic encephalopathy. Neonatology 2013;103:261.

46. Kracer B, Hintz SR, Van Meurs KP, et al. Hypothermia therapy for neonatal hypoxic ischemic encephalopathy in the state of California. J Pediatr 2014;165(2): 267–73.

47. Massaro AN, Murthy K, Zaniletti I, et al. Short-term outcomes after perinatal hypoxic ischemic encephalopathy: a report from the Children's Hospitals Neonatal Consortium HIE focus group. J Perinatol 2015;35(4):290–6.

48. Rao R, Trivedi S, Distler A, et al. Neurodevelopmental outcomes in neonates with mild hypoxic ischemic encephalopathy treated with therapeutic hypothermia. Am J Perinatol 2019;36(13):1337–43.

49. Kumar V, Singla M, Thayyil S. Cooling in mild encephalopathy: costs and perils of therapeutic creep. Semin Fetal Neonatal Med 2021;26(3):101244.

50. Chawla S, Bates SV, Shankaran S. Is it time for a randomized controlled trial of hypothermia for mild hypoxic-ischemic encephalopathy? J Pediatr 2020;220: 241–4.

51. Tagin MA, Gunn AJ. Neonatal encephalopathy and potential lost opportunities: when the story fits, please cool. Arch Dis Child Fetal Neonatal Ed 2021.

52. Mani Singla LC, S Thayyil, S Mehta, et al. International survey on current practices of therapeutic hypothermia in neonates with mild hypoxic-ischaemic encephalopathy. Paper presented at: PAS 2021.

53. Thayyil S. Cooling therapy for the management of hypoxic-ischaemic encephalopathy in middle-income countries: we can, but should we? Paediatr Int Child Health 2019;39(4):231–3.

54. Amstutz A, Schandelmaier S, Frei R, et al. Discontinuation and non-publication of randomised clinical trials supported by the main public funding body in Switzerland: a retrospective cohort study. BMJ Open 2017;7(7):e016216.
55. Schandelmaier S, Tomonaga Y, Bassler D, et al. Premature discontinuation of pediatric randomized controlled trials: a retrospective cohort study. J Pediatr 2017;184:209–214 e201.
56. Kasenda B, von Elm EB, You J, et al. Learning from failure–rationale and design for a study about discontinuation of randomized trials (DISCO study). BMC Med Res Methodol 2012;12:131.
57. Carlisle B, Kimmelman J, Ramsay T, et al. Unsuccessful trial accrual and human subjects protections: an empirical analysis of recently closed trials. Clin Trials 2015;12(1):77–83.
58. Glass HC, Soul JS, Chang T, et al. Safety of early discontinuation of antiseizure medication after acute symptomatic neonatal seizures. JAMA Neurol 2021.
59. Guttmann KF, Wu YW, Juul SE, et al. Consent related challenges for neonatal clinical trials. Am J Bioeth 2020;20(5):38–40.
60. Giesinger RE, Levy PT, Lauren Ruoss J, et al. Cardiovascular management following hypoxic-ischemic encephalopathy in North America: need for physiologic consideration. Pediatr Res 2020.
61. O'Dea M, Sweetman D, Bonifacio SL, et al. Management of multi organ dysfunction in neonatal encephalopathy. Front Pediatr 2020;8:239.
62. McPherson C, Miller SP, El-Dib M, et al. The influence of pain, agitation, and their management on the immature brain. Pediatr Res 2020;88(2):168–75.
63. Garcia-Alix A, Arnaez J, Herranz-Rubia N, et al. Ten years since the introduction of therapeutic hypothermia in neonates with perinatal hypoxic-ischaemic encephalopathy in Spain. Neurologia 2020.
64. El-Dib M, Munster C, Szakmar E, et al. Late onset oxygen requirement following neonatal therapeutic hypothermia. Acta Paediatr 2020.
65. Massaro AN, Tsuchida T, Kadom N, et al. aEEG evolution during therapeutic hypothermia and prediction of NICU outcome in encephalopathic neonates. Neonatology 2012;102(3):197–202.
66. Thoresen M, Liu X, Jary S, et al. Lactate dehydrogenase in hypothermia-treated newborn infants with hypoxic-ischaemic encephalopathy. Acta Paediatr 2012; 101(10):1038–44.
67. Thoresen M, Hellstrom-Westas L, Liu X, et al. Effect of hypothermia on amplitude-integrated electroencephalogram in infants with asphyxia. Pediatrics 2010;126(1):e131–9.
68. Thoresen M. Supportive care during neuroprotective hypothermia in the term newborn: adverse effects and their prevention. Clin Perinatol 2008;35(4): 749–63, vii.
69. Shankaran S, Natarajan G, Chalak L, et al. Hypothermia for neonatal hypoxic-ischemic encephalopathy: NICHD Neonatal Research Network contribution to the field. Semin Perinatol 2016;40(6):385–90.
70. Chalak L, Kaiser J. Neonatal guideline hypoxic-ischemic encephalopathy (HIE). J Ark Med Soc 2007;104(4):87–9.
71. Patterson JK, Pant S, Jones DF, et al. Informed consent rates for neonatal randomized controlled trials in low- and lower middle-income versus high-income countries: a systematic review. PLoS One 2021;16(3):e0248263.
72. Montaldo P, Vakharia A, Ivain P, et al. Pre-emptive opioid sedation during therapeutic hypothermia. Arch Dis Child Fetal Neonatal Ed 2020;105(1):108–9.

73. Liow N, Montaldo P, Lally PJ, et al. Preemptive morphine during therapeutic hypothermia after neonatal encephalopathy: a secondary analysis. Ther Hypothermia Temp Manag 2020;10(1):45–52.

74. Szakmar E, Smith J, Yang E, et al. Association between cerebral oxygen saturation and brain injury in neonates receiving therapeutic hypothermia for neonatal encephalopathy. J Perinatol 2021;41(2):269–77.

75. Szakmar E, Jermendy A, El-Dib M. Correction: respiratory management during therapeutic hypothermia for hypoxic-ischemic encephalopathy. J Perinatol 2019;39(6):891.

76. Szakmar E, Jermendy A, El-Dib M. Respiratory management during therapeutic hypothermia for hypoxic-ischemic encephalopathy. J Perinatol 2019;39(6):763–73.

77. Neville KL, McCaffery H, Baxter Z, et al. Implementation of a standardized seizure action plan to improve communication and parental Education. Pediatr Neurol 2020;112:56–63.

78. Tsuchida TN, Wusthoff CJ, Shellhaas RA, et al. American clinical neurophysiology society standardized EEG terminology and categorization for the description of continuous EEG monitoring in neonates: report of the American Clinical Neurophysiology Society critical care monitoring committee. J Clin Neurophysiol 2013;30(2):161–73.

79. Shellhaas RA, Barks AK. Impact of amplitude-integrated electroencephalograms on clinical care for neonates with seizures. Pediatr Neurol 2012;46(1):32–5.

80. Shellhaas RA, Chang T, Tsuchida T, et al. The American clinical neurophysiology Society's guideline on continuous electroencephalography monitoring in neonates. J Clin Neurophysiol 2011;28(6):611–7.

81. Gundersena JK, Chakkarapanib E, Jaryb S, et al. Morphine and fentanyl exposure during therapeutic hypothermia does not impair neurodevelopment. EClinicalMedicine 2021;. https://www.sciencedirect.com/science/journal/25895370.

82. Spencer APC, Brooks JCW, Masuda N, et al. Disrupted brain connectivity in children treated with therapeutic hypothermia for neonatal encephalopathy. Neuroimage Clin 2021;30:102582.

83. Wood TR, Gundersen JK, Falck M, et al. Variability and sex-dependence of hypothermic neuroprotection in a rat model of neonatal hypoxic-ischaemic brain injury: a single laboratory meta-analysis. Sci Rep 2020;10(1):10833.

84. Lee-Kelland R, Jary S, Tonks J, et al. School-age outcomes of children without cerebral palsy cooled for neonatal hypoxic-ischaemic encephalopathy in 2008-2010. Arch Dis Child Fetal Neonatal Ed 2020;105(1):8–13.

85. Mir IN, Leon R, Chalak LF. Placental origins of neonatal diseases: toward a precision medicine approach. Pediatr Res 2021;89(2):377–83.

86. Machie M, Weeke L, de Vries LS, et al. MRI score ability to detect abnormalities in mild hypoxic-ischemic encephalopathy. Pediatr Neurol 2021;116:32–8.

87. Chalak L. Historical perspectives for therapeutic hypothermia in the newborn: a life worth saving. Pediatr Res 2021.

88. Pavageau L, Sanchez PJ, Steven Brown L, et al. Inter-rater reliability of the modified Sarnat examination in preterm infants at 32-36 weeks' gestation. Pediatr Res 2020;87(4):697–702.

89. Chalak LF, Adams-Huet B, Sant'Anna G. A total Sarnat score in mild hypoxic-ischemic encephalopathy can detect infants at higher risk of disability. J Pediatr 2019;214:217–221 e211.

90. O'Shea A, Lightbody G, Boylan G, et al. Neonatal seizure detection from raw multi-channel EEG using a fully convolutional architecture. Neural Netw 2020; 123:12–25.
91. Raurale SA, Nalband S, Boylan GB, et al. Suitability of an inter-burst detection method for grading hypoxic-ischemic encephalopathy in newborn EEG. Conf Proc IEEE Eng Med Biol Soc 2019;2019:4125–8.
92. Murray DM, Boylan GB, Ryan CA, et al. Early EEG findings in hypoxic-ischemic encephalopathy predict outcomes at 2 years. Pediatrics 2009;124(3):e459–67.
93. Hellstrom-Westas L. Amplitude-integrated EEG–useful for early outcome prediction after birth asphyxia? Nat Clin Pract Neurol 2008;4(2):74–5.
94. Chalak LF, Zhang R. New wavelet neurovascular bundle for bedside evaluation of cerebral autoregulation and neurovascular coupling in newborns with hypoxic-ischemic encephalopathy. Dev Neurosci 2017.
95. Tian F, Sepulveda P, Kota S, et al. Regional heterogeneity of cerebral hemodynamics in mild neonatal encephalopathy measured with multichannel near-infrared spectroscopy. Pediatr Res 2021;89(4):882–8.
96. Das Y, Wang X, Kota S, et al. Neurovascular coupling (NVC) in newborns using processed EEG versus amplitude-EEG. Sci Rep 2021;11(1):9426.
97. Toet MC, Hellstrom-Westas L, Groenendaal F, et al. Amplitude integrated EEG 3 and 6 hours after birth in full term neonates with hypoxic-ischaemic encephalopathy. Arch Dis Child Fetal Neonatal Ed 1999;81(1):F19–23.
98. Weeke LC, Groenendaal F, Mudigonda K, et al. A novel magnetic resonance imaging score predicts neurodevelopmental outcome after perinatal asphyxia and therapeutic hypothermia. J Pediatr 2018;192:33–40.e2.
99. Walsh BH, Inder TE. MRI as a biomarker for mild neonatal encephalopathy. Early Hum Dev 2018;120:75–9.
100. Trivedi SB, Vesoulis ZA, Rao R, et al. A validated clinical MRI injury scoring system in neonatal hypoxic-ischemic encephalopathy. Pediatr Radiol 2017;47(11): 1491–9.
101. Robertson NJ, Thayyil S, Cady EB, et al. Magnetic resonance spectroscopy biomarkers in term perinatal asphyxial encephalopathy: from neuropathological correlates to future clinical applications. Curr Pediatr Rev 2014;10(1):37–47.
102. Thayyil S, Chandrasekaran M, Taylor A, et al. Cerebral magnetic resonance biomarkers in neonatal encephalopathy: a meta-analysis. Pediatrics 2010;125(2): e382–95.
103. Shankaran S, McDonald SA, Laptook AR, et al. Neonatal magnetic resonance imaging pattern of brain injury as a biomarker of childhood outcomes following a trial of hypothermia for neonatal hypoxic-ischemic encephalopathy. J Pediatr 2015;167(5):987–99.e3.
104. Barkovich AJ, Hajnal BL, Vigneron D, et al. Prediction of neuromotor outcome in perinatal asphyxia: evaluation of MR scoring systems. AJNR Am J Neuroradiol 1998;19(1):143–9.
105. Rutherford M, Ramenghi LA, Edwards AD, et al. Assessment of brain tissue injury after moderate hypothermia in neonates with hypoxic-ischaemic encephalopathy: a nested substudy of a randomised controlled trial. Lancet Neurol 2010;9(1):39–45.
106. Maitre NL. Neurorehabilitation after neonatal intensive care: evidence and challenges. Arch Dis Child Fetal Neonatal Ed 2015;100(6):F534–40.
107. Benninger KL, Inder TE, Goodman AM, et al. Perspectives from the Society for Pediatric Research. Neonatal encephalopathy clinical trials: developing the future. Pediatr Res 2021;89(1):74–84.

108. Shankaran S, Laptook AR, Pappas A, et al. Effect of depth and duration of cooling on death or disability at age 18 Months among neonates with hypoxic-ischemic encephalopathy: a randomized clinical trial. JAMA 2017;318(1):57–67.
109. Laptook AR, Shankaran S, Tyson JE, et al. Effect of therapeutic hypothermia initiated after 6 hours of age on death or disability among newborns with hypoxic-ischemic encephalopathy: a randomized clinical trial. JAMA 2017;318(16): 1550–60.
110. Dubowitz L, Mercuri E, Dubowitz V. An optimality score for the neurologic examination of the term newborn. J Pediatr 1998;133(3):406–16.
111. Novak I, Morgan C, Adde L, et al. Early, accurate diagnosis and early intervention in cerebral palsy: advances in diagnosis and treatment. JAMA Pediatr 2017; 171(9):897–907.
112. Romeo DM, Bompard S, Cocca C, et al. Neonatal neurological examination during the first 6h after birth. Early Hum Dev 2017;108:41–4.
113. Ricci D, Romeo DM, Haataja L, et al. Neurological examination of preterm infants at term equivalent age. Early Hum Dev 2008;84(11):751–61.
114. Ricci D, Romeo DM, Serrao F, et al. Application of a neonatal assessment of visual function in a population of low risk full-term newborn. Early Hum Dev 2008; 84(4):277–80.

Moving?

Make sure your subscription moves with you!

To notify us of your new address, find your **Clinics Account Number** (located on your mailing label above your name), and contact customer service at:

Email: journalscustomerservice-usa@elsevier.com

800-654-2452 (subscribers in the U.S. & Canada)
314-447-8871 (subscribers outside of the U.S. & Canada)

Fax number: 314-447-8029

Elsevier Health Sciences Division
Subscription Customer Service
3251 Riverport Lane
Maryland Heights, MO 63043

*To ensure uninterrupted delivery of your subscription, please notify us at least 4 weeks in advance of move.

ELSEVIER